HEALTH STUDIES
DEPT.

D0754952

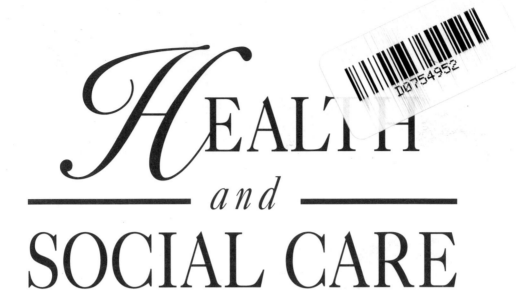

HEALTH
and
SOCIAL CARE

HEALTH STUDIES
DEPT.

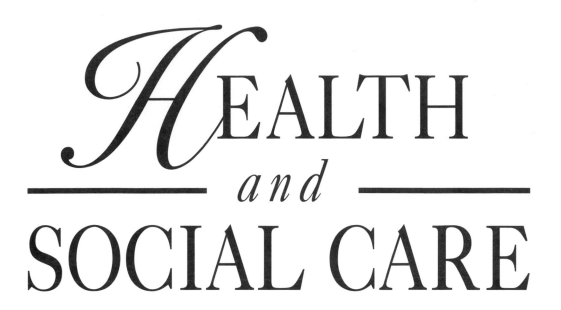

HEALTH
and
SOCIAL CARE

Hilary Thomson

Caroline Holden

Gillian Hutt

Carolyn Meggitt

Jean Manuel

Hodder & Stoughton

A MEMBER OF THE HODDER HEADLINE GROUP

Cataloguing in Publication Data is available from the British Library

ISBN 0 340 58538 2

First published 1994
Impression number   10 9 8 7 6 5 4 3 2 1
Year   1998 1997 1996 1995 1994

Copyright © 1994 Hilary Thomson, Caroline Holden,
Gillian Hutt, Carolyn Meggitt, Jean Manuel

All rights reserved. No part of this publication may be reproduced
or transmitted in any form or by any means, electronic or
mechanical, including photocopy, recording, or any information
storage and retrieval system, without permission in writing from
the publisher or under licence from the Copyright Licensing
Agency Limited. Further details of such licences (for reprographic
reproduction) may be obtained from the Copyright Licensing
Agency Limited, of 90 Tottenham Court Road, London W1P 9HE.

Typeset by Wearset, Boldon, Tyne and Wear.
Printed in Great Britain for Hodder & Stoughton Educational, a
division of Hodder Headline Plc, 338 Euston Road, London
NW1 3BH by Thomson Litho Limited.

CONTENTS

ACKNOWLEDGEMENTS

We would like to thank the following for their help and advice during the preparation of this book: Chrissie Rycroft for the correlation exercise; Sylvia Aslangul (NESCOT) for careers and work experience assignments; Sneh Kapoor for contributing some case studies in Chapter 4; Julie Rzezniczek for contribution on M.E.; Margaret Evans for information from hospitals; Freda Dudfield for the exercise on listening skills; Nicola Crabbe and Tanya Grogan, students, for contributions to material on child abuse.

Our special thanks go to our families for their support and encouragement.

Every effort has been made to obtain permission to use quoted material in this book. If copyright holders wish to contact Hodder & Stoughton, they should do so at the publisher's address.

INTRODUCTION

There were two reasons why it was essential to produce this book: first, because no other suitable health and social care textbook was available to school or college students; and second, because the recent development of General National Vocational Qualifications (GNVQs) called for a new approach to study in this field.

Up until now, students on health or social care courses (for example, BTEC or other courses aimed at preparing future caring professionals) have had to select relevant material from a variety of sociology, psychology, biology and statistics texts. This book, however, combines the relevant areas of these subjects and includes, in addition, a comprehensive guide to the structure of the health and social care systems, their operation, and experience in the workplace.

The book covers, chapter by chapter, the eight mandatory units of the Advanced GNVQ 'Health and Social Care'. These mandatory units were set centrally and are the same irrespective of the awarding body offering the qualification (BTEC, RSA or City and Guilds). The mandatory units, and therefore this book, cover the fundamental skills, knowledge, understanding and principles common to a wide range of 'caring' occupations.

The GNVQ also requires four additional units to be completed; these are to be chosen from a list of eight options. As these units are not centrally devised they vary from one awarding body to another, and therefore cannot be covered within this book.

Advanced GNVQ units are comparable in educational standard to A and AS Level, and it is possible for an A Level student to take one or more units which may be useful for his or her intended career. This book is ideal for such students as it will cover their chosen unit(s) as well as giving them essential background reading.

The GNVQ programme sets outcomes but does not prescribe the course. The reader will find that the number of suggested activities within this book gives scope for a programme of learning to be devised that suits the availability of resources and the circumstances of the student. In line with GNVQ practice, the use of project assignments, surveys, investigations of processes and services, and case studies is encouraged.

As well as completing eight mandatory units and four additional units, a student aiming at Advanced GNVQ must show the following 'Core Skills': 'Communication', 'Application of Number' and 'Information Technology', all of which are formally assessed, and 'Problem Solving' and 'Personal Skills', which are encouraged and may be recorded in the National Record of Achievement, but are not formally assessed and certified. The numerous activities suggested in this book provide ample opportunity for students to develop and practise all these skills; with reference to information technology skills, it is assumed that students will have the facilities to produce written reports on a word processor at least occasionally.

The Advanced GNVQ is assessed in two ways: through external tests, and from a 'Portfolio of Evidence' derived from projects carried out within the course. This book will help with both elements. An external written test, consisting of short answer or multiple choice questions and lasting for one hour, is taken for each mandatory unit. Each chapter will help students to master the necessary underpinning knowledge, understanding and principles to reach the required high pass mark in the corresponding test. Because the tests can be sat at different times of the year, and students may repeat the tests until they pass, a text which allows students to study independently is obviously very useful.

The student-centred approach and the many activities allow the student to take a leading role in the collection and presentation of evidence to be used for project-based assessment. On the basis of the Portfolio of Evidence, a Merit or a Distinction may be awarded if a level of performance above the basic requirement is demonstrated. Within the book activities are suggested which give the student ample opportunity to develop and demonstrate the abilities on which the criteria for awarding grades focus. These are the ability to plan, to seek and handle information and to evaluate approaches, outcomes and alternatives. The Portfolio of Evidence can also be used by people outside the scheme to examine the quality of a student's work.

Chapter 1 provides an introduction to the social influences on attitudes and behaviour and applies the concepts discussed to the ways in which people's behaviour and attitudes may lead to prejudice and discrimination towards others. A critical and comprehensive guide to anti-discrimination legislation is presented, along with detailed advice and guidance for students undertaking assignments and projects.

In Chapter 2 communication with other individuals and in groups is investigated. The treatment goes beyond straightforward communication with others of the same age and social and educational background (such as student-to-student communication) to cover communication with those from very different social backgrounds, outlooks and educational levels, necessary in any profession involving social care. Verbal and non-verbal forms of communication are considered, as are the different styles of the English language used in our society, which may cause confusion if not understood. Active listening and responding skills are analysed, as well as factors which inhibit communication. Types of groups, and the way in which group behaviour develops, are also analysed. This chapter includes a section on the values which underpin health and social care work. Activities for project work suggested in this chapter cover the four common skills in 'communicating' that are formally assessed in the Advanced GNVQ.

Chapter 3 is an introduction to human anatomy and physiology. After opening sections on molecular and cellular organization, tissue structure and function are discussed, together with organ systems. The cardiovascular and respiratory systems are studied in more detail, from a health perspective. Human disease and its main causative agents are covered, and prevention of disease is emphasized. The socio-economic factors affecting incidence of disease are recognized. The topic of diet is included as being fundamental to health.

In Chapter 4 the psychological and social development of the individual is investigated through the life cycle. Erikson's eight psychosocial stages of development have been been used as a basis for considering the emotional and social needs of each age group. This chapter includes an introduction to attachments, classical and operant con-ditioning and social learning theory, and stereotyping. The life events that threaten individual identity at each stage of the life cycle are also considered. These include disruption of attachment bonds, child abuse, substance abuse, major changes in social role (for example, unemployment), bereavement and loss of health and mobility.

Chapter 5 aims to raise health awareness by highlighting the areas in which people have genuine choices in following a healthier lifestyle: smoking, drug abuse in its widest sense, sexually transmitted diseases, HIV and AIDS, and personal safety. Students are given up-to-date background information on all these topics and activities are structured towards health promotion.

In a rapidly changing area such as health and social care it is essential to have really up-to-date information on the structure of the system and practices within it. This is provided in Chapter 6, along with many suggestions for activities both in the classroom and in the workplace. The opportunity is provided for students to find out about their chosen careers.

Chapter 7 is an introduction to the development and implementation of care plans, which are an increasingly important aspect of care provision. It should be read in conjunction with Chapter 2, which covers some of the skills necessary for producing a care plan. Students are given guidance on the investigation of care plans within the workplace.

Chapter 8 gives a comprehensive guide to research methods used in health and social care. The reader will find this chapter useful for reference when carrying out many of the pieces of research suggested throughout the rest of the book.

The National Council for Vocational Qualifications states that 'Work placements can provide invaluable experience and a context for project work. Careful planning is required to exploit the full potential of learning opportunities provided by placements.' For these reasons an appendix

has been included to give students and lecturers advice on how to go about setting up a work placement, and suggesting activities to be carried out before, during and after the placement. There are also activities throughout the book which can be carried out in the workplace. These have been indicated with the symbol **W** for easy reference.

The GNVQ requires students to demonstrate an understanding of the 'value base' in health and social care work. The components of the value base are: freedom from any type of discrimination; maintaining confidentiality of information; promoting and supporting individual rights and choice; and supporting individuals through effective communication. All of these components are comprehensively covered within the book to give students the in-depth knowledge they will need.

Each chapter is followed by a short list of suggested further reading and useful resources, as well as details of works cited in the text.

ACCESS, EQUAL OPPORTUNITIES AND CLIENT RIGHTS

ATTITUDES AND OTHER SOCIAL INFLUENCES ON BEHAVIOUR

All of us spend time wondering why people think and behave in the way they do. We puzzle over those nearest to us – our parents and our children; our neighbours; our teachers, fellow students or workers; our employers; our friends – as well as politicians and people we hear or read about.

Some people, particularly those working in occupations related to health and social care, generally have serious and pressing reasons for being concerned about people's behaviour and attitudes. A child is being abused; a schoolboy is truanting from school; a nursery-school toddler is crying and upset; a mother is severely depressed and suicidal; a young woman is losing weight rapidly as a result of drastically limiting her diet; a teenager has run away from his foster-home; a man has just hit a nurse in Accident and Emergency . . . These and a thousand other such situations regularly confront workers in health and social care. Problems need to be tackled and the care, safety and welfare of patients and clients protected.

The search for possible explanations of why people think and behave in the ways they do draws on the theories, perspectives and research of social science. The work of sociologists and psychologists is studied, evaluated and, to a greater or lesser degree, applied to specific situations. Until we have a wider understanding of behaviour than that gained solely on the basis of our own personal experience, we may be unsure how

Parents sue church over sexual abuse

Pressures at work 'fuel suicides'

Policeman and two others hurt in market square knife attack

Man who snatched Lamplugh sister 'ill'

Concern for missing man is growing

to care for and help others with different experiences from our own. While the social sciences are unlikely to provide all the answers, they may enable us to ask more appropriate and critical questions, to understand the social context of people's lives and to have some appreciation of the perspectives through which others view their worlds. We can also use what we learn from social scientists to reflect upon our own experiences, so that we are more able to empathize with others seeking help and using services.

In this chapter the theories and research of social scientists will be used to explore some of the fundamental questions which health and social care workers will continually need to ask of themselves and of others:

- Where do our attitudes towards and ideas about other people come from?
- How do these attitudes, beliefs and ideas affect our behaviour towards others?
- How are people in societies affected by the attitudes and behaviour of other people around them?
- In what ways can the attitudes and behaviour of people in societies lead to prejudice, discrimination and the unfair treatment of others?
- How have people in this society sought to overcome the unfair treatment of others?

Beliefs, ideas and values: the influence of socialization

However helpless and dependent they may seem, within a few weeks of being born, babies will show signs of their need for emotional contact and INTERACTION with others. They smile, they cry, they babble, they reach out and they are particularly fascinated with the human face. As they grow and develop, they learn more about interacting with others, they acquire language and they begin to understand how others behave and how they, in turn, are expected to behave in particular situations. Learning the meaning of

social behaviour and the values and beliefs of others is the way CULTURE is learned, re-learned and shared by each new generation. Culture is a 'set of guidelines – both implicit and explicit – which the individual inherits as a member of a particular group, and which tells him how to view the world, and how to behave in it in relation to other people, to the natural environment and to supernatural forces and gods' (McAvoy and Donalson 1990).

The process of learning the culture of a society (and/or of a sub-group within that society) is called SOCIALIZATION. It is a continual process, lasting throughout our lives and involving the use of language, symbols and ritual. As we join different groups in society we learn new things; the initially strange becomes more familiar as we become accustomed to the new situation. At the same time as we adapt to or absorb values from the people around us we also contribute as individuals, however minutely, to the culture of our group and/or the wider society. We may challenge ideas, question attitudes or join with others in diverging from usual patterns of behaviour. As a result, changes in society inevitably occur.

There is a debate about whether our experience of socialization during childhood and the attitudes, values and ideas we encounter in our families, friends and neighbours (PRIMARY SOCIALIZATION) is a much more powerful and influential one than any subsequent experience and socialization gained from a wider variety of contexts – the family, friends, schools, the media, colleagues at work, etc. (SECONDARY SOCIALIZATION). Are ideas and values learned in the early years of life more difficult to alter or change later? Why should this be the case?

ACTIVITY

1 The process of socialization can be grasped by thinking back to a time and a situation which was *new* to you, such as your first days at a new school, in a new

job, in a new country, staying with a family other than your own for the first time . . .

What were your initial impressions and feelings? Did initially strange and difficult situations gradually become more familiar? How did this happen? What were you learning that made you gradually change the way in which you viewed this situation?

2 Do you think that early childhood experiences are particularly important? Why or why not? Interview several people older than yourself, asking them this question. Have their attitudes, values and beliefs altered significantly during their lives?

How do our attitudes, beliefs and ideas affect our behaviour towards others?

In many western, industrialized societies, the beliefs, ideas and values people absorb from others and test out through their own experiences as they grow up from childhood to adulthood are unlikely to be completely coherent, a neat package which never varies. Even if a child learns a consistent set of moral and religious ideas from his or her family, sooner or later that child will hear contrary, different ideas and will understand that other people may have other perspectives. Hence the basis on which we adopt or reject certain values and ideas and make them our own is an interesting process for study.

ACTIVITY

Make a list of ten values, ideas or beliefs about life in this society which you hold, for example:

'I don't believe in stealing'
'I believe that it is important to care for others'

When your list is complete, think about where those ideas, values and attitudes came from. Have you always held those attitudes? Has a particular experience led you to hold a certain belief ?

Discuss your list with other people.

Look again at your list. If you were asked 'How do your attitudes, values and beliefs influence your behaviour', what would be your response?

You may well find that several problems arise in trying to answer the last question in the Activity on this page. For example:

- Not all our ideas and values are always fixed and 'set'. We may be unsure about what we think on many issues. For example, we may be 'toying' with the idea of joining a church or a religious organization.
- We may hold ideas and attitudes but not act on them. For example, we may 'believe' that working hard is a virtue but may often avoid doing it ourselves.
- Our attitudes may be reinforced and strengthened if people we are close to or people we associate with share them. For example, we may decide to protest at something we regard as unjust if others are also doing so.
- We may hold certain ideas but feel prevented from acting upon them by the behaviour of others around us or others we perceive to be more powerful than ourselves, and perhaps threatening. For example, we may wish to declare our teachers boring and incompetent but feel worried about how such a protest might affect our grades!
- We may simply be unaware or only half-aware of the reasons for our behaviour and the ideas which shape it. Many cultural factors influence us without our conscious knowledge, and we may not know what hidden ideas and prejudices we carry around with us and how they play a role in our lives. For example, a student nursery

teacher may suddenly realize that she has been telling off the children in her class in the same way that she was reprimanded as a child.

- The material circumstances of our lives and certain experiences can be positive or negative or a mixture of both. Negative, traumatic episodes in our lives may leave us with views and beliefs we might rather not have but which we find difficult to abandon. For example, a woman who has been raped may feel uneasy in the presence of all men and see all men as a possible threat to her safety.

- We may express certain ideas overtly (openly to others) while simultaneously holding different and often contradictory attitudes. For example, a patient may say to the doctor, 'I've come to ask you for advice about these bouts of colds and 'flu I seem to keep getting,' while thinking, 'I know what's wrong with me really: I'm over-worked and need a holiday but I bet he won't give me a prescription for that!'

Even if there were universal agreement upon what 'acceptable' behaviour was, and children grew up into societies learning and adopting accepted and socially approved ways of behaving, it is highly unlikely that every individual would always conform to the written or unwritten rules of social life. Social relationships are problematic. Many experiences – a disability, a traumatic accident, the move to a new country or area of a country, the break-up of a family through divorce or bereavement – may lead people to behave towards and relate to others in unconventional, unexpected and therefore sometimes socially disapproved-of ways. In addition, we all bring to every social situation our unique personalities.

However, it is sometimes the case that the values, attitudes and ideas which we question the least are the ones which appear to us to embody 'common sense', ones which appear 'given' and 'natural'. Problems regarding the impact of these common-sense ideas on others may arise when:

- different groups of people from different cultural, religious, economic or social backgrounds evolve different ideas of what constitutes common sense;
- certain groups in society have the power to, and do, attempt to persuade others that their versions of common sense are the only correct ones;
- different views of common sense come into conflict.

ACTIVITY

1 Romantic love is a natural part of human experience and is therefore found in all societies, in close connection with marriage.

2 How long people live is dependent upon their biological make-up and cannot be strongly influenced by social differences.

3 In previous times the family was a stable unit, but today there is a great increase in the proportion of 'broken homes'.

4 In all societies some people will be unhappy or distressed; therefore rates of suicide will tend to be the same throughout the world.

In small groups or pairs, discuss each of the four statements above. With which (if any) does your group tend to agree most strongly? What reasons do people in your group give for agreeing with these statements? Are there any statements with which your group tends to disagree? What reasons do people in your group give for disagreeing with these statements?

Now read the following comments on these statements:

Each of these assertions is wrong or questionable, and seeing why will help us to understand the questions sociologists ask – and try to answer – in their work.

1 As we have seen, the idea that marriage

ties should be based on romantic love is a recent one, not found either in the earlier history of Western societies, or in other cultures. Romantic love is actually unknown in most societies.

2 How long people live is very definitely affected by social influences. This is because modes of social life act as 'filters' for biological factors that cause illness, infirmity or death. The poor are less healthy on average than the rich, for example, because they usually have worse diets, live a more physically demanding existence, and have access to inferior medical facilities.

3 If we look back to the early 1800s, the proportion of children living in homes with only one natural parent was probably as high as at present, because many more people died young, particularly women in childbirth. Separation and divorce are today the main cause of 'broken homes', but the overall level is not very different.

4 Suicide rates are certainly not the same in all societies. Even if we only look at Western countries, we find that suicide rates vary considerably. The suicide rate of the United Kingdom, for example, is four times as high as that of Spain, but only a third of the rate in Hungary. Suicide rates increased quite sharply during the main period of industrialization of the Western societies, in the nineteenth and early twentieth centuries.

(Giddens 1989, p. 14)

The Activity on this page suggests that a useful skill for anyone working in health and social care is to be prepared to ask of any of our beliefs: 'Is this really so? What evidence is there for this idea or belief ?'

This leads us into asking perhaps the most controversial question so far. If it is useful to question and examine our beliefs and ideas (particularly in the light of the possible impact they may have on others), how do we EVALUATE them? How can we tell if we are 'right' or 'wrong'? The study of the social sciences is often an unsettling experience in itself because of this focus on questioning and because of the variety of possible ways of seeing things and of theories and explanations which it provides. This will be illustrated in the next section of this chapter, which considers one of the eternal areas of social concern:

- In what ways can the behaviour and attitudes of people in society lead to prejudice towards and the unfair treatment of others?

In exploring this issue, the focus will be on two questions:

- What sort of evidence indicates that people are being treated less equally than their circumstances justify?
- Where this occurs, how does it happen?

DISCRIMINATION AND ITS EFFECTS ON INDIVIDUALS

ACTIVITY

The following pages present some groupings of statistics, results of research studies and other information. Bearing in mind the limitations associated with data gathered from primary and secondary sources (see the section of Chapter 8 on 'Research Methods'), discuss the implications of each grouping of information.

What does this information indicate about life in Britain?

How can this information be explained?

RACE/ETHNICITY

ONE IN TEN NON-WHITE FAMILIES SUFFER RACIAL HARASSMENT

One in ten ethnic minority households in London have suffered racial abuse, threats or

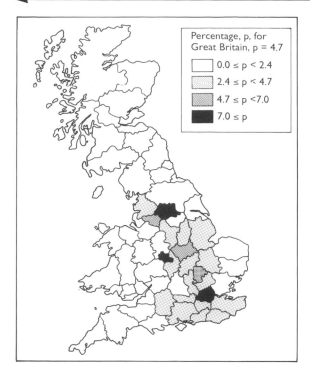

Figure 1.1 inside map legend:
Percentage, p, for Great Britain, p = 4.7
$0.0 \leq p < 2.4$
$2.4 \leq p < 4.7$
$4.7 \leq p < 7.0$
$7.0 \leq p$

Figure 1.1 Estimated minority ethnic group population as a percentage of total population, by county or region, 1986–8
Source: Population Trends 63, OPCS, HMSO (1991).

physical attacks, according to recent research.

The study by the independent London Research Centre found that 48,000 households have experienced racial harassment: 64 per cent of those say family members have been verbally abused, 24 per cent report physical assault and 17 per cent have members who have been threatened because of the colour of their skin. The study also found that 10,000 white families had suffered harassment.

- Of London's 480,000 ethnic minority households 10 per cent say they have suffered racial harassment (sample: 6,500)
- 64 per cent of victims claim a member of the household was verbally abused; 24 per cent claim physical assault, and 17 per cent threats.
- Incidents were reported to the police in 51 per cent of all cases and 59 per cent of assaults.

- 32 per cent of households said they still felt threatened.
- 55 per cent of victims were owner-occupiers, 38 per cent council or association tenants, 7 per cent private tenants.

(The Independent, 11 March 1993)

The European Parliament is increasingly encouraging member states to act against racism. The Committee of Inquiry into Racism and Xenophobia made the following points in 1990:

- there were 7,000 racial attacks in the UK in 1989;
- institutional racism is prevalent in British society and ethnic minorities continue to be discriminated against in the justice system, job opportunities and recruitment;
- it is twice as difficult for black people to get jobs as whites;
- management can manipulate formal rules to their advantage to hinder, rather than help, blacks in their efforts to get jobs;
- without positive action, ethnic minorities may forever fail to join mainstream economic life;
- in 1988, more than half the ethnic minority population of Strathclyde had experienced racial attacks.

(European Parliament 1990)

. . . racial discrimination has indeed continued to have a great impact on the employment opportunities of black people. . . . At least a third of the employers recruiting people to the jobs covered in this study discriminate against Asian applicants or West Indian applicants or both.

(C. Brown and P. Gay 1986, Policy Studies Institute)

We now have 4 black or Asian MPs out of 650, 1 senior Asian judge out of 500 at circuit level or above and 1 Asian Civil Servant out of 668 at under-secretary level or above, that is 0.15% compared to an economically active ethnic minority population of 4.7%.

(The Independent, 7 June 1991)

Thirteen of every 1,000 Asian babies die in their first year, compared with the national rate of five out of 1,000.

(Race Through the 90s, CRE and BBC 1992)

Compulsory detention under the Mental Health Act is twenty-five times more likely for 16–25-year-old blacks than for whites.

(Observer, 1 January 1987)

In 1985 DHSS figures showed that while overseas-born doctors in the NHS formed 28% of all hospital doctors, they were confined to the lower professional ranks.

(DHSS 1986)

In a survey entitled 'Equal Voice' carried out by Portsmouth University's social services research and information unit in 1992, it was revealed that most black and ethnic minority households interviewed in south-east Hampshire had not heard of the local council's Social Services Department; and more than one-third of those who had, did not know what services were on offer.

(Community Care, 28 March 1993)

SEX/GENDER

Women take overwhelming responsibility for domestic duties in Britain. Work mainly done by women in households includes washing and ironing (88%), preparing the evening meals (77%), looking after sick children (67%); the only work done mainly by men is repairing household equipment (82%).

(Social Trends, 1989)

Table 1.1 Employment by occupation: Great Britain, 1991

Occupational group	Females 000s	% of group	Males 000s	% of group	Total 000s
1 Managers & administrators	1,118	30.7	2,527	69.3	3,644
Bank, building society & post-office managers	23	21.9	83	78.1	106
2 Professional occupations	915	38.4	1,470	61.6	2,385
Medical practitioners	32	32.3	67	67.7	99
Solicitors	17	23.3	57	76.7	75
3 Associate professional & technical occupations	1,112	49.3	1,146	50.7	2,257
Computer analysts/programmers	41	20.6	157	79.4	198
Nurses	**397**	**89.7**	**46**	**10.3**	**443**
4 Clerical & secretarial	3,047	75.2	1,007	24.8	4,054
Computer operators	146	70.1	62	29.9	208
5 Craft & related	414	10.7	3,462	89.3	3,876
Bakers, flour confectioners	16	35.5	29	64.5	44
6 Personal & protective services	1,530	65.4	809	34.6	2,340
Police officers (Sgt & below)	17	12.1	124	87.9	141
Hairdressers, barbers	**100**	**86.7**	**15**	**13.3**	**115**
7 Selling	1,242	62.0	760	38.0	2,002
Sales assistants	867	77.6	251	22.4	1,118
8 Plant & machine operatives	570	22.1	2,011	77.9	2,581
Assemblers/lineworkers	113	48.8	119	51.2	233
9 Other occupations	1,178	51.8	1,079	48.2	2,276
Postal workers, mail sorters	32	17.6	150	82.4	182
Cleaners, domestics	**709**	**87.4**	**103**	**12.6**	**811**
Inadequately described/not stated	19	34.5	35	65.5	55
All occupations	11,145	43.8	14,324	56.2	25,470

Source: Labour Force Survey 1991.

Majorities of both sexes still regard certain occupations as being mainly suitable for men or women, but not suitable for both. For instance, majorities regard being a car mechanic as an exclusively male occupation, and substantial minorities of both sexes believe the same of the job of bus driver, police officer and bank manager. Similarly, substantial numbers of both sexes think women more suitable than men to be nurses and secretaries.

(*Social Trends*, 1990)

The average part-time working woman earns little over half as much per hour as a full-time working man while 4 out of 10 women are below the 16 hour threshold which legally denies them major employment rights. 82% of part-time workers are women.

(*Options*, November 1991)

Of those women who were in employment in 1990 (both employees and the self-employed), 81% were employed in three service sectors: 1. distribution, hotels, catering and repairs; 2. banking, finance, insurance, etc.; 3. other services which include nursing and education. (The corresponding figure for men was 53%). A further 14% of women were employed in manufacturing, compared with 28% for men. . . . Clerical and related occupations constituted the largest single category of women's employment (31%), followed by managerial and professional occupations (29%).

(*Labour Market Quarterly Report*, November 1991)

OLD AGE

NEGATIVE ATTITUDES TOWARDS OLD AGE

Although old age is a status that all of us might expect to reach, negative attitudes about old age

Table 1.2 School examination results, 1990/1991 (000s)

Subject	England GCSE Grades A–C		Scotland SCE Ordinary and Standard Grades 1–3		Wales GCSE Grades A–C	
	Females	Males	Females	Males	Females	Males
English	158.7	120.5	19.3	15.1	9.3	6.4
Mathematics	98.0	108.1	12.2	12.9	5.4	5.5
Biology	31.5	25.3	8.3	3.5	2.5	1.7
French	72.0	47.6	9.4	5.3	3.6	1.8
History	53.6	45.6	5.1	3.6	2.5	1.7
Chemistry	25.2	33.5	7.9	8.9	1.6	1.9
Physics	18.6	39.5	5.4	10.8	1.1	2.2
Computer Studies	12.4	15.9	2.0	3.7	1.2	1.6

Source: Department for Education; Scottish Examination Board Report 1991; Welsh Office.

Table 1.3 First destinations of school leavers, 1989/1990 (000s)

Leavers entering:	England		Scotland*		Wales	
	Females	Males	Females	Males	Females	Males
Degree courses and teacher training courses	35.2	37.9	3.9	4.1	2.5	2.1
Other full-time further and higher education courses	84.0	58.4	7.9	4.9	5.3	4.3
Labour market/destination unknown	162.7	199.9	24.9	29.1	9.4	12.1
All leavers	281.9	296.2	36.7	38.1	17.2	18.5

*1988/9 figures.
Source: Department for Education; Scottish Office; Welsh Office.

Table 1.4   The over-65s in the UK population

	Numbers (millions)		% of total population	
	Aged 65–79	Aged 80+	Over 65	Over 80
1901	1.3 (65–74)	0.5 (75+)	4.7	1.3 (75+)
1921	1.9 (65–74)	0.7 (75+)	5.9	1.5 (75+)
1951	4.8	0.7	10.9	1.4
1971	6.1	1.3	13.4	2.3
1981	6.9	1.6	15.0	2.8
1989	6.9	2.0	15.6	3.5
Males	3.0	0.6	6.3	1.1
Females	3.9	1.4	9.3	2.4
Projected 2001	6.7	2.5	16.0	3.8

Source: Social Trends 1986 (Table 1.1) and 1991 (Table 1.2).

Table 1.5   Percentage of the population aged 65 and over in selected countries

	1980	2010	2030
Canada	9.51	14.61	22.39
France	13.96	16.26	21.76
Germany	15.51	20.35	25.82
Italy	13.45	17.28	21.92
Japan	9.10	18.62	19.97
UK	14.87	14.61	19.24
USA	11.29	12.79	19.49

Source: OECD 'Ageing populations: the social policy implications', Demographic Change and Public Policy, 1988.

and 'the elderly' are common. To use Goffman's terminology, old age is a weakly stigmatised, discreditable status. Old age is not directly and inevitably discrediting for a number of reasons. Most importantly, it is often not immediately apparent how old someone is. In any case definitions of 'old' are indeterminate and so although negative attitudes and stereotypes are prevalent it is often difficult to know who is or is not 'old'. Hence old people who are fit, active and who look young are not stigmatised in the ways in which frail elderly disabled people may be. Indeed, the negative stereotypes of old age seem to be based upon the association between old age, sickness and dependency. Negative stereotyping highlights dependency, sickness and the inability to perform socially. A review by Lehr (1983) of studies of negative attitudes towards old age in industrial societies summarises the evidence as follows: 'Generally the image of the aged, aside from a few positive traits is defined by negative characteristics such as decline and loss of functions and capacities. The aged are perceived as ill, retarded, tired, slow, and inefficient in their thinking; they are seen as asexual, or if even showing sexual interests, as ridiculous.'

Such negative, stereotypical attitudes are widespread in British society and are constantly reinforced in the media and everyday conversation. . . . Because an old person has difficulty with her walking and eyesight, she or he is also presumed to have difficulty in understanding others, to be unable to make everyday decisions, and to have lost interest in world affairs and their own sexuality. As with other stereotypes the contradictory evidence of able and competent old people who manage their lives successfully is explained away by, for example, claiming they are 'exceptions'.

Most older people do not accept the stereotype of old age as applying to themselves, although there may be self-stigmatisation among some older people. Research shows that old people differentiate between how they look and their chronological age, and that their self-image is often that of being a younger person. . . .

Not all old people are able to resist the negative label of 'being old', especially if they are dependent upon other people for a range of physical and social support. . . . In such circumstances the attitudes of others can be said to create social handicaps for the old person and to create a 'self-fulfilling prophecy'.

(Field 1992)

DISABILITY

Government statistics . . . independent research projects and personal experiences show that on nearly every indicator of participation in mainstream life disabled people come out extremely badly: for example on employment statistics, income levels, suitable housing and access to public transport, buildings, information (newspapers, radio and television) and leisure facilities.

(Vic Finkelstein, in Swain et al.)

Poverty is also a restriction on the lives of people with learning difficulties. Those who live independently often rely on state benefits which are low: Flynn (1989) found that the average weekly income of 88 people in her study was £39 in 1985.

(Jan Walmsley, Swain et al.)

After over a century of state-provided education disabled children and young people are still not entitled to the same kind of schooling as their able-bodied peers, nor do they leave with equivalent qualifications . . . The majority of British schools, colleges and universities remain unprepared to accommodate disabled students within a mainstream setting.

(Mike Oliver and Colin Barnes, in Swain et al.)

Disabled people are more likely to be out of work than non-disabled people, they are out of work longer than other unemployed workers, and when they do find work it is more often than not low-paid, low-status work with poor working conditions.

(Mike Oliver and Colin Barnes, in Swain et al.)

The NHS does not publish statistics about the employment of disabled women in the National Health Service. However, the statistics collected by the Employment Service from Health Authorities in 1990 showed that only 4 out of 215 District Health Authorities and Boards and one out of 17 Regional health authorities have more than 1% of staff in employment who are registered disabled. Eight Authorities and Boards employed no registered disabled staff at all. NUPE's survey of nurses showed that disabled nurses tend to be employed in the lower grades and that their disability has resulted from injury sustained in the course of their employment. NUPE points to a need for greater preventative measures and imaginative efforts to integrate nurses with disabilities into satisfying work.

(Equal Opportunities Commission 1992, p. 40)

Your discussions of these groupings of statistics and information should have produced some interesting ideas. They may well have involved some conflict or disagreement among members of your group in attitudes, ideas and beliefs expressed. There may have been considerable confusion in trying to find appropriate explanations for some of the trends illustrated. Social scientists involved in the production and evaluation of the kind of information illustrated above have been concerned to *make sense* of it – to relate it to the way people interact and to changes in the social, economic and political structures of the society in which we live. Just as yours may have done, their interpretations of the data differ in many respects; but certain common themes can be described.

The bases of discrimination

Social scientists have suggested that data such as those presented above can be explained by using the concept of DISCRIMINATION to refer to the unfair treatment or neglect of certain groups of people in society. They suggest that discrimination in societies such as Britain can arise in several ways:

1 At the level of *individual prejudice*, where people may have personal attitudes and beliefs which they use to prejudge other groups negatively (or, in some instances, positively). There are many forms of prejudice; the following are some of the major 'isms' we will consider in this chapter:

- *racism*: a belief in the inherent superiority of one race over all others and thereby its right to dominance;
- *sexism*: a belief in the inherent superiority of one sex over the other and thereby its right to dominance;
- *ageism*: a belief in the inherent superiority of one age-group over all others.

And, of course, people may express a variety of prejudices towards people with disabilities.

These categories are not mutually exclusive. They may interlink, as in prejudice towards 'old women' or 'black youth'.

2 At the level of *institutional discrimination*, where there is public legitimation of prejudice. Within the structures and hierarchies of organizations, power can be used to exclude certain groups from access to resources, and to form (or to contribute to the formation of) general beliefs that such exclusion is justifiable.

3 At a *cultural* level, where people's 'common-sense' values, beliefs and ideas (i.e. those rarely questioned or challenged) can endorse and reinforce both individual prejudice and institutional discrimination. Here discrimination can be transmitted through history, through daily language and interaction and through media influences.

Strategies of discrimination

It has been argued that these bases or types of discrimination (which may produce undesirable, painful or life-threatening experiences for people) are reinforced by the strategies which people use to deny, ignore and minimize the presence of discrimination in their own institutions, culture and personal behaviour. This COVERT discrimination contrasts with OVERT discrimination, which is openly practised, acknowledged and even justified. Covert discrimination may take the following forms (adapted from Dominelli 1992):

- *Denial strategies*, based on the idea that there is no such thing as cultural and institutional racism/sexism, etc., only personal prejudice in its crude manifestations.
- *Colour- or gender-blind strategies*, which focus on the idea that all people are the same – members of one human race with similar problems, needs and objectives.
- *Dumping strategies*, which rely on placing the responsibility for eliminating racism, sexism, etc. on the shoulders of the groups discriminated against.
- *Omission strategies*, which rest on the view that racism, sexism, etc. are not important parts of social interaction and can be safely ignored in most situations.
- *Devaluing strategies*, which acknowledge the presence of discrimination in general terms but fail to 'see' it in specific instances involving daily routines/interaction and in the testimonies and accounts of family, friends, colleagues, etc.
- *Avoidance strategies*, where it is accepted that discrimination exists but there is a refusal or denial of the particular responsibility of the individual or institution to do something about it.

Theories relating to discrimination

Most social-psychological and (in sociology) interactionist theories of prejudice and discrimination have focused upon the following two ideas:

- that prejudice may arise from early socialization and learning experiences, personality traits and the general psychological processes involved in attitude formation;
- that prejudiced attitudes and adverse 'labelling' may result in low self-esteem and a 'self-fulfilling prophecy' of low achievement.

These theories are discussed in much greater depth in Chapter 4 on 'Psychological and

Social Aspects of Health and Social Care'. In this chapter we will examine theories relating to institutional and cultural discrimination.

Institutional and cultural discrimination

By growing up in this society, by incorporating its culture and history and by being exposed to the mass media, many people will become familiar with negative racial and sexual stereotypes and with stereotypes relating to people with disabilities and older people.

ACTIVITY

Whether or not we believe in the stereotyped views of race, gender, age and disability, their existence can be readily demonstrated. Working in groups, draw up lists of the most common negative stereotypes you have encountered.

These negative ideas and assumptions are reinforced when dominant organizations in society (local and central government, the legal system, schools, the health and welfare services, private companies) conduct their affairs in ways resulting in distinctive patterns of social disadvantage. Discriminatory practices become part of general routines and rules. The discrimination may not necessarily be recognized or intended (although it would be naïve not to believe that some forms of discrimination are deliberate). Institutional racism can also persist through the omission of serious and active attempts within such organizations to overcome the unfair treatment of certain groups within the population. For example, racial discrimination has no central place in the EC Social Charter and there are no EC race equality directives.

ACTIVITY

If you are doing a project on racism not exclusively based on Britain, you might consider looking at

- the experiences of migrant workers in EC countries;
- the conflict in the former Yugoslavia and the notion of 'ethnic cleansing'.

THE MEDIA'S ROLE IN CULTURAL DISCRIMINATION

PRESS 'GIVES SLANTED VIEW OF DISABLED PEOPLE'

National newspapers are presenting a partial and distorted view of people with disabilities and those who care for them, sometimes breaching the Press Complaints Commission's guidance on discrimination, according to a report published by the Spastics Society.

The choice of stories covered, and the language used, combine to portray disabled people – one in ten of the population – in a stereotyped and detrimental way, undermining their individuality, the society said.

It was easier to find bad examples in the tabloids, but the broadsheet press was also prone to sensationalising or marginalising the issues, it added. Both concentrated on fundraising, charity stories and personal interest medical stories, while disabled people are most affected by political and social issues. Community care, of profound interest to disabled people, was not covered by the tabloids in the periods studied, while stories about carers, sport, employment or local authority provisions for disabled people received little attention.

The report says that too often newspapers write about 'the disabled' or 'the handicapped' implying there is one homogeneous group, and that all disabled people are victims. It says newspapers often patronise, by referring to disabled people by their first name, as if they are small children in need of help. Conversely, anything a disabled person achieves, however minor, is heralded as worthy of congratulation.

Brian Lamb, head of campaigns at the Spastics Society, said that distorted reporting cut disabled people off from mainstream society. 'We hope this report will stimulate debate . . . and help point the way to good journalistic practice in the future,' he said.

The report, which analysed stories on disabilities over an eight-week period in late 1990, and two weeks last February, says the commission should ensure the Press 'avoids' prejudicial and perjorative reference to the person's race, colour, religion, sex or sexual orientation, or to any physical or mental illness or handicap'.

(The Independent, 3 December 1991)

INSTITUTIONAL DISCRIMINATION?

RICHMOND COUNCIL IS IGNORING THE DISABLED

Richmond Council came under fire this week for failing to appoint any disabled staff this year.

Cllr Malcolm McDougall, chairman of the Personnel Sub-Committee which published the findings, claimed that few from either group had applied for the jobs.

'If they don't apply, they can't be appointed', he explained, and claimed that 'the council goes out of its way to show its equal opportunities policy'.

Asked about the legal requirement that disabled people should form three per cent of all workforces, Cllr McDougall revealed: 'this requirement is not generally regarded as being an obligation, but the council plays its part in encouraging equal opportunities'.

Cllr McDougall said the council is looking into adapting its premises for disabled workers, should it be necessary, and that 'the council is always willing to pursue any positive initiative'.

But local disabled leaders are not impressed. Alan Pinn, Chairman of Thames Valley's Disabled Drivers Association, told the *Times* 'it's an absolute disgrace'.

He went on: 'I believe that comments like those made by Cllr McDougall are out of touch with current thinking, and don't help the situation.'

(Richmond and Twickenham Times, 9 October 1992)

Language and discrimination

One way in which discrimination enters culture is through the association between language and thought. The following is adapted from the publication of the National Association of Teachers in Further and Higher Education *Equal Opportunities Guide to Language* (NATFHE 1993), which offers a useful discussion of the issues in this area.

Overtly discriminatory and offensive language is an obvious problem, and can be a disciplinary issue related to harassment and discrimination. Beyond this obvious area, however, there are problems in laying down guidelines, because language is a fluid and dynamic medium, and reflects the society in which it is used. It is constantly changing in response to changes in society, and to the perceptions of people within society.

However, language is not neutral, neither is it a simple transparent medium for conveying messages. Language can help to form, perpetuate and reinforce prejudice and discrimination. Because of prejudice, negative feelings and attitudes may come to be associated with a word or phrase which was originally coined with positive intention. No word is good or bad in itself. Its use can be judged on two criteria: the intention of the person using it; the effect on the person about whom it is used. Few of us would have any hesitation about condemning words used with the intention to abuse or offend. But because of the frequent changes of terminology for describing groups which are the subject of prejudice, some people may use words which many now find offensive, although they have no intention of causing offence. The most positive line in these situations is to accept the wishes of the person/people offended, and use the terminology they would prefer.

GENDER

Sexist language is language that promotes and maintains attitudes that stereotype people according to gender. Non-sexist language treats all people equally, and either does not refer to a person's sex at all when it is irrelevant, or refers to men and women in symmetrical ways when their gender is relevant. It is accepted that stereotyping of the masculine can often affect men adversely. But the main problem with sexist language remains that generally it assumes that the male is the norm. The words 'man', 'he', 'him' are often used in referring to human beings of either sex. This gives a distinct impression to the reader or hearer that women are absent, silent, or of no importance. This problem can be overcome by:

1 Avoiding the use of he, his, him, by:

adding the female:	she or he, his or hers, s/he
using the first person:	I, me, mine, we, our, ours
using the second person:	you, your, yours
using the plural:	they, them, theirs.

2 Avoiding composite words containing the word 'man', e.g.:

Instead of:	Try:
manpower	workforce, staff
manning	staffing, running
man-made	artificial, synthetic
to a man	everyone, without exception, unanimously
man hours	work hours

In the workplace, biased language reinforces the stereotyping of men and women, and the fact that they are often typecast as being suitable for particular jobs. The gender description in such terms as 'male secretary', 'woman carpenter', 'male nurse', 'female director', reveals this typecasting. Linking jobs to gender can be avoided by using alternative expressions.

Instead of:	Try:
chairman	chair
headmaster	headteacher
businessman	business manager, executive
foreman	supervisor
policeman	police officer
salesman/girl	shop assistant/worker
stewardess/air hostess	airline staff/flight attendant

RACE

Racist language is language that promotes and maintains attitudes that stereotype people according to their skin colour and racial origin. It often involves stereotyped attitudes to culture and religion. Non-racist language treats all people equally, and either does not refer to a person's race when it is not relevant, or refers to black and white people in symmetrical ways when their race is relevant. Although there may be examples of language which negatively stereotypes white people, the main problem with racist language in our society is that it is either deliberately offensive to or abusive of those who are not part of the Anglo-Saxon majority, or it assumes that majority is the norm, and superior to all minorities. For examples, the term 'non-white' is directly exclusive, and implies deviation from the norm.

The controversies that surround the terminology in this area can be illustrated by the fact that even the term 'race' itself is loaded in the way it can be interpreted, and it does not carry the same meaning for all people. 'Ethnic minority', although widely used and accepted, is seen by many as containing both cultural and religious bias (the dictionary definition of ethnic is 'pertaining to nations not Christian or Jewish; Gentile, heathen, pagan'). However, most institutions use 'ethnic monitoring', and until some alternative is found the term will remain in use. The term 'immigrants' is inappropriate to describe people who were born or have settled in Britain, although the word is frequently used inaccurately to refer to black people.

In the first part of this century, the terms 'Negro', 'coloured', etc. were widely used. The development of Black movements in the 1960s led to the use of the word 'Black' as a proud and assertive term, and for many people, from then until now, this has been the preferred term. However, its use is seen by some as restricted to those of African origin, and some people from Chinese or Asian backgrounds may prefer to describe themselves, and be described, as such. Although for many years the term 'coloured' has been regarded as offensive, the expression 'people of colour' to cover those who are not members of the white majority has recently become fashionable in America, and its usage is now appearing in Britain. The principle remains to follow the wishes of the person/people concerned before deciding what terminology to use.

A number of phrases and terms used in everyday speech can cause offence. Some, like 'nigger in the wood pile' and 'working like a black' have their roots in a more openly racist past, and should be avoided. There is also a problem with the use of the word 'black' as an adjective. It is parody to object to 'black' as a purely descriptive colour adjective, as in such terms as 'black coffee', 'blackboard', 'black car', etc. The problem arises because so many uses of 'black' involve negative and sometimes evil connotations, e.g. 'black magic', 'black mark', 'black sheep', etc.

DISABILITY

The term 'disability' is now widely used to cover people who may have a physical disability, a mental illness, emotional, behavioural, or learning difficulties. The term 'disability', though contested by some, is more acceptable to many organizations controlled by disabled people than 'handicapped'. It takes into account that people may be disabled (i.e. prevented from being able to do something) not only by accidents (of birth, or otherwise) but by social organization which takes little or no account of such people and thus excludes them from participating in the mainstream of society's activities.

Again we find that what is acceptable in

one period causes offence in another, and there is a need to update our language on a regular basis. In education, for example, expressions such as 'ESN (Educationally Sub-Normal)', 'retarded', 'maladjusted' were once widely used. The expression 'special needs' was coined as an attempt to get away from those negative labels, and is still the coherent usage, although not acceptable to all disabled people. The term 'special educational needs' is not accurate, as in many cases the needs are not educational, but involve problems of access, etc. It can be dehumanizing to use blanket expressions such as 'the deaf' and demoralizing for disabled people to hear themselves constantly described as unfortunate victims.

Instead of:	Try:
mentally handicapped/ backward/dull	learning difficulty
spastic	cerebral palsy
mongol	Downs syndrome
cripple	person with disability/ mobility impaired
Idiot/imbecile/ feeble-minded	development disability
crazy/maniac/insane	emotional disability
The deaf	deaf person/person with impaired hearing
The blind	blind person/partially sighted person

AGE

It is now accepted that ageism is a form of prejudice and discrimination which must be taken seriously. In employment practices, although most managers now trumpet their equal opportunity policies and credentials, they are increasingly discriminating on the grounds of age. Language must be carefully constructed so as to combat this. The use of terms such as 'old fogey', 'dead wood', 'out of the Ark', 'geriatric', 'too old to change', 'over the hill', 'out of date', creates an environment in which it is possible to intimidate people into premature retirement. If we talked of 'more experienced', 'long-serving' instead of 'middle-aged' and 'the old guard', the intimidation could be avoided.

Effects of discrimination

Research into the effects of discrimination in the contexts of early education, health and welfare, and work is so wide-ranging that it would be impossible to summarize all the issues covered in the space available in this book. Instead, some of the main areas of concern raised by studies of the effects of racism, sexism, ageism and discrimination against people with disabilities are summarized below along with ideas for student assignments or projects and examples of key texts which students might find helpful. Work experience placements may provide opportunities for students to investigate some of these issues.

SEXISM

Early education

Important issues to consider in the study of sex and gender in the context of early education at home/at playgroups or nurseries/within other childcare arrangements/in primary schools are:

- sex-role stereotyping and socialization;
- the formation of gender identities and gender-linked labelling processes;
- the interaction between parents and children/carers and children/teachers and children, and between children themselves;
- the influence of cultural forms such as books, the mass media, songs, stories and play.

ACTIVITY

Ideas for projects and assignments

1 Carry out a content analysis of children's books, analysing the images of male and female characters which appear and the language used to describe them or which they are given to use. Interview children about their perceptions and

understanding of sex roles and gender in the books they read.

2 Observe children's play in a setting such as a nursery, playgroup, infant school or playground. Are boys and girls playing different games in different ways? Is this reinforced by the organization of the school/group/playground and the attitudes and behaviour of the adults caring for the children?

3 Interview parents or childcare workers about their perceptions of the differences between boys and girls and their approaches to caring for and working with each sex.

Key texts

Grabrucker, M. (1988), *There's a Good Girl: Gender Stereotyping in the First Three Years of Life*. London: Women's Press.

Best, L. (1993), 'Dragons, Dinner Ladies and Ferrets: Sex Roles in Children's Books', *Sociology Review*, vol. 2, no. 3, February 1993.

Health and social care

Studies of health, welfare and sex dis-crimination have looked at areas such as:

- why women form the largest proportion of 'carers' for elderly or disabled relatives and what implications this has for their lives;
- reproductive rights – access to abortion, contraception, fertility and IVF pro-grammes; ante- and post-natal care; pregnancy and childbirth;
- access to adequate maternity and child benefits as well as other state benefits;
- the response of the authorities and organizations to women suffering sexual abuse, rape or other physical abuse;
- how social and health services might be provided in non-sexist and non-hierarchical ways so that divisions between the service providers and service users are minimized and prejudice and discrimination therefore lessened.

ACTIVITY

Ideas for projects and assignments

1 Contact any voluntary 'carers' organization in your area (such as the 'Crossroads' scheme) to investigate their views about the pressures on women (and men) with regard to caring for elderly or disabled relatives.

2 Investigate the history of legislation relating to abortion, contraception and IVF in this and one other country, contrasting the development it has taken in the two examples chosen.

3 Carry out a survey among women with children, asking them about their views on maternity and child benefits and investigating whether they feel that the current system leads to prejudice and/or discrimination against women when they return to work.

4 Find out what facilities and services exist in your area for women (or men) suffering from sexual or physical abuse. Are they adequate?

5 Write to your local health and social services organizations asking for details of any equal opportunities they are carrying out and ask to talk to some of the key workers involved.

Key Texts

Abbot, P. and Wallace, C. (1990), *An Introduction to Sociology: Feminist Perspectives*. London and New York: Routledge (contains a useful chapter on 'Women, Health and Caring').

Faludi, S. (1991), *Backlash: The Undeclared War against Women*. London: Vintage (contains an excellent chapter on reproductive rights).

Work

Studies of gender and discrimination in the context of work have addressed:

- the reasons why women remain concentrated in the lower-status, less well-paid strata of occupations;
- whether there is a 'glass ceiling' for women at work which forms a barrier to promotion;
- how popular images of female employers in the 'caring professions' such as nursing contribute to prejudice and discrimination against them;
- problems and possibilities of part-time work and flexible working hours for women;
- the effects of attempts to combine paid work with domestic responsibilities and childcare.

ACTIVITY

Ideas for projects and assignments

1 There are many studies documenting the concentration of women in low-status, low-paid occupations, so there is the possibility here of carrying out an interesting overall survey of the issues using secondary sources.

2 Interview a particular category of women in one type of job to find out whether they think a 'glass ceiling' operates in their organizations.

3 Take one category of occupation in the health and welfare field and investigate the images and stereotypes that people hold about that form of work.

4 Carry out a survey of men and women working in the caring professions, asking what their ideal working arrangements would be and why.

Key texts

Equal Opportunities Commission, *Equality Management: Women's Employment in the NHS*. London: EOC. (Almost all EOC publications are of course useful; for address see list at end of chapter.)

Savage, J. (1985), *The Politics of Nursing*. London: Heinemann.

RACISM

Early education

As with sex and gender, important issues to consider in relation to the effects and implications of prejudice and discrimination in dealing with younger children are:

- the learning of racial stereotypes and images and the implications for 'labelling' and 'self-concept';
- the unintentional and sometimes intentional teaching of racist ideas, attitudes and cultural beliefs;
- structures of family life which reinforce an 'us and them' mentality and may contribute to hostility and lack of understanding between different groups in society.

ACTIVITY

Ideas for projects and assignments

1 Conduct an investigation into the way children see people from cultures and ethnic groups other than their own.

2 Visit a branch of a national chain of shops which sells books for children, such as The Early Learning Centre or W.H. Smith, and assess how many of the books on sale contain images of black or ethnic minority children or adults.

3 Hold discussions with a school or a playgroup which has a race equality policy to find out how that policy is implemented and what the attitudes and feelings of the staff and the children are towards it.

Key texts

Commission for Racial Equality (1989), *From Cradle to School: A Practical Guide to Race Equality and Childcare*. London: CRE (for address see list at end of chapter).

Milner, D. (1983), *Children and Race Ten Years On*. London: Ward Lock Educational.

Health and social care

Here studies have looked at:

- the extent to which Area Health Authorities and Social Services Departments have drawn up and/or implemented race equality policies;
- the issues of transracial adoption and fostering of ethnic minority children;
- the disproportionately large numbers of ethnic minority children taken into care in Britain;
- why most black elders in Britain today maintain themselves either on the level of income support rates or below the poverty level.

ACTIVITY

Ideas for projects and assignments

1 Write to your local Area Health Authority or Social Services Department asking if they have a race equality policy and if so, whether you can have a copy . Your teachers or lecturers may be able to arrange for you to interview any key personnel in these organizations concerned with equal opportunities.

2 Investigate the issue of transracial adoption and fostering.

Key texts

Leicester City Council (1990), *Earnings and Ethnicity*. Leicester: LCC.

CRE publications generally; a list may be obtained from the address given at the end of this chapter.

Community Care magazine (Reed Publishing Monthly Ltd, published monthly). Your local, school or college library should stock this.

Work

There are a large number of concerns here, which include:

- why qualified black social workers remain relatively scarce – although there has been a small rise in successful applicants for professional social work courses, from 7.9% in 1981 to 11.8% in 1984 (Bhat et al. 1988, p. 226);
- prejudice and discrimination against black and ethnic minority workers in the fields of health and social care.

ACTIVITY

Ideas for projects and assignments

1 Use secondary sources (the publications of the CRE and the Runnymede Trust are very helpful in this respect) to investigate the employment position of black and ethnic minority workers in this country.

2 Interview black or ethnic minority nurses, doctors and other health and social services professionals about their views on and experiences of racism. (You may find it helpful here to refer to the material on 'Interviews' in the section of Chapter 8 on 'Research Methods'.)

Key texts

Skellington, Richard and Morris, Paulette (1992), *'Race' in Britain Today*. London: Sage.

Richardson, John and Lambert, John (1985), *The Sociology of Race*. Ormskirk: Causeway Press.

The publications of the Commission for Racial Equality will be useful; for address see list at end of chapter.

DISABILITY

Early education

Important issues here are:

- the integration of children with special needs into mainstream schools;
- the 'STATEMENTING' of children with special needs so their needs might be met;
- the stresses faced by families with under-fives with a disability and the services

which would alleviate some of those stresses;
- the prejudice towards, labelling and self-image of children with disabilities;
- advocacy and EMPOWERMENT – i.e. that adults ensure that the wishes of the child are heard and considered and that the child is enabled (empowered) to make his or her wishes known to adults.

ACTIVITY

Ideas for projects and assignments

1 If a placement can be found in a school which has successfully integrated children with special needs, then it may be possible to investigate how this occurred.

2 Research into the stereotypes and images children hold of children with special needs or disabilities could be carried out.

3 If you know someone well who has a young child with a disability, it might be possible to use an unstructured interview to find out more about what the experience of having a child with a disability in the family can mean.

Key texts

Stow, L. and Selfe, L. (1989), *Understanding Children with Special Needs*. London: Unwin Hyman.

HMSO (1991), *The Children Act Guidance and Regulations*, vol. 6: *Children with Disabilities*. London: HMSO.

Health and social care

Many studies here look at:

- The experiences, including those of prejudice and discrimination, and the situations of people with disabilities, *from their own perspective*. There is much criticism and questioning of the very categories used in terms such as 'disabilities' and 'disabled person'. The essential focus of many studies is therefore on the social barriers to full participative citizenship which people with disabilities may face.

- Images of disability and concepts of 'normal' and 'abnormal' and how they may have furthered the disadvantages faced by people with disabilities.
- The extent to which disabled people can participate in and/or control the provision of services and facilities intended for their use.
- The experiences of older people with disabilities who are noticing the effects of ageing.

ACTIVITY

Ideas for projects and assignments

1 Interview people with disabilities about how they view the terms and labels applied to them.

2 Get in touch with voluntary and self-help organizations for people with disabilities in your area and talk to the people who are involved in these about the issue of participation in the running of services and facilities.

3 Investigate the images and stereotypes of disability which appear in the mass media.

Key texts

O'Hagan, Maureen and Smith, Maureen (1993), *Special issues in Child-Care*. London: Ballière Tindall (contains a very good chapter on children and special needs).

Work

Important issues here are:

- the absence to date of anti-discriminatory legislation for people with disabilities along the lines of that already provided in terms of race and sex;
- the discrimination faced by people with disabilities in applying for jobs;
- positive examples of where people with disabilities have been enabled (sometimes

through the use of information technology) to obtain work.

ACTIVITY

Ideas for projects and assignments

1 Write to your local council, asking what proportion of registered disabled employees they have. Visit your local job centre to ask how many vacancies advertised by them have been filled by registered disabled people in the last year.

2 Find out more about the kinds of facilities which would make it easier for people with disabilities to find employment.

Key texts

Skett, Alan (1993), *Caring for People with Disabilities*. London: Pitman Publishing.

AGE

Early education

Studies here have concentrated on:

- the lack of state-funded nursery and childcare provision in this country and the possible implications for children's emotional, social and intellectual development as well as for equal working opportunities for working parents (especially women and single parents);
- the prejudice and discrimination faced by women who breast-feed their babies in public and the attitudes towards women and children implied by these reactions;
- the prejudice and discrimination faced by parents and carers towards children in general in public places, e.g. restaurants;
- the lack of inexpensive leisure facilities for young people.

ACTIVITY

Ideas for projects and assignments

1 Survey the provision of playgroup and nursery places in your area. (Your local

council or community health clinic should be able to provide a list of playgroups/nurseries in the area.) What facilities are available? What do parents with under-fives in the area where you live think of these facilities?

2 Interview women who have breast-fed their babies in public places about their experiences.

3 Investigate the provision of leisure facilities for young people in your area. What do young people think of these facilities? Are they adequate?

Key texts
Contact the following organizations for useful reading material:

Association of Breast Feeding Mothers
Order Department
Sydenham Green Health Centre
Holshaw Close
London SE26 4TH

Pre-School Playgroups Association
61–63 Kings Cross Road
London WC1X 9LL

Health and social care
Studies here have covered issues such as:

- general prejudice and discrimination towards older people in society;
- child poverty.

ACTIVITY

Ideas for projects and assignments

1 Carry out a survey of young people's attitudes and perceptions of older people. You may wish to refer to the material on questionnaires in Chapter 8 for advice on constructing an appropriate survey.

2 Contact the Child Poverty Action Group for information relating to this issue.

Key texts
All publications from the Child Poverty Action Group will be helpful. Write to:

Child Poverty Action Group
4th Floor
1–5 Bath Street
London EC1V 9PY

Field, David (1992), 'Elderly People in British Society', *Sociology Review*, vol. 1, no. 4, April 1992.

Work
- A major concern is the barriers to employment and promotion faced by older people and the lack of any legislation to protect them from discrimination in this respect.

ACTIVITY

Ideas for projects and assignments

Find out if the local Job Club or employment training programmes in your area include groups for older people wishing to return to work. Find out if it would be possible to talk to some of the people who attend these sessions about their experiences.

Key texts
Family Policy Studies Centre (1991), Fact Sheet 2 'An Ageing Population'. London: Family Policy Studies Centre.

HOW EQUAL OPPORTUNITIES ARE MAINTAINED

Combating prejudice and discrimination: equal opportunities legislation

The problems faced by the NHS in Britain are well publicized; as budgets are cut, hospital wards and clinics are forced to close, waiting lists for operations grow longer and services are run down. These events are given prominence on TV and in the press, especially when highlighted by charity campaigns to raise money for machinery and buildings previously funded by the NHS. In contrast, over the past ten years there has been considerable growth in the availability of and advertising for private medicine, promoted by images of luxury very different from the dingy wards and ramshackle facilities of the public sector.

It is therefore not surprising to have found that *inequality of access is a commonplace theme in accounting for health and illness, articulated out of both the political ideology of socialism and a broader-based expectation in Britain that the sick deserve the best of treatment, irrespective of their ability to pay.*

(Stainton Rogers 1990, emphasis added)

The previous section of this chapter looked at the bases and forms of discrimination existing within a society. Just as there are different explanations for prejudice and discrimination, so there are different suggested 'solutions'. In highlighting the issue of 'inequality of access', the question of EQUAL OPPORTUNITIES becomes crucial, directing attention as it does to three fundamental questions:

1 In what areas of social and political life is it unjustified to treat men and women, members of different ethnic, cultural or religious groups, people of different ages, people with special needs or learning difficulties differently?
2 Are there any areas of social and political life where it *may* be justified to treat anyone differently?
3 How could access to and treatment within education, housing, employment and in the provision of goods and services be made equitable and fair?

Key legislation in this country such as the 1976 Race Relations Act, the 1975 and 1986 Sex Discrimination Acts and the 1981 Education Act (which laid down that local authorities must draw up STATEMENTS assessing the needs of children with physical and mental disabilities or learning difficulties, with the implication that these needs should be met) paved the way for the issue of equal opportunities to be addressed by organizations and employers around the country. Figures 1.2–1.4 outline the major equal opportunities legislation now in place and the role of the Commission for Racial Equality (CRE) and the Equal Opportunities Commission (EOC) in implementing it. Figure 1.5 summarizes the legislative measures introduced since the Second World War relating to people with a disability.

Public support for equal opportunities at work for men and women has grown in recent years. A survey by the Family Policy Studies Centre in 1992 found that 85% of their respondents favoured laws against sex discrimination but only 23% believed that opportunities are, in fact, equal. According to the 1992 Annual Report of the Equal Opportunities Commission, the number of women reporting sex discrimination at work rose by 40% in 1991–2. However, it is important to recognize that while equal opportunities legislation has generally been welcomed as a good thing, there are other perspectives on the issue of prejudice and discrimination which deserve serious consideration.

Some people have argued that the right-wing Conservative governments in power in this country since 1979 have not embraced and promoted the idea of equal opportunities quite so enthusiastically as they might. Organizations such as the CRE and EOC, which have focused upon legal initiatives as a way of making progress, suggest that these governments have failed to respond to proposals to strengthen and improve race relations and sex discrimination legislation. They point out that while discrimination continues to be a widespread phenomenon in Britain today, only a handful of discrimination cases succeed each year in industrial tribunals or courts. The CRE has said that when it first reviewed the 1976 Race Relations Act in 1985, it 'suggested many ways of making the

THE SEX DISCRIMINATION ACTS 1975 AND 1986

With some exceptions in certain circumstances (and the Act does not apply to Northern Ireland), the 1975 and 1986. Sex Discrimination Acts make discrimination unlawful in:

- employment and training
- education
- the provision of goods, facilities and services

These acts give people a right of access to the civil courts and industrial tribunals for legal remedies for unlawful discrimination.

Types of discrimination

DIRECT DISCRIMINATION: DEFINITION AND EXAMPLE

This occurs when one person is treated less favourably, on the grounds of their sex, than a person of the other sex is or would be treated in similar circumstances.

Example:

A child is refused a place in a nursery class and the only reason given is that there are 'already too many girls'.

INDIRECT DISCRIMINATION: DEFINITION AND EXAMPLE

This occurs when a requirement or condition, which cannot be justified on grounds other than sex, is applied to men and women equally but has the effect in practice of disadvantaging a considerably higher proportion of one sex than the other.

Example:

A girls' school insists that no pupils should be allowed to wear trousers as part of a school uniform. This indirectly discriminates against Asian girls in the school who follow a religious code of conduct requiring that they wear garments which conceal all the lower part of the body (usually a fabric 'shift' dress

The 1975 Act also set up

THE EQUAL OPPORTUNITIES COMMISSION

This has a statutory duty to enforce the Sex Discrimination Act 1975 and the Equal Pay Act 1970 (which came into force in 1975).

The EOC produces leaflets and guidelines on all types of issues related to equal pay and sex discrimination. It carries out research, awards grants to other groups for research, advises employers and trade unions on 'working towards equality' and assists individuals or groups to fight cases of discrimination.

The Sex Discrimination Acts do not apply to work outside Great Britain; to cases where sex can be a 'genuine occupational qualification; to the armed forces. There is special provision for the police, prison officers, ministers of religion and competitive sport.

VICTIMIZATION

This occurs when an employer treats an employee (of either sex) less favourably than other employees are or would be treated on the grounds that the employee has or intends or is suspected of:

- bringing proceedings against the employer under the SDA or EPA
- helped another to do so or took part in an EOC formal investigation or tribunal hearing
- alleged that the employer or anyone else had contravened the SDA or EPA

Example:

A social worker in a residential home gives evidence in proceedings under the SDA against a co-worker who has been accused of sexual discrimination against other employees. She is subsequently refused promotion.

Types of discrimination (only applicable in employment matters)

DIRECT MARRIAGE DISCRIMINATION: DEFINITION AND EXAMPLE

This occurs when a married person is treated less favourably, because he/she is married, than a single person of the same sex is or would be treated in similar circumstances.

Example:

An employer rejects all applications for posts from married people.

INDIRECT MARRIAGE DISCRIMINATION: DEFINITION AND EXAMPLE

This occurs when a requirement or condition which cannot be justified on grounds other than marital status is applied equally to married and single persons (of either sex) but has the effect in practice of disadvantaging a considerably higher proportion of married than single people (of the same sex).

Example:

A health authority issues application forms for student midwife posts on which applicants are required to state their sex and dates of birth of their children. Married female applicants for the posts with pre-school children subsequently receive letters stating they cannot be considered for 5 years because of their pre-school children. This arrangement is indirectly discriminatory because the requirement or condition that an applicant must not have children of pre-school age is such that the proportion of married female applicants who can comply with it is considerably smaller than the proportion of female applicants who can do so.

(The EOC found southern Derbyshire health authority discriminating in this way in 1988. See EOC 1990.)

Figure 1.2

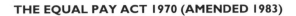

THE EQUAL PAY ACT 1970 (AMENDED 1983)

The most important provision of this legislation is that an employee is entitled to equal pay (and other contractual terms and conditions) with an employee of the opposite sex if:

(i)   they are doing work which is the same or broadly similar;

(ii) they are doing work which has been rated as equivalent by an analytical job evaluation scheme; or

(iii) they are doing work of equal value in terms of the demands made on the worker (whether or not there has been a job evaluation scheme).

THE EMPLOYMENT PROTECTION ACT 1975

This gave women the right to paid maternity leave and the opportunity of returning to work afterwards.

Figure 1.3

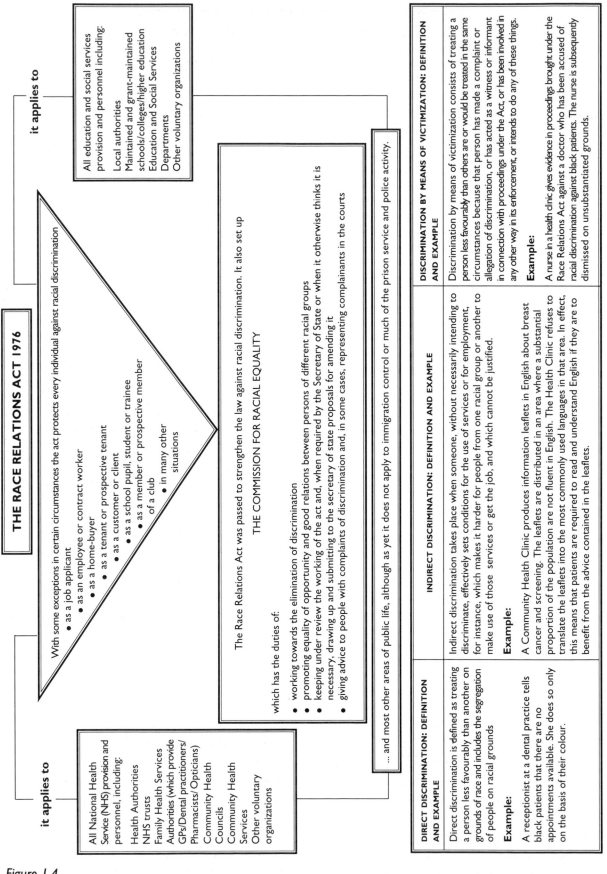

Figure 1.4

LEGISLATION RELEVANT TO DISABILITY

Disabled Persons (Employment) Act 1994	Attempted to secure employment rights for disabled people.
Education Act 1944	Specified that disabled children should be educated alongside their peers in primary and secondary education.
National Assistance Act 1948	Laid a duty on local authorities to 'arrange services for people'.
Chronically Sick and Disabled Persons Act 1970	Listed the services local authorities should provide and made it compulsory for local authorities to compile a register and publicize services (which only need to be provided 'where practical and reasonable' to do so).
Education Act 1981	Sets out the requirements for the integration of children with special needs into the mainstream school system.
Disabled Persons (Services, Consultation and Representation) Act 1986	Provided professional and administrative approaches to the provision of services. Gives the person with disability the right to have an 'advocate', e.g. a social worker, to be present when needs are being assessed.

Figure 1.5

law more effective. The Government never responded formally, and little has changed.'

There are fears, too, that as the European Community (EC) has not so far adopted a formal ban on racial discrimination, Britain's laws could be weakened when the single market comes fully into effect.

These arguments have led some to suggest not only that the powers of the CRE and the EOC are far too limited but also that a focus on 'equal opportunities' alone is too weak and will not bring about the wider and more fundamental social changes in attitudes and in social and economic structure in society necessary to eliminate institutional prejudice and discrimination. For example, where people do not start out from an equal base, offering fair treatment may do little to redress more fundamental disadvantages faced by certain social groups, such as the experience of poverty and long-term unemployment. The following extract is from *The Independent*'s report on the first national survey of the blind:

MOST BLIND PEOPLE 'LIVING IN POVERTY'

Most blind people 'live at the extremes of poverty', are unemployed and do not go out on their own, according to the first national survey of people with visual handicaps, published yesterday by the Royal National Institute for the Blind.

Ian Bruce, the director-general of the RNIB, said the report showed that the blind 'are poorly served by hard-pressed social services departments, with fewer than one in five being visited even once at the time of their sight loss'.

The survey reveals that nearly 1 million people are eligible for registration as blind or partially-sighted – far higher than government estimates. There are 300,000 completely blind people in Britain, 119,000 more than previously thought.

The report, which was based on 600 interviews, says four out of five blind people of working age are unemployed. More than half have been out of work for five years. In both respects, the blind fare worse than the general disabled population, in which 31 per cent have found employment.

(The Independent, 16 October 1991)

While some writers have been critical of the implementation and effectiveness of equal opportunities legislation, others have noted how the debate over social class, income and 'equality of access' to services and treatment is expressed in the public debate about private versus public health and social care services, an area where differential treatment has not been seen by governments as a form of discrimination comparable to sexism or racism. The treatment of the public as 'consumers' of health care is reflected in the following extract from the St Helier NHS Trust Publication, *Health Extra +, May 1993*.

The Maternity Wards at St Helier Hospital have seen the birth of over 3,500 new babies in the last year.

Over this year, the Maternity Wards have continued to improve their service, for example, new developments in the out patients service. 'Some mums find it difficult to get to the hospital during the day, so we have been setting up appointments for them, "out of working hours" ' said Shermane Peters, Clinical Midwife Manager on the Maternity Wards.

Tours of the Maternity Unit have also proved very popular with mothers and their partners. 'It gives an opportunity to meet the midwives, ask any questions and allows us to allay any anxieties or concerns' added Shermane.

Also available in St Helier Hospital, is the Private Ward, which has proved particularly attractive to women who would like a higher degree of privacy during their time on the ward. Maternity care is provided by an independent team of midwives and doctors are always available. Peace of mind is added to, as the ward is at the centre of a large hospital, with all its high technology equipment.

Whichever option chosen by the mother and her partner, The Trust will care for the whole family in the considerate and compassionate manner, which women have come to expect, from this leader in the field of maternity care.

(Health Extra +, May 1993)

SHORTCOMINGS OF THE LEGISLATION

In itself, legislation to maintain equal opportunities has not proved sufficient to ensure:

- That the existence of the law is recognized or that it is understood.
- That 'loopholes' in the legislation have not been used to discriminate.
- That individuals can discover whether they are victims of unlawful discrimination in the first place. For instance, if an individual is turned down for a job or promotion, how can he or she be certain that this is because of his or her sex, race, cultural background, disability, etc.?
- That organizations, employers and

individuals change their long-term practices, even if they have been proved to have been discriminating in a particular area or against a particular individual. Many organizations may choose to respond to a situation such as this by paying costs or damages to the individual who has brought the case to a tribunal or to the courts, as in the following example:

PC Joginder Singh Prem, the Sikh constable who won £25,000 damages from Nottinghamshire Constabulary for racial discrimination and victimisation, was turned down for promotion to sergeant five times, despite passing the sergeant's and inspector's exams.

When he was rejected for the fourth time in 1991, he lodged a complaint with Nottingham industrial tribunal. After a fifth rejection in 1992, he filed a second complaint.

A month later, the force started disciplinary proceedings against him over his investigation of an assault.

PC Prem said: 'I was called a turban-headed git.

'I could tolerate that sort of slogan from junior officers, but life got difficult when they started saying it in front of senior officers who seemed to be supporting them.

'Nobody could ever touch my work effort. But instead of getting encouragement, all I had was discouragement and ridicule.'

Yesterday's settlement, which avoided a six-week tribunal hearing, included £10,000 for each of his two last rejections, which the force admitted were the result of racial discrimination.

The case, which comes more than two years after the force paid a total of £30,000 damages for race discrimination to another Sikh constable, Surinder Singh, and two sergeants, raises questions about the effectiveness of the equal opportunities policy set up in the wake of that case.

(Guardian, 5 May 1993)

Nevertheless, in some organizations, it does seem that the allegation of and investigation into discriminatory practices can provide the spur for long-term change. For example, a formal CRE investigation into admissions for medical training at St George's Hospital in London found direct racial discrimination. The computer program which was used for initial selection of applicants for interview gave differential and less favourable weighting to women and ethnic minority candidates. The admissions policy has since been changed to eliminate discrimination.

• That the law is implemented. For example, the 1981 Education Act was accompanied by government guidelines that recommended that children with special needs should be assessed for 'statementing' within six months. A report in 1992 by the Audit Commission and Her Majesty's Inspectors found that some pupils were having to wait for up to three years and that the average wait was twelve months.

Robert Clay should be starting school next term, but has yet to be assessed for his educational needs.

Robert is almost five and physically disabled. A year ago his mother, Catherine, wrote to her local county council's education department asking for a statement on his needs, and was refused.

Several attempts later the assessment has been agreed, but may be too late for him to start school.

'He should be going after Easter, but the school is waiting to see how many hours' help he will get,' said Mrs Clay.

If a school thinks that a child who has not been assessed needs extra help, it has to apply to the Mainstream Support Group, set up by the education authority, to fund special needs sessions.

But there are many schools applying for a limited amount of money, so not all schools get what they say they need. Had Robert been assessed, he would automatically receive the help he needs.

'At the moment the school doesn't even know if it will be able to take him, because if it doesn't get funding for extra help, it can't afford to take him on.

The council could not comment on individual cases, said a spokeswoman.

(Guardian, 29 March 1993)

• That the law is interpreted in the same way by everyone concerned. There is a legal requirement that disabled people should form 3% of all workforces of twenty or more people. This requirement is rarely regarded as an obligation.

ACTIVITY

1 Write to the EOC and the CRE (for addresses see list at end of chapter) for further information about sex discrimination and race relations legislation. These organizations publish many useful and free guides.

2 Test 'awareness' of the legislation by designing a small-scale survey and carrying it out in your school or college or on the general public (see Chapter 8 for guidance). There may also be opportunities to interview the people you meet during a work experience placement. How familiar are people with the laws? What are their attitudes towards the legislation?

By the early 1980s it was clear that laws against unequal pay and sex discrimination would do nothing to tackle the entrenched patterns of inequality that had built up over centuries . . . people have begun to insist that POSITIVE measures are needed in order to compensate for past discrimination.

(Coote and Campbell 1982)

There has been a growing recognition that the legislation on racial equality, sex discrimination and special needs provided a starting point, but that there are other areas which organizations, employers and individuals need to address:

• Organizations (schools, local authorities, employers, hospitals, etc.) need to formulate equal opportunities policies of their own, specific to their own needs and concerns as well as complying with the law.

• Training and education in equal opportunities and race awareness needs to be provided; there should be agreed procedures and policies which need to be monitored and evaluated.

• Recruitment and selection procedures need to be non-discriminatory.

• More flexible working arrangements and facilities (e.g. workplace nurseries) should be considered to encourage the recruitment and retention of women with children or carers looking after elderly or disabled relatives.

• Positive action policies to improve employment prospects for disadvantaged groups could be carried out where monitoring showed that particular groups have been under-represented in certain types of work or grades of work (positive discrimination at the point of selection remains unlawful). Training for work in which one particular group had previously been under-represented may lawfully be provided and employers may encourage members of that group to take up work. One way of doing this is through job advertisements which encourage applications from a particular sex or ethnic group to apply for the post. Some examples are given opposite. The advertisement for a manager for an Asian women's refuge is allowed specifically to request an 'Asian woman' because her ethnic background and sex constitute a 'genuine occupational qualification' for the job – i.e. she will provide services to particular groups in the community that may be done most effectively by an Asian woman. Similar

COUNTY COUNCIL
WORKING TOWARDS
EQUAL OPPORTUNITIES

SOCIAL SERVICES DEPARTMENT
INSPECTION UNIT

INSPECTORS
£18,615 – £20,238

A number of opportunities arise for Inspector appointments during the period April to July 1993 owing to the cessation of fixed term contract employees, retirement and career progression.

The duties of these posts include registering and inspecting private and voluntary residential care homes for adults and inspecting Local Authority homes. Applicants should have: experience of the practice and management of residential care; a recognised social services qualification; a commitment to promoting high standards of care and quality of life for residents.

Personal skills and abilities required include: a well organised approach to your work; good presentation, oral and written communication; negotiation; evaluation; confident manner in dealing with owners, managers and residents and working with colleagues in other agencies. Keyboard skills will be an advantage and training will be provided in the use of the Unit's computerised register, work processing and inspection management system.

You must be a car driver, an essential car user allowance is payable. Applicants must be prepared to work unsocial hours as necessary to meet the requirements of the work.

The Social Services Department particularly welcomes applications from Afro-Caribbean and Asian people and people with disabilities as they are under represented in the department. (Race Relations Act 1976 Section 38(1)(b) applies).

Job sharers welcome

County Council

 An Equal Opportunities Employer welcoming applications from all sections of the community.

TEMPORARY SOCIAL WORKERS FOR MINORITY ETHNIC COMMUNITIES
(2 POSTS – FULL-TIME OR PART-TIME)

Salary: **Social Work Grade (Qualified)**
£12,810 (Scp 23) – £16,194 (Scp 38) (Review)
£18,615 per annum (Scp 35)
(Pro rata if part-time)

Desirable qualifications: CQSW, CSS or equivalent qualifications in field related to Social Work.

We are seeking to recruit two temporary social workers who will assist in the County Council's aims to ensure that members of the ethnic communities from the New Commonwealth are provided with a social work service and that this service is developed in accordance with their needs.

Due to the specialised role it is essential that applicants are able to understand and communicate clearly in spoken and written English and spoken Gujerati and Urdu. It is also desirable to have a knowledge of Afro-Caribbean cultures and communities, and therefore members of this community would be welcome applicants.

Due to the funding arrangements of these posts, contracts will be offered on a fixed term basis until 31st March, 1995. The County Council offers the following:

* a major commitment to training
* optional superannuation scheme
* car user allowance payable; facilities available for car loan or lease
* professional supervision
* re-location expenses up to £4,400
* a real commitment to Equal Opportunities
* attractive Local Conditions of Services complementing the National Scheme which can include additional annual leave, enhanced sickness provisions, etc.
* creche facilities
* It is essential that postholders possess a full driving license and have access to a vehicle during working hours.

For an informal discussion, please contact the Practice Manager.

CHILDREN AND FAMILIES SERVICE

TEAM LEADER – Hospital based

£22,008 – £24,275 p.a. inc.

A full time (35 hours) fieldwork team leader is sought.

The Children and Families fieldwork service is divided into teams undertaking assessments or long term work. There is a vacancy for a team leader in the assessment team, which has special links with all hospital paediatric services.

We are looking for social workers/ managers with at least 3 years post qualification experience, most of which should be in children's fieldwork. Candidates should have experience of working in a hospital setting and preferably some managerial experience.

The ethnic minorities population of Harrow is under-represented at this level and applications from black and other ethnic minorities would be particularly welcomed.

an equal opportunities employer

MANAGER FOR ASIAN WOMENS REFUGE

in Birmingham. The successful applicant will be an Asian woman with a professional social work qualification, who is committed to developing services to Asian women and families in need. She will:

* speak Punjabi and at least one other South Asian language;
* be experienced in family and child care work;
* have some experience of management and/or supervising staff.

The post involves familiarity with the Benefits system; counselling of residents and their families; carrying overall control of the domestic budget; and understanding and implementing an Equal Opportunities policy.

The post is non-residential. Salary £16,500 – £18,500.

The post is exempt from the requirements of the Sex Discrimination Act under Section 52D and Section 7.

criteria apply to the County Council Advertisement for temporary social workers for minority ethnic communities.

- Ethnic monitoring, which involves employers finding out how many people from ethnic minorites are employed with the aim of giving everyone an equal chance, can be controversial unless visible progress on these issues is subsequently made. At present, however, ethnic monitoring is carried out by only a small number of employers and public services.

ORGANIZATIONAL RESPONSES TO THE LEGISLATION

The late 1970s and 1980s saw a wave of projects and programmes initiated in local authorities (particularly the Inner London Education Authority, ILEA), in individual schools and colleges, and in health and social services organizations in inner-city and urban areas. Some legislation of the 1980s, however, seemed contrary to the spirit of these initiatives. For example, Clause 28 of the Local Government Act 1988 stated that there would be a

prohibition on promoting homosexuality by teaching or by publishing material.

(i) A local authority shall not:
 (a) intentionally promote homosexuality or publish material with the intention of promoting homosexuality;
 (b) promote the teaching in any main-tained school of the acceptability of homosexuality as a pretended family relationship.

A persistent theme in this political context has been the relationship between LOCAL GOVERNMENT and CENTRAL GOVERNMENT, including aspects such as the crisis in local government funding; local democratic initiatives; and central government powers. Conservative governments have preferred the language of 'equal opportunities' to the more radical 'anti-racist' and 'anti-sexist' policies and programmes which have emerged in health, welfare and social work contexts.

ACTIVITY

Compare these two articles from *Community Care* (published within a month of each other in 1992). In the first extract, Tim Yeo is critical of 'anti-discriminatory' policies. In the second, Baroness Cumberlege calls on health authorities to promote 'equal opportunities'.

Devise a role-play in which these two junior health ministers are called on to explain and discuss their views.

BLACK STAFF WELCOME ANTIRACIST STANCE

Black social workers expressed concern this week at the government's criticisms of the social work training council's anti-discriminatory policies.

In a statement released shortly before its annual conference this weekend the Association of Black Social Workers and Allied Professions welcomed the growing prominence of race.

Supporting CCETSW's anti-racist guidelines, the association said it deplored the actions of those 'seeking to destabilise the process'. Junior health minister Tim Yeo has complained of CCETSW's emphasis on anti-discriminatory policies.

EQUALITY OPTION

Baroness Cumberlege, a junior health minister, has called on health authorities to promote equal opportunities and provide appropriate services for black and ethnic minority communities. Speaking at an open day of the London Chinese Health Resource Centre, she praised the work of Chinese social workers, doctors and nurses in care provision.

A TORRENT OF NEW LEGISLATION

An extraordinary 145 pieces of legislation affecting local government have been passed by Conservative governments since 1979. What follows is just the tip of the legislative iceberg which has affected local government in the past few years. It includes some of the most controversial and most significant for social services.

- Housing Act 1988
- Local Government Act 1988 – included Clause 28
- Local Government Finance Act 1988 – introduced poll tax
- Local Government and Housing Act 1989 – restrictions on 'political activity' by local authorities
- Children Act 1989
- NHS and Community Care Act 1990
- Local Government Act 1992 – local government structures
- Local Government Finance Act 1992 – introduces council tax

The 'torrent of new legislation' outlined in this extract from *Community Care* (6 May 1993), together with the Education Acts passed in the 1980s and 1990s, in the political climate in which it has been implemented, has undoubtedly had an impact upon the financial and organizational commitment to positive action on equal opportunities in many health and social care contexts. A 'momentum for change' has, arguably, been slowed down.

ACTIVITY

Invite speakers/representatives from the main political parties to talk to your class about their views on how organizations should implement equal opportunities legislation.

Four interesting reports highlight the progress which has been made and the problems which remain.

1 The study *Racial Equality in Social Services Departments: A Survey of Equal Opportunities Policies*, carried out by the CRE in 1988 and published in 1989, focused particularly on equal

opportunities and service delivery, that is, whether all users of Social Services Departments could be said to be treated fairly. It provided the CRE with a 'snapshot of the state of development of equal opportunities practice in social services delivery in 1988 as reported by just over a third of the departments in England, Scotland and Wales'.

The survey found that 66% of those departments had no written equal opportunities policy and most were not meeting their duties in law under section 71 of the Race Relations Act 1976, i.e. they were not ensuring that unlawful racial discrimination was not taking place and not promoting equality of opportunity and good relations between persons of different racial groups.

The CRE suggested that there was a need for departments to use a formal written policy rather than simply a general intention to treat all service users fairly.

In the survey, Social Services Departments were asked whether they had:

(a) adopted particular measures to meet the needs of ethnic minorities;
(b) adapted existing services to meet the needs of a multi-racial community.

In answer to (a), the particular measures most often cited were:

- the translation of social services information into relevant community languages;
- the use of an interpreting service;
- race relations training for staff;
- the appointment of specialist race advisers for services.

In reply to (b), the adaptations most frequently mentioned were:

- recruitment campaigns for ethnic minority foster and adoptive parents;
- guidelines for staff on the needs of ethnic minority children in care;
- training for staff involved in child care;
- involving members of the ethnic minority

communities in planning for care, the translation of leaflets and in outreach work;

- adapting the dietary requirements of meals-on-wheels services to ethnic minorities;
- changes to day centres to make them more attractive to ethnic minority users;
- the funding of ethnic minority groups who provided social services to the community.

ACTIVITY

The replies given by Social Services Departments to the CRE's survey questions provide a useful indication of the practical ways in which the needs of ethnic minorities might be taken into account when planning social services. Can you think of other ways in which services could become more responsive to needs in this way?

2 A report by the EOC entitled *Equality Management: Women's Employment in the NHS*, carried out in 1990 and published in 1992, concluded that discrimination against women in the NHS is 'deeply engrained'. The report suggested that 'High labour turnover and staff shortages are the inevitable consequence of the failure of the NHS to address issues of sex and marital discrimination, and to promote good quality equal opportunities employment practices.'

3 *The Work of the Equal Opportunities Task Force 1986–1990: A Final Report*, published in March 1991 by the King Edward's Hospital Fund for London, pointed to 'glaring' racial inequalities in the NHS and called on the NHS to implement equal opportunity policies.

The task force found that while most health authorities had set up equal opportunity policies, relatively few had translated their policies into a timetabled programme for action, or had allocated responsibilities or sufficient resources. Most had failed to produce data about the ethnic composition of their workforce or monitor the outcome of selection decisions, especially in

regard to promotion procedures and outcomes. Few health authorities complied with the recommendations of the CRE code of practice, while equal opportunities had not yet become part of the formal and routine duties of health service managers. The report concluded that action was needed immediately even to maintain the limited progress made during the 1980s, but that the new market-style NHS, effective from April 1991, could not alone be relied upon as the means of achieving racial equality in the NHS.

The King Edward's Hospital Fund for London Task Force was established in 1986 to help health authorities to implement equal opportunities policies for all racial groups in the health service, with the greatest emphasis upon employment. During its research, many authorities asked the Task Force for guidance on writing their equal opportunities policies. As a result the Task Force produced a 'model policy' on race and discrimination.

4 The *Guardian* of 19 July 1993 reported on a study of equal opportunities in Southwark Council. This study appears to highlight some of the confusion and ambiguity surrounding equal opportunities issues in public services today.

RACE RANKLES COUNCIL STAFF

After interviewing more than 130 council staff, an outside consultant found that 'without any doubt' race was their main concern. 'Angry statements were recorded,' says the report. The council declared its opposition to all forms of racism and sexism nearly 10 years ago.

Disturbingly high numbers of staff said that colleagues made sexist or racist comments. A quarter of staff members had been made to feel uncomfortable or upset at work, and more than a fifth, disproportionately black and female, claimed that they had been discriminated against. But few felt able to make a formal complaint.

The report notes that more than 70 per cent of staff members felt that existing training and support under the equal opportunities provisions was inadequate, though most had little or no interest in receiving such training.

The consultants said that almost half the council staff had not received a copy of the council's equal opportunities policy statement. The statement and the council's recruitment procedures needed revision and overhaul.

ACTIVITY

1   What criticisms of the NHS and Social Services Departments are made in the four reports quoted above?

2   Does the institution in which you are studying have a formal, written policy on 'equal opportunities', 'anti-sexism', 'anti-racism', disability or special needs? If so, ask for copies of the policies and use these as a basis for discussion of the following questions (and if not, ask why not!):

   • What general areas do these policies cover?
   • Do you think that the policies should be rewritten in any way?
   • Are these policies widely publicized in your institution?
   • What practical changes/developments/ initiatives are being taken in your institution as a result of these policies?
   • Who in your institution is responsible for the implementation of these policies?
   • Are there working parties, committees, informal or formal groups of people concerned with equal opportunities in your institution? If so, what are they doing?
   • Are there particular equal opportunities or race equality issues which you think your institution should be addressing?

3   Working individually or in groups, make a list of the practical issues within social

and health care contexts which you think equal opportunities and race equality policies should be trying to address.

4   What would you include in equal opportunities and race awareness training for staff working in a health or social care context?

5   A recent study of Asian women in North London found that only 3% of respondents said that they could turn to their GPs, social workers or health visitors and many were not aware of these services. What practical proposals and policies could be made to ensure better COMMUNICATION in health and social care contexts?

Systems of redress: enforcement of the legislation

CONCILIATION AND TRIBUNALS

Cases of sex or racial discrimination not involving employment are dealt with in the courts. However, anybody who feels that he or she has been discriminated against unlawfully in employment or equal pay cases has a number of other courses of action open to them:

• The COMPLAINANT, as an individual, may bring a case before an INDUSTRIAL TRIBUNAL.
• Before doing so, the complainant can try two other courses of action. He or she may ask the employer concerned to

   (a)   complete a questionnaire giving reasons for the treatment which caused the complaint, or
   (b)   answer a letter to the same effect.

If there is no reply or the answers are unsatisfactory, this can be used as evidence during a hearing at an industrial tribunal.

- The complainant (or the employer) may ask a CONCILIATION OFFICER from the Advisory, Conciliation and Arbitration Service (ACAS) to attempt a settlement.
- If no settlement is reached and the complaint is still unresolved, an industrial tribunal will hear the case.

An industrial tribunal is an independent judicial body whose hearings are relatively informal. It consists of three people (see Figure 1.6). Tribunals sit in most areas and usually no costs or fees are charged.

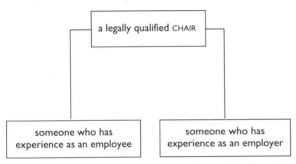

Figure 1.6 **Composition of an industrial tribunal**

Complainants can present their own cases, employ a lawyer to act for them or ask another person to present the case.

There are time limits on presenting some cases to industrial tribunals: this must be done no later than three months from when the act complained of occurred for sex discrimination cases, but equal pay complaints can be made at any time.

The burden of proof is on the complainant to show evidence that he or she has been discriminated against.

REMEDIES

If a tribunal upholds a complaint it may:

- declare the rights of both parties;
- award compensation, including special damages where there has been, for example, loss of earnings and general damages for other situations such as injury to feelings. In very serious cases exemplary or aggravated damages can be awarded.

- recommend that the complained-against person should, within a specified time limit, take a particular course of action to reduce or stop the effect of any discrimination.

If an industrial tribunal hearing goes against a complainant, she or he may appeal to the Employment Appeal Tribunal if she or he feels that the law was misinterpreted. This appeal is heard by a high court judge and two lay members.

Further appeals can be made to the Court of Appeal (or Court of Sessions in Scotland) and finally to the House of Lords.

In certain cases the CRE and the EOC can take action to support individual complainants and/or conduct formal investigations into discriminatory practices.

Example of a case taken to a tribunal

In 1992 four male coroner's officers investigating sudden deaths in Birmingham's city coroner's office took a sex discrimination case under the Equal Pay Act to an industrial tribunal. They claimed that they were being paid about £1,000 a year less than a newly appointed female coroner's officer for doing the same job. The new female employee was appointed to her post on a top scale, even though she was still training, and the four men involved had been doing the job for several years but were paid on a lower scale.

West Midlands Police Authority agreed to a substantial cash settlement with the men. One of the men involved said: 'It was sexual discrimination against men.'

PREPARING A CASE

Race through the 90s, a magazine produced jointly by the CRE and the BBC, produced some useful summary notes on preparing a complaint of discrimination:

Remember –

- **No one will openly admit that they discriminated against you.**

- It's not always easy to get the evidence you need.
- If your complaint is about promotion or unfair treatment at work, people you work with, managers and others may get resentful and label you a troublemaker.

It is important to –

- make detailed notes of conversations as soon as possible after the incident you are complaining about;
- keep copies of all letters and documents concerning your case;
- contact possible witnesses; keep in touch with them, in case they move;
- make sure you have a strong case. The law is very complicated. Your chances of winning are best if you have good legal advice and help throughout. Remember, the other side will usually have lawyers!

OTHER AVENUES FOR REDRESS

The Government has also published the 'Patient's Charter' which outlines patients' rights and avenues for complaints in general terms and also refers to special needs and 'respect for' religious and cultural beliefs. Copies are available from:

The Patient's Charter
FREEPOST
London SE99 7XU

Establishing and implementing equal opportunities policies: examples of local initiatives

Nirveen Kalsi and Pamela Constantinides, in their report *Working Towards Racial Equality in Health Care: The Haringey Experience* (1989) provide a clear demonstration of the difficulties and achievements involved in establishing and implementing equal opportunities policies. Nirveen Kalsi was appointed by the London Borough of Haringey to lead an ethnic minorities development worker project as part of a three-

year development post. She describes the difficulties faced:

Establishing an equal opportunities policy, let alone getting it fully implemented, can take longer than anticipated, with unforeseen setbacks along the way. Similarly, changing patterns and methods of service delivery, and setting up structures through which the views of service users can be incorporated into the planning process can be lengthy tasks.

Community organisations and health service managers can have quite different perspectives on the time-scales involved. Community groups, impatient for change, can become frustrated by the early lack of visible results, and this can lead to accusations of 'token' appointments, 'the appearance of activity', and 'marginalisation' of the issues. To community activists the health authority processes – set up a sub-committee, carry out a survey – can look like recipes for delayed action. Health service managers of the 1980s, on the other hand, sometimes feel almost swamped by the number and scale of changes and impending changes with which they have to contend. They feel beset by financial constraints. They want time – to become better informed, to be consulted, to assess budget implications. There can also of course be more trenchant resistance. Both management and staff may wish to avoid facing up to the uncomfortable issues surrounding health, race and inequality. They may prefer to cling to the notion that a 'colour-blind' service is by definition an equitable service and may wish to deny evidence which makes it clear that this is not so. There can be marked resistance to altering established practices in employment and promotion and a refusal to accept that these practices may be discriminatory.

(Kalsi and Constantinides 1989)

Despite these problems Kalsi, working as a 'linkworker' with other health professionals, was able to develop specific priority areas for change in terms of race and health. These included:

- services for the growing numbers of elderly

people of black/ethnic minority origin;
- mental health services;
- the setting up of a sickle-cell and thalassemia counselling centre;
- the writing of health promotion material in community languages other than English;
- the development of teams of 'linkworkers'.

The concept of a 'linkworker' has been adopted by other health authorities. In the following extract from its 1991 Annual Report, Wandsworth Health Authority sets out its linkworker scheme.

Most health promotion programmes and resources, especially those developed nationally, have been based on the needs of white individuals and groups.

Often these resources are not appropriate for use locally. The Linkworker Service largely works with non-English speaking clients and has been proactive in terms of providing advice and consultancy and in-service education to NHS staff, as well as a service to clients using NHS services.

The aims of the Linkworker Service are listed below:

- To assist the Department of Public Health and the Health Promotion Service to identify health needs in the local ethnic and cultural minority community.
- To facilitate and improve communication between non-English speaking clients and health professionals.
- To facilitate understanding of cultural and other factors which need to be taken into account when care and advice are being given.
- To facilitate provision of health care which is appropriate to the needs of the different cultural groups within Wandsworth Health Authority.
- To undertake proactive health promotion programmes in line with the Health Authority strategy and to contribute to the strategy.
- To identify opportunities and networks in support of local health promotion initiatives.
- To identify gaps in service provision.

Linkworkers are trained to participate in a three-way communication process involving the health professional, client and themselves to enable everyone to get the best from the consultation.

Another of their roles is to identify the different views of health expressed by the various ethnic and cultural groups.

There is a continuing need for the Health Authority to listen to these views and to find ways of actively involving people from all races in assessing the service needs of the population.

ACTIVITY

1 Find out, by writing for information to the various organizations involved, what local initiatives on equal opportunities, race equality, disability and special needs exist in the areas where you live and/or study. You could write to:

- local hospitals;
- the Area Health Authority;
- the local Social Services Department;
- the local county or borough council;
- the local Race Equality Council;
- community organizations, voluntary organizations and charities in your area.

2 If possible try to arrange for someone working on an initiative in this area to talk to your group or class.

ACTIVITY

Consider and discuss these situations:

Jane is admitted to hospital via casualty. She walked in declaring that she had just taken an overdose of paracetamol. She is seventeen. Two days later, while recovering from her treatment, Jane spits at one of the black nurses attending her and shouts racial abuse at her.

How should a situation like this be handled?

Jaswinder came to England to join her husband and his family. Her ordeal began when her husband threw her out with the four children.

'It was hard when I came here from Pakistan, what with young children, and not knowing anybody or anything, and the neighbours always watching us and muttering to themselves when we passed.

'Then suddenly, one day, my husband just told me to leave this house and to take the children. I was stunned. I didn't know what to say, where to go, who to talk to. I have no relatives in England, and his relatives all took his side and didn't even want to see us. It was like it was my fault, even though I had done nothing wrong.

'I wasn't able to do anything, not even look after my children properly . . . I thought I was going mad . . . I saw the doctor and he gave me vitamin tablets and sleeping pills . . . but I didn't tell him about my problems at home . . . he couldn't change the way my husband and his family had behaved . . . They finally sent me to hospital.'

(Race through the 90s, CRE and BBC Radio, 1992)

Could Jaswinder and her children have been helped in any other ways?

Working in groups, write 'case studies' like these, involving other instances where equal opportunities issues need to be considered. These might be based on your own experiences and observations or on situations you envisage might arise in health and social care contexts.

Swap these case studies with another group in your class and discuss the ones you have been given.

GENERAL SOURCES OF HELP AND ADVICE

Most trade unions have equal opportunity policies of their own and can provide advice and support for anyone wishing to pursue a complaint. A useful exercise would be to write to the national headquarters of trade unions in the health and social care field, asking them for information on the help that they can provide in this area. Relevant unions might include GMB, NUPE, UNISON.

Other organizations you could usefully contact might be:

- the Citizen's Advice Bureau;
- a local law centre;
- a local Racial Equality Council.

There is also a Health Information Service helpline run by the Department of Health, which can be reached on 0800 66 55 44 (a Freephone number).

SOURCES FOR ASSIGNMENTS, INVESTIGATIONS AND PROJECTS

The best general reference/address/telephone number directory of all health and social services organizations, including those dealing specifically with equal opportunities, is the *Social Services Year Book* published annually by Longman Community Information and Reference. If your school or college library does not have a copy of this, your local public reference library will.

Commission for Racial Equality (CRE)
10–12 Allington St
London SW1E 5EH
Tel.: 071 828 7022

Equal Opportunities Commission (EOC)
Overseas House
Quay Street
Manchester M3 3HN
Tel.: 061 833 9244

The King's Fund (King Edward's Hospital Fund for London) publishes an extremely useful list of publications. Write for a booklist to:
Bournemouth English Book Centre
9 Albion Close
Parkstone
Dorset BH12 3LL

Policy Studies Institute
100 Park Village East
London NW1 3SR
Tel.: 071 387 2171

Child Poverty Action Group
4th Floor
1–5 Bath St
London EC1V 9PY
Tel.: 071 253 3406

Citizen's Advice Bureaux: see your local
telephone directory.

Runneymede Trust
11 Princelet Street
London E1 6QH
Tel.: 071 375 1496

REFERENCES AND RESOURCES

Bhat et al. (1988), Race in Britain Today. London:
Sage.

Commission for Racial Equality, Act for Equality:
Strengthening the Race Relations Act. London: CRE.

Commission for Racial Equality (1989), Racial
Equality in Social Services Departments: A Survey of
Equal Opportunities Policies. London: CRE.

Commission for Racial Equality (1992), Race
Relations: A Code of Practice in Primary Health Care
Services. London: CRE.

Coote, A. and Campbell, B. (1982), Sweet
Freedom: The Struggle for Women's Liberation.
London: Picador.

Equal Opportunities Commission (1990),
Formal Investigation Report: Southern Derbyshire
Health Authority (March). Manchester: EOC.

Equal Opportunities Commission (1992a),
Equality Management: Women's Employment in the
NHS. A Survey Report. Mancester: EOC.

Equal Opportunities Commission (1992b), A
Guide for Employers to the Sex Discrimination Acts
1975 and 1986. Manchester: EOC.

Field, David (1992), 'Elderly People in British
Society', Sociology Review, vol. 1, no. 4, April.

Giddens, A. (1989), Sociology. Cambridge:
Polity Press.

Kalsi, Nirveen and Constantinides, Pamela
(1989), Working towards Racial Equality in Health
Care: The Haringey Experience. London: King's
Fund Centre for Health.

King Edward's Hospital Fund for London
(1991), The Work of the Equal Opportunities Task
Force 1986–1990: A Final Report. London:
King's Fund.

McAvoy and Donalson (1990), Health Care for
Asians. Oxford: Oxford Medical Publications.

National Association of Teachers in Further
and Higher Education (1993), Equal
Opportunities Guide to Language. London:
NATFHE.

Race Through the 90s (magazine). London:
CRE/BBC Radio.

Stainton Rogers, W. (1991), Explaining Health
and Illness: An Exploration of Diversity. Hemel
Hempstead: Harvester Wheatsheaf.

Swain, J., Finkelstein, V., French, S. and
Oliver, M. (1993), Disabling Barriers: Enabling
Environments. London: Sage.

TVEI (1992), The Equal Opportunities Fact Pack.
London: Department of Employment
Group.

Wandsworth Health Authority (1991), Working
Together for Health: Annual Report 1991. London:
Wandsworth Health Authority, Department
of Public Health Medicine.

2

INTERPERSONAL INTERACTION

COMMUNICATING WITH INDIVIDUALS

The health or social care worker must be able to communicate effectively with a wide range of other people: with patients or clients, who may be children, adolescents, young adults, middle-aged or elders; and with many different professionals (for example doctors, nurses, physiotherapists, teachers, the police), each of whom will have their own angle of perception and the jargon of their profession.

Lack of proper communication between the health or social care worker and the patient or client will mean that the patient/client will not receive the help he or she needs. Lack of proper communication between professionals can mean that a vulnerable client, for example a child 'at risk' or a frail old person, who is totally dependent for his or her safety and well-being on a carefully designed network of care and supervision, can be exposed to danger or accident, perhaps with tragic consequences.

The two following case studies illustrate various aspects of communication.

Case Study 1: Ivy Trent

Mrs Ivy Trent is 76 years old and a widow. She has had a stroke and is now in a wheelchair. She is remaining in hospital while her future is considered. She is rather deaf. Her progress is slow, but medical staff think she will be able to walk with aids in time. She is rather afraid of going home and managing alone. She lives alone in a low-rise block of council flats, on the first floor. There are working lifts. She has one good neighbour/ friend. Her daughter lives quite near and visits

once a week. Her son lives a long way away but could offer some financial help. Mrs Trent feels that her children should help more. They haven't even suggested that she should live with them.

HOSPITAL STAFF

The *consultant* has done what can be done medically for Mrs Trent. Now it is time for her to leave hospital and continue physiotherapy as an outpatient. He urgently needs the bed for new cases.

The *ward sister* agrees with the doctor that Mrs Trent ought to leave hospital. She has become quite 'institutionalized' – she depends on ward routine. The ward sister thinks that Mrs Trent likes the security of being in hospital. She finds her rather demanding.

The *occupational therapist* has noticed that Mrs Trent's progress is slow physically but that she has the strength to start walking again once the will is there. Mrs Trent has enjoyed occupational therapy sessions, chatting with the other patients, and her right hand has improved sufficiently for her to try various crafts. She has also practised household tasks from her wheelchair – boiling a kettle, making tea and toast, boiling an egg. The occupational therapist feels that perhaps Mrs Trent would enjoy a day care centre if there is one locally.

The *physiotherapist* finds that Mrs Trent's progress has been rather slow. She doesn't seem all that motivated. But the physiotherapist is convinced that in time, with continued physiotherapy, Mrs Trent will be able to walk with a tripod or a zimmer frame. Outpatient physiotherapy is available.

FRIENDS AND RELATIVES

Mrs Trent's *daughter*, Mrs Baker, lives nearby and will visit once a week, but she is married with children, and has a job, and is very busy. Her relationship with her mother has not always been that good. She says very strongly that she cannot have her mother to live with her, it would not work (though she does not say this directly to her mother). However, she will continue to visit once a week. Her children like to see their grandmother.

Mrs Trent's *son*, Mr Trent, lives a long way away. He cannot have his mother to stay with him (he makes various excuses). But he can give a little financial help – enough for some aids around the flat, perhaps an electric wheelchair. He can only stay around for a few more days while his mother's future is decided, because of the pressure and demands of work.

Mrs Smith, an *elderly neighbour and friend*, can go round for a chat every day and make a cup of tea. She and Mrs Trent have been friends for years. But she would be too frail to lift Mrs Trent if she fell.

SERVICES

The *home care service* provides help with personal care, such as help with getting up, washing and dressing. Care at home is available seven days a week, as well as evenings and weekends. The personal care worker will sometimes give practical help with shopping or cooking.

The *meals on wheels organizer* can have frozen or hot meals delivered to the home five days a week. What about the weekends?

The *day care centre* provides company and activities and helps clients cope with day-to-day problems that might arise at home. Transport can be arranged. Chiropody and hairdressing are available. Day care can be provided one or two days a week including weekends.

The *district nurse* will call once a week at first to help the patient with any incontinence and prevention of pressure sores.

STAGES IN PLANNING MRS TRENT'S DISCHARGE FROM HOSPITAL AND FUTURE CARE

1 At a multidisciplinary ward meeting, the consultant, ward sister, physiotherapist, occupational therapist and social worker give their assessment of the patient.
2 The social worker talks to Mrs Trent. She cannot stay in hospital; what does she really want to do?
3 The social worker talks to relatives – Mrs Trent's son and daughter – to hear their views.
4 Home visit with patient. Present at this multidisciplinary meeting will be the social worker (acting as co-ordinator), the physiotherapist, the occupational therapist, Mrs Trent and her elderly neighbour. Calling in briefly will be the home care organizer, meals on wheels organizer and the district nurse. A thorough physical assessment of the patient in her own home will be made and suggestions of aids and gadgets to help her will be put forward by the physiotherapist and occupational therapist. A careful plan, going through every hour of the patient's day, will be made and special plans will be made for Sundays and bank holidays when services may not be available. A decision will be taken whether Mrs Trent could cope alone while still in her wheelchair, or whether discharge should be postponed until she can take several steps unaided.

Case Study 2: Tracy Congdon (*suitable for role-play*)

Characters involved in the inquiry into the future of Tracy Congdon, aged 8:

Jean North	Tracy's mother
Frank North	Jean's husband and Tracy's stepfather
William Beatty	Tracy's uncle and previous foster-father

Susan Beatty	Jean's sister and Tracy's aunt and previous foster-mother
Alison Greene	Tracy's teacher at Harville Junior School
Terry Hill	social services

THE SITUATION

Frank and Jean North have been married for one year. They have taken their six children (three each) from previous marriages out of care, with the council's approval of course, and are living in a council house in Harville. Tracy, who is the subject of this inquiry, used to live with the Beattys, who took her when she was nine months old, when Jean left her first husband, Alan Congdon, Tracy's father. Mrs Beatty is Jean's sister. Tracy is now 8 years old and has been at home with Frank and Jean for a year.

The family appear to live quite happily together, but neighbours have gossiped about Tracy's appearance. They say she frequently has bruises and a black eye; she has been seen carrying heavy sacks of shopping up the steep hill to her home; and one neighbour is reported as seeing all the North children except Tracy being bought ice-cream. One of the children ate his ice and gave Tracy the dry cornet. Frank North has been heard shouting and swearing in the house. He used to drink regularly and rather heavily. Jean North is quiet and withdrawn, but has no time for the 'authorities'.

Nevertheless, the North family is now complete again, and with Tracy they might hope to resume normal life.

THE BRIEF

You are all attending a Social Services Department meeting held to consider the case.

It is the brief of the reporting groups to interview each character and to decide whether Tracy should be returned to care, or whether she should remain at home. In the latter case you may make recommendations as to future action (regular social worker visits, etc.). Each member of the group should take notes on the progress of the interviews, and one member should be elected to report on these and to communicate to the rest of the class the decision of the group. Remember that whatever you decide will have a lasting impact on the life of this child.

Your only concern is for the health and well-being of Tracy.

SOME THOUGHTS TO HELP YOU

It may be detrimental to move Tracy again; she has been in this environment for one year and will only just be settling in.

The natural bond of blood between mother and child has always been regarded by the courts as important, and it has been their practice to encourage families to live together wherever possible, provided that the child's life does not appear to be in danger.

There is no positive evidence of ill-treatment; but hearsay suggests that Tracy might be punished harshly, and that she is more familiar with the Beattys.

Terry Hill is a qualified and experienced social worker.

There are two main alternatives: (a) leave her at home under the eye of the social services, or (b) return her to the Beattys. You may, though, recommend she be placed in council care under a care order.

Remember: You must be able to justify your decision, with reference to the characters you have interviewed. Do not try to trip them up with questions about intricate details of family life; you should judge them by their feelings about Tracy, their past record and your assessment of their reliability in the future.

THE CHARACTERS

Jean North

You are 38 years old and have been married once before. You and Frank, the three children of your first marriage and the three of Frank's first marriage, aged between 1 and 11, live quite happily together. You are not over-houseproud, but the home is kept reasonably clean and the children are all well fed. You do not go out to work. The only problem is that Frank drinks rather heavily at times and then picks on your daughter Tracy. He does not mean to do this, but appears not to be able to control himself. Tracy is rather an annoying child. She does not eat properly, wets her bed, is moody and quiet. She daydreams a lot and does not immediately do as she is told. You insist, however, that she should not return to your sister's home, as a family should stick together and a girl's place is with her mother. You must persuade the committee of this. The neighbours are nasty-minded and have spread rumours of the ill-treatment of Tracy deliberately to cause trouble. Tracy's teacher, Miss Greene, is just as bad – school is a waste of time anyway, the children just play with sand all day. The social services have no business to interfere with your private life. Tracy must stay with you.

Frank North

You are 42 years old and have been married once before, your first wife having divorced you. You are now quite happy with Jean and you and she, the three children of your first marriage and Jean's three, live on your wages as a factory-hand. In the past you have shown a weakness for drink and, when drunk, tend towards violence. However, you mean to turn over a new leaf, to work harder and to look after your family better. You try very hard to treat all the children alike, but somehow Tracy gets on your nerves. You tend to smack her more often than the others but you have never really hurt her. You hope very much that the family can be kept together so that a stable home can be built up. It would break Jean's heart to lose Tracy now, and you must convince the committee that you and she are good parents.

You also strongly resent the interference of busybodies like the social services people, your sister-in-law and her husband, and so on. 'Live and let live' is your motto.

William and Susan Beatty

Susan is Jean North's sister, and the two of

you cared for Tracy from when she was nine months old, when Jean divorced her first husband, Alan Congdon. Tracy's return to her mother one year ago caused you and the child great distress. Until then she had been a normal, happy girl. Now, on the very few occasions Jean has let you see her (the three of you are hardly on speaking terms) she has been quiet and looked depressed. She always seems to be crying. You have heard from neighbours that she is ill-treated; you know that Tracy's stepfather, Frank, drinks heavily and is a 'bad lot'. You cannot understand what Jean sees in him. You are very anxious that Tracy should come back to you and to what you regard as her real home, and you will go to any lengths to achieve this.

Alison Greene

You have been Tracy's teacher at Harville Junior for two years. When she first came to you she seemed a normal, happy child. Her foster-parents, Mr and Mrs Beatty, though not very 'bright', were interested in her education and clearly looked after her well. However, when Tracy returned to her real mother, all that changed. She lost weight, became quieter and sadder, and was often absent without excuse. Mrs North takes no interest in the school and is not concerned for Tracy's education, although this is not unusual in the best of families.

You are convinced that Tracy is ill-treated at home and have mentioned this often to the Education Welfare Officer. He has told you that this information has been passed on to Terry Hill who is in charge of Tracy's case, but nothing else has happened about it. You are very worried about Tracy, but have no evidence to support your beliefs.

Terry Hill

You work for the Harville Social Services Department and you are responsible for Tracy Congdon, aged 8. One year ago you were responsible for returning her, against her will, to her mother and stepfather, under a court decision. However, she seems to have settled down reasonably well. On your fairly infrequent visits to the house, you have thought she looked pale and perhaps rather thin, but otherwise well cared for. You have heard rumours from neighbours about Tracy being ill-treated, but have no evidence that these are true; the area is well known for its gossips and scandal-mongers. You know nothing against the stepfather, Frank North, except that he has been 'short' with you on your visits. He does not like social workers interfering in his private life – but then, few people do.

You have over 60 other cases to deal with, and among these Tracy's is far from the most urgent. The time taken to investigate her case in detail might be better spent saving old people's lives (from the cold) and dealing with urgent child abuse cases where lives are in danger. In your experience, this sort of minor family problem sorts itself out as the child settles down. It always takes some time to get used to the change, but it is worth it in the end to see a child with her real mother.

The initial interview between health/social care worker and patient/client

The first interview with a client is of crucial importance. The client may well be in a state of acute anxiety and distress, and may, depending on the problem, feel shame about asking for help at all. The way in which the worker handles the initial interview will therefore determine whether the client will receive help and return. From the point of view of the health or social care worker, the purpose of the first interview is threefold:

- *screening*, to find out whether the person is eligible for the service offered;
- *information gathering*: amassing of concrete facts about the situation and what led to it;
- *assessment or 'diagnosis'* of the problem and assessment of the client/patient – general physical health, personality strengths and weaknesses, and the strength of his or her social support network in the community.

Care workers will naturally take in first impressions from the posture, dress, manner and speech of a client. But their professional training will have taught them the importance of self-knowledge, so that they will be aware of any stereotypes and prejudices they might hold, and so be able to keep an open mind (see Chapter 1). People are far too complex to be summed up rapidly, and though workers might make a tentative assessment of a client's personality, they will be prepared to change and adapt it as the interview, and subsequent interviews, progress.

Workers should be well acquainted with the physical, social and psychological needs of the various age groups (Chapters 3 and 4) and will have specialized knowledge of some of these, depending on their profession. They should be aware that at a time of acute anxiety people will look, dress and act differently from normal, that they must use listening skills (see page 57) and that clients who have painful material to reveal may talk about something else entirely, only to reveal the true nature of the trouble just as they are leaving.

Individual needs

Health or social care workers should be able to assess the needs and abilities of each client and adjust their level of communication to fit these needs.

PHYSICAL NEEDS

First of all, before communication can be established, any handicaps in hearing and sight must be ascertained. This is especially important with the elderly, who may have difficulties seeing or hearing that are not immediately obvious.

In the case of elderly people about to be discharged home from hospital (like Mrs Trent – see Case Study 1 on page 43), multidisciplinary health assessments are often made, with the social worker acting as co-ordinator. Assessments might be made by a physiotherapist, an occupational therapist, a district nurse and a social worker, each of whom will have different areas of concern.

In 1989 a study of Runciman described the factors that different professional groups perceived as important to check in an assessment. The areas to be checked, and their practical applications, were:

mobility	inside, outside, steps, balance, etc.
exercise	on exertion, e.g. chest pain, leg pain
lower limbs	feet, circulation, ankles, ulcers
skin	pressure areas, itching
vision	reading, glasses
hearing	door-bell, conversation, aids
self-care	washing, bathing, toileting, dressing
continence	bladder, bowels, day, night, frequency
house and household tasks	garden, heating, hazards, security
nutrition	diet, appetite, cooking, weight, teeth/dentures
finance	benefits, pensions
medication	drugs prescribed/taken, side effects
medical history	
services	voluntary/private, health visitor, GP, home help, meals on wheels
mental status	memory, orientation, mood, sleep, grief
attitudes	to health, housing, help, carers
social support	relatives, friends, neighbours, amount, stress
aids	walking, toileting, bathroom, kitchen
communication	telephone, emergency help

ACTIVITY

1 Read Case Study 1 on Ivy Trent (see page 43).

2 Divide into groups and take one role each of:

- physiotherapist
- occupational therapist
- district nurse
- home care worker

3 Find out what are the responsibilities and special concerns of your profession with regard to the elderly.

4 Refer to the checklist in the text. What questions would you ask Mrs Trent on the home visit? Write a list.

5 Go through each room of her flat – kitchen, toilet and bathroom, bedroom, living room. Think of each part of the day. What help would she need? What aids or equipment could you help her with?

COGNITIVE NEEDS

The mental processes of each client/patient must be assessed: the way they perceive things and the way they handle problems. The client's intelligence and level of education is relevant. The worker must make an immediate assessment of the client's mental abilities in order to communicate effectively at the right level, meanwhile taking into account the life stage of the client.

It is obvious that communication between two individuals will be hampered if one of the parties has a poor grasp of English, for example if they come from an ethnic minority group.

However, it is also possible for people who speak the same language not to understand each other.

Language and social class

In 1961 Bernstein, an English sociologist, put forward his theory of *restricted* and *elaborated* codes of language.

Bernstein claimed that working-class and middle-class children in England speak two different kinds of language. The working-class style of speech tends towards a *restricted* code, which:

- is syntactically crude;
- is repetitive;
- is rigid;
- is limited in its use of adjectives and adverbs;
- uses more pronouns than nouns;
- involves short, grammatically complete and incomplete sentences;
- is context-bound;
- makes frequent use of uninformative but emotionally reinforcing phrases such as 'you see', 'you know', 'wouldn't it' and 'don't I';
- tends to emphasize the present, the here and now;
- is poor at tracing causal relationships;
- does not permit the expression of abstract and hypothetical thought;
- rarely uses 'I' and conveys much meaning non-verbally.

The *elaborated* code, as used by the middle class:

- is syntactically more complex and flexible, with longer and more complicated sentences;
- makes use of a range of subordinate clauses, as well as conjunctions, prepositions, adjectives and adverbs;
- allows the expression of abstract thoughts;
- makes frequent use of 'I';
- uses more nouns than pronouns;
- is context-independent;
- makes the meaning explicit;
- emphasizes the precise description of experiences or feelings;
- tends to stress the past and future rather than the present.

Stones (1971) gave examples of imaginary conversations on a bus between a mother and child:

Mother: hold on tight
Child: why?
Mother: hold on tight
Child: why?

Mother: you'll fall
Child: why?
Mother: I told you to hold on tight, didn't I?

This is a fairly typical restricted code type of conversation, with very little attempt by the mother to explain or reason. Contrast this with an elaborated code mother and her child:

Mother: hold on tight, darling
Child: why?
Mother: if you don't you'll be thrown forward and you'll fall
Child: why?
Mother: because if the bus suddenly stops, you'll jerk forward onto the seat in front.

Bernstein's theory has been criticized as making a value judgement, implying that middle-class speech is 'superior' or closer to the 'Queen's English' than working-class speech. But, this debate aside, those working in the health or social care professions should be aware of the difference between restricted and elaborated codes of speech. It is very possible that a worker speaking the elaborated code and a client speaking the restricted code may misunderstand each other and fail to communicate properly at all (see page 50).

Black English

Similarly, but more obviously, English black children and adults speak in dialogues which show a restricted code. It has been found that they do not speak fully and comfortably in their own language when with whites.

Labov (1970) demonstrated this:

A young black boy, Leon, was asked by a friendly white interviewer to tell him everything he could about a toy.

The 8-year-old boy said very little and remained silent for most of the time.

In a second situation Leon was interviewed by a black interviewer. This time he answered the questions with single words or sounds.

On these first two episodes, Leon would have

been labelled 'non-verbal' or 'linguistically retarded'.

However, in a third situation he sat on the floor, shared a bag of crisps with his best friend, and with the same black interviewer asking questions in the local dialect, conversed in a lively way.

In 1972 Williams devised the BITCH test (black intelligence test of cultural homogeneity), which was specially designed to measure the true abilities of black children, written in the dialogue in which they are skilled, instead of the usual Standard English. When white children were tested using only black dialect sentences they did very badly indeed.

Language differences and communication in the caring professions

In the 1970s, J.E. Mayer and Noel Timms studied the views of 61 clients who had requested help from the Family Welfare Association. The clients were predominantly working class. Social workers at the FWA had access to limited funds to help clients with pressing debts, but mainly their aim was to help people with relationship problems, particularly marital difficulties.

Some clients approached the FWA for help with paying, for example, an electricity bill.

Typically, the social worker, who was trained to look behind a 'presenting' problem for an 'underlying' problem, would sort out some financial help and then try to find out if there was an underlying problem, by asking about the past, or about present relationships.

In the case of dissatisfied clients it seems that the workers were using the elaborated code – they were trying to take the problem out of context and relate it to past difficulties, trying to get the client to look for causes behind getting into debt so that the situation would not recur.

But the client, using the restricted code, could not see any point in looking to the past, trying to make causal relationships, or talking hypothetically.

The result of this failure in communication meant that the worker felt frustrated, while the client felt that the worker's questions were irrelevant, time-wasting and 'nosey'.

For health workers, similar communication problems can arise if, for example, a doctor talks to a patient as if the patient had also received a medical education and describes symptoms and treatments in technical terms. This will often leave the patient bewildered and anxious.

SOCIAL NEEDS

Social support network

The social support network of each individual must be assessed. Isolated people are more at risk from mental, physical and social problems. A strong social support network can prevent many problems and is greatly conducive to mental health and life satisfaction at all stages of the life cycle. Research has shown, predictably, that people who are more isolated tend to turn to formal agencies for help in times of trouble.

One way of clearly showing a person's social support system is by an 'eco map'. Figure 2.1 shows such a map for the case of Mrs Trent (see Case Study 1 on page 43).

Culture and gender matching

Ideally 'culture and gender matching' should be achieved between the helper and the person in need: that is, the helper should be of a similar class background and racial type and of the same gender as the person in need.

As this is often not possible, the worker must use empathy and attempt to communicate with the client on the client's level.

ACTIVITY

1 Draw an eco map to show Tracy's social support system.

2 Draw an eco map to show Jean North's social support system.

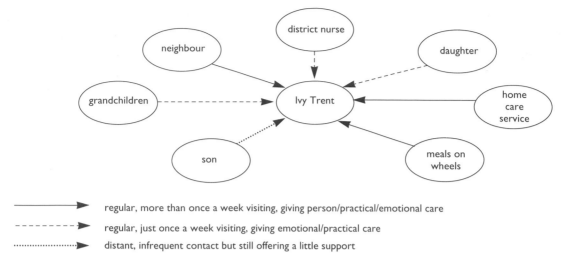

regular, more than once a week visiting, giving person/practical/emotional care

regular, just once a week visiting, giving emotional/practical care

distant, infrequent contact but still offering a little support

Figure 2.1   Eco map for Mrs Trent

3 Find out from your local social services department what facilities are available for the elderly in your area: Is there an occupational therapist attached to the Social Services Department? Are there specialist social workers who can supply equipment such as telephone and TV aids to help with communication for the deaf or hard of hearing, and help with mobility and communication for the blind or partially sighted? Is day care available? Is respite care for short periods in a residential home available? Are personal alarms available? What kind of home help service is available and can hot or frozen meals be delivered?

EMOTIONAL NEEDS

All those who work in the caring professions notice in the course of their work that there are some people who cope courageously with incredible hardships and difficulties in their lives, while at the other end of the spectrum there are those who 'break down' in the face of a relatively minor crisis. It is thought that everyone has their breaking point, but what is it that gives such inner strength to some individuals?

Some psychologists, who believe in nature rather than nurture, would propose that personality types are inherited and inborn.

Eysenck (1991) wrote:

It is nothing short of tragic that so many mothers (and perhaps fathers too) worry about the bringing up of their children and blame themselves for anything that seems to have gone wrong, as if their actions in looking after their children were primarily responsible for their character and their abilities and achievements. The truth, of course, is simply that the influence of parents is strictly limited; their major contribution to the future of their child is made when they join their chromosomes and shuffle their genes into the unique pattern that will for ever after determine the looks, the behaviour, the personality and the intellect of the child. How much more relaxed the parents could be if only they realized the limitations which nature has put on their later contributions!

But many psychologists and psychiatrists would disagree with this, believing that mental health and strength is due to nurture, particularly in the first years of life.

Maslow's hierarchy of needs

The psychologist Maslow proposed in 1954 that there is a hierarchy of needs, ascending from the basic biological needs to more complex psychological needs that become important only after the basic needs have been satisfied. This hierarchy can be represented in a pyramid diagram (see Figure 2.2).

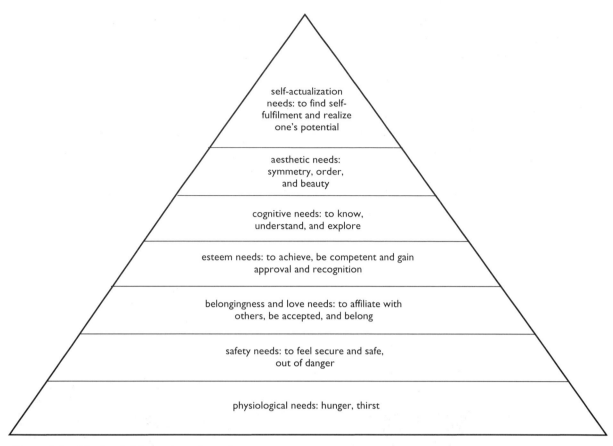

Figure 2.2   Maslow's hierarchy of needs
Source: Maslow in *Psychology: an introduction*, Hayes, N. and Orrell, S. (Longman Group UK Ltd, 1993).

The needs at one level must be at least partially satisfied before those at the next level start to motivate behaviour. When food and safety are difficult to obtain, the relief of those needs will dominate a person's actions and higher motives are of little importance. Artistic and scientific efforts do not flourish in societies in which people have to struggle for food, shelter and safety. The highest motive, self-actualization, can be fulfilled only after all other needs are satisfied.

Carl Rogers: self-concept and positive regard

Carl Rogers (1902–87) developed his theory from his work with emotionally troubled people. He was impressed with what he saw as the individual's innate tendency to move towards growth, maturity and positive change. He argued that human beings have a need to develop their potential as fully as possible. From his clinical work, he saw neurotic or psychotic problems developing when this aspect of a person's personality is consistently denied.

Everyone has an ideal self-concept, a way they would like to be, and people are troubled if their self-concept does not measure up to their ideal. In mentally healthy people, their self-concept is close to their ideal self-concept.

All individuals have a need for positive regard from other people. Rogers believed that people are likely to show greater mental health, and live more fully, if they are brought up with unconditional positive regard. This means that they feel themselves specially valued by one or two people even when their feelings, attitude and behaviour are less than ideal.

Rogers insisted that most, if not all, of his neurotic clients had parents who did not give their children a strong sense of being loved and approved of unconditionally. The child got the message he or she wasn't really loved at all – the parents would have liked some other, ideal child, who never misbehaved. Therefore, these children grow up striving for approval from others and ignoring their own self-actualization in the process. People like this tend to have very unrealistically high standards for their own behaviour, that is, their ideal self-concept doesn't correlate strongly with their own self-concept.

Rogers developed the idea of ENCOUNTER GROUPS. Personal growth is achieved by unconditional positive regard from other members of the group. Once defences are broken down, people can help each other. People are able to sort out their own problems, he felt, if put in a situation in which they had unconditional positive regard from someone else. A therapist could provide that relationship, so long as the therapist was warm, accepting, genuine and non-directive. This relationship is central to the healing process.

'Difficult' clients

A client approaching a social care worker may feel one or more of the following: low self-esteem, a feeling of failure, high anxiety, shame, guilt, fear or grief.

By use of defence mechanisms (see page 140) these negative emotions may come across as belligerence or aggression, or perhaps flippancy. Professional workers will be able to interpret this behaviour, at first to themselves, and later, when the time is right, to the client. They will use calming and listening skills (see page 57) to reduce the client's anxiety and lower his or her defences.

The effects of strong emotion

A sudden shock can produce physical and psychological symptoms. Trembling, shaking, temporary loss of memory, sleeplessness, lack of concentration are common symptoms of shock or stress that may be quite long-lasting.

See Chapter 4 for discussion of grief and stress.

Care workers will be aware of the symptoms of stress and realize that the client is not acting in his or her 'normal' manner. They will also know that a time of crisis, when a person is thrown into a state of disorganization and remembers other times of crisis in his or her life, may also be a significant opportunity for personal growth and change.

Behavioural/emotional needs and life stages

At each life stage an individual has certain emotional and behavioural needs. If these are not met, behavioural disturbances may result. Table 2.1 overleaf sets out these stages in schematic form.

ACTIVITY

Refer to the two case studies at the beginning of this chapter.

1 Ivy Trent
   What are the emotional needs of Mrs Trent?
   What behaviour might she show if these are not met?

2 Tracy Congdon
   What are Tracy's emotional needs?
   What behaviour does she show that indicates emotional problems?

3 Frank North
   What are Frank North's emotional needs?
   What behaviour does he show that indicates emotional problems?

Forms of communication

In the initial interview between health or social care worker and client, when the individual needs of the client are being tentatively assessed, the worker will be

Table 2.1   Life stages and emotional/behavioural needs

Life stage	Life event threats	Behavioural needs	Examples of behaviour disturbances if needs are not met
Infant	Frequent changes of carer; indifferent carer, abuse	Security; attachments; physical comfort	Withdrawn; passive
Young child	Neglect; deprivation; abuse (emotional, physical, sexual)	As for infant; also space and permission for play and self-expression in a safe environment. Stimulation, encouragement and friendships	Failure to thrive, clinging dependent behaviour, indiscriminate friendliness, aggression, enuresis, recurrent nightmares
Adolescent	Peer group pressure into substance abuse, petty crime Family discord or breakdown may lead to delinquency or eating disorders Feeling of failure at school may lead to truancy	Enough freedom for expression of own developing identity but also caring control Friendships, good relationships with adults, encouragement, achievement	Confusion, aggression, moodiness, substance abuse, eating disorders (anorexia nervosa and bulimia), truancy, delinquent behaviour
Adult	Infertility (for those who feel the need for children) Separation and divorce Ill-health Unemployment Mental illness, especially depression Homelessness	Intimate, long-lasting relationships Reproduction and nurturing Employment, which provides identity, security, social contacts and the ability to provide for dependants	Depression Regression Loss of self-esteem Alcoholism Shop lifting Gambling Wife- or husband-battering
Elder	Bereavement and loss Ill-health and loss of mobility Reduced income Isolation	Maintained contacts with family members, social contacts, interests, good health and mobility, sufficient income	Depression Withdrawal Self-neglect

expressing a desire to help, both verbally and non-verbally.

The worker will, for example, greet the client using appropriately friendly and welcoming words, and matching the words with non-verbal signals – welcoming gestures and tone of voice. If a client has a communication difficulty, a great deal more non-verbal communication will be used.

NON-VERBAL COMMUNICATION

Non-verbal communication refers to all the body signals which we deliberately or inadvertently make when we are with other people.

It has been calculated that, on average, the total impact of a message owes 7% to the actual words, 38% to the 'paralanguage' (how we say the words) and 55% to our non-verbal signals. Argyle et al. 1972 demonstrated that, where the non-verbal message contradicts the verbal message, the latter tends to be discounted. They found that the non-verbal style in which a message is communicated has five times more effect than the actual verbal message itself. Our non-verbal behaviour is the more reliable guide to our real feelings.

There are roughly eight kinds of non-verbal communication:

- paralanguage – the way we say things, tone of voice, timing
- eye contact
- facial expression
- posture
- gesture
- touch
- proxemics – how close we come to the other person/people
- dress

Paralanguage

This includes the way things are said, the tone of voice, and the timing of speech.

Research in paralanguage has shown that:

- People are very accurate in assessing which emotion is being expressed by a speaker. The assessment is made from paralanguage cues such as loudness, pitch, rate of speaking, rhythm and inflection.
- These patterns of speech can be recorded and analysed on a machine called a speech spectograph. People who suffer from mental disorders tend to show unusually flattened speech patterns.
- When someone is in a highly emotional state, for example angry or anxious, they tend to stutter, repeat themselves and make more slips of the tongue than usual.
- When someone is not sure of what they are saying, or uncertain of how what they say will be received, they will say 'er' and 'um' more often than usual.
- The timbre of the voice, its softness or harshness, is also different in different emotional states.
- The timing of speech is important in communication. Very slow speech may indicate that a person is uncertain of what they are saying. Fast speech can indicate that a person is anxious or excited.

The listener will unconsciously register all these signals from the speaker, and from them guess his or her state of mind. In the active listening undertaken by those in the caring professions (see page 57), the signals from the speaker will be more consciously noted, and from them an appropriate assessment of the speaker's emotional state may be made.

Eye contact

Eye contact powerfully indicates emotion. The more eye contact someone has with another person, the closer they tend to feel to them. People who don't like each other tend to avoid eye contact.

Research has suggested that eye contact has four important functions in communication:

1. it regulates the flow of conversation;
2. it gives feedback to the speaker on what he or she has communicated;
3. it expresses emotion;
4. it informs both the speaker and the listener of the nature of the relationship they are in.

Other studies have shown that people who have strong emotional needs for approval make more eye contact than others; and that speakers feel that if people are not looking at them, they are not attending to what they are saying.

A care worker who is listening to a client will therefore use eye contact to express sincerity and concern and to show that he or she is attending carefully.

Facial expression

Research has shown that there are some facial expressions which have the same meaning all over the world. An example is the 'eyebrow flash' in which, when people greet each other, they rapidly raise and lower their eyebrows. This has been observed throughout human societies (and also among the great apes).

There are seven major groups of facial expressions, which are recognized in virtually all human societies: happiness, surprise, fear, sadness, anger, interest, and disgust/contempt. However, some cultures inhibit the expression of certain emotions, for example anger, which is perhaps allowed expression more in the West than in parts of the East.

ACTIVITY

Facial Expressions

Write the names of different emotions on pieces of paper and put them in a hat. Take it in turns to take a piece of paper and mime the emotion written there. Which emotions are most easily recognized?

Posture

People may want to appear to others in a certain way. But how they really feel is often given away by body posture, or small unconscious gestures which demonstrate nervousness or anxiety. This is called emotional leakage.

Gesture

People who are communicating together often show 'postural echo', that is, they copy the gestures and posture of the person they are talking to. This demonstrates attentiveness and empathy.

Many gestures, for example head nodding, bowing, raising a thumb, are culture-specific: that is, they mean something to people from one culture, but may mean nothing, or something entirely different, to those from another culture.

ACTIVITY

1 Choose one of the minority racial groups living in England.

2 Research their traditions and customs. What behaviour is expected of the women? What behaviour is expected of the children? How do they express joy and anger? What are their customs regarding touch, of family members and friends? What are the common gestures of their culture? Do they have special customs regarding eye contact and proxemics?

3 Analyse how these customs differ from British customs.

4 Discuss how the cultural differences could inhibit communication between a British care worker and a client from this minority racial group.

Touch

The amount of everyday touch which we will allow people to have with us is again culturally determined.

Those who work with distressed people, who are in fear, shock, pain or bereavement, know that there are times when touch, holding or hugging, is expressive and comforting when there are no suitable words.

Proxemics

This is another culturally determined method of communication. Each society has its own idea of personal space. For example, in Western Europe the normal conversational distance is 1–1.5 metres, but in some Arab countries it is very much closer than that.

ACTIVITY

How do you, in the library, on a crowded tube train, protect your own personal space? Do care arrangements, for example in hospitals or residential homes, take account of this need?

Dress

The clothes of the health worker may be a uniform which will convey its own important/official/reassuring message. If a uniform is not worn, the clothes of the worker should not make an extreme statement expressing, for example, wealth, membership of a cult, sexual invitation. On the other hand, very drab and dowdy clothes reflect a lack of confidence and poor self-esteem, which might equally unconsciously deter clients, who will inevitably carry a set of stereotypes in their own minds.

Manner

This is extremely important and includes paralanguage, eye contact, facial expression, gestures and proxemics.

A warm smile and open, welcoming gestures with a friendly tone of voice, will convey warmth and sincerity to an anxious client.

A care worker's manner is one of his or her professional tools and must always be used, even if he or she is rushed and under pressure.

Example: Non-verbal factors in the interview situation

The interview room should, if possible, be a comfortable temperature and free from distracting noises.

The arrangement of the furniture is significant. One chair higher than the other, or a large desk as a barrier are non-verbal symbols of power and dominance, which are unhelpful in the caring context as the client probably already has low self-esteem and may feel fear. Therefore the worker and the client should sit on chairs of equal height. If a desk is used it should be made clear that this is so that the worker can take essential notes. It is best if interviewer and interviewee sit on two sides of the desk (an arrangement used by many GPs).

Sackeim *et al.* 1978 found that the left side of the face is far more expressive of emotion than the right side. They suggest that the reason for this is that the left half of the face is controlled by the right side of the brain, which is thought to deal with artistic, emotional and intuitive skills, while the left side of the brain is thought to deal with logical reasoning and language. So perhaps the interviewer should have a good view of the left side of the client's face.

ACTIVE LISTENING AND RESPONDING

On the whole we are poor listeners. Research shows that we tend to listen in short 30-second spurts before losing attention. We tend to hear items we are interested in and not attend to others. If we are bored, if we dislike the speaker's personality, mannerisms, accent or appearance, we may 'switch off', and follow more interesting thoughts of our own.

Active listening, the listening required in a caring context, calls for concentration; it is hard work and tiring.

Eye contact

Typically the interviewee, the person talking, looks away at times, then looks back now and then to check that the interviewer is still attending.

The listener's eye contact tends to be stronger.

Posture

The listener should keep the body and hands neat and relaxed.

An occasional nod acts as positive reinforcement; that is, it can encourage the client when he or she is saying something useful or helpful.

Conveying warmth

Conveying warmth in the initial stages of the interview is very important. The client may have personal and painful data to reveal and will decide not to do so if the worker is in any way cold and rejecting.

Warmth may be conveyed non-verbally:

- a warm smile (facial expression);
- open welcoming gestures;
- friendly tone of voice (paralanguage);
- confident manner – this reassures the client that something can be done;
- offering physical help – for example a guiding arm to an elderly or distraught person;
- general appearance of care worker;
- physical arrangement of the chairs in the interview room;
- calm movements.

And verbally:

- use of friendly words that nevertheless show appropriate respect;

- expression of a desire to be of help;
- clear explanation of how long the interview will last;
- reassurance about confidentiality;
- clear assessment at end of interview about what has been achieved and arrangement of a follow-up, if necessary.

Conveying understanding

A care worker conveys understanding through empathy, acceptance and a non-judgemental attitude. These are values which underpin social care work and are described in full in the third part of this chapter.

A client often experiences great relief at being able to tell his or her truth without getting an emotional reaction from the other person. This process, sometimes called 'ventilation', lowers anxiety and can, if the worker provides warmth and acceptance, be sufficient in itself to let the client see his or her own solution to the problem without further help. (This is the therapeutic value of the confessional.)

Understanding is also conveyed where the care worker shows knowledge and acceptance of the particular physical, cognitive and social needs of the client. Understanding is also shown when the worker can paraphrase what the client has just said (see nos. 3 and 4 in the 'micro-skills of interviewing' listed opposite).

Conveying sincerity

Warmth, understanding and sincerity are all communicated by the use of eye contact, which shows interest and attention.

Sincerity is also conveyed by:

- the worker clearly stating at the outset how long the interview will last;
- reassurance about confidentiality, while explaining its boundaries;
- clear assessment at the end of the interview about what has been achieved.

Interview skills

The '5WH Test' is a useful standby formula to obtain information in a fact-finding interview. This stands for sentences that start with why (use this sparingly), who, what, when and where? A sixth useful question word is how? Sensitive use of these key words can elicit a lot of fundamental information.

For example: what is the problem, when did it start, who could help, where should we begin to sort it out, how have you managed so far?

Effective counsellors should demonstrate the following seven qualities:

1 Empathy or understanding: the effort to see the world through the other person's eyes.
2 Respect: responding in a way which conveys a belief in the other's ability to tackle the problem.
3 Concreteness or being specific, so that the interviewee can reduce confusion about what he/she means.
4 Self-knowledge and self-acceptance. The interviewer should have these qualities and should be ready to help others to gain them.
5 Genuineness: being real in a relationship.
6 Congruence: so that the words we use match our body language.
7 Immediacy: dealing with what is going on in the present moment of the counselling session, as a sample of what is going on in someone's everyday life.

The skills of interviewing may be broken down into 20 points or 'micro-skills'. Skills 1–13 are the more basic skills of interviewing:

1 Let a person finish talking without reacting.
2 Be able to reflect back accurately to the interviewee the content of what they have said and their feelings.
3 Be able to paraphrase what the interviewee has just said.
4 Be able to summarize what has been said in order to move the interview forward.
5 Be able to define your own role clearly to the interviewee.
6 Be able to use open questions, rather than closed questions which lead to a yes or no answer and tend to close the topic.
7 Be able to use prompts to encourage the

person to continue, especially if an important area has been reached and the interviewee suddenly goes quiet.

8 Be able to tolerate silences of about five seconds. Silences are often the client's best thinking times, in which she/he is deciding what is the best thing to do.

9 Be able to control your own anxiety at what the client is revealing, which may strike some personal chord with you, and be able to relax.

10 Be able to provide direction and keep the interview in focus.

11 Be able to set mutual goals.

12 Be able to discuss and generate alternative plans of action.

13 Be able to begin, sustain and end the interview well.

Skills 14–20 are more advanced skills, and time and practice are needed to develop them.

14 Be able to draw out feelings from the interviewee.

15 Be able to offer tentative understanding and interpretation of what has been happening.

16 Be able to see how the interviewee affects your own emotions.

17 Be able to focus on the 'here and now' as well as 'there and then'.

18 Be able to recognize and confront ambivalence and inconsistencies.

19 Be able to tolerate painful topics.

20 Be able to evaluate the costs and gains of what was achieved.

ACTIVITY

A In this task you will learn what it feels like not to be listened to.

1 Divide into groups of three.

2 One of the group talks to the other two on a subject, for example 'one good thing that has happened to me this week'.

3 The other two listen intently for one minute. They then switch off and stop listening until given a sign to stop the exercise.

4 Repeat the exercise twice with each member of the group taking the role of the speaker.

After this exercise, you should each answer the following questions:

- For the listeners – was it easy or difficult to stop listening?
- For the speaker – how did the two students show with their body language that they had stopped listening?
- What did it feel like to be listened to intently?
- What did it feel like not to be listened to?
- What do you think makes a good listener?

B In this task, you will attempt to tap into the emotion behind a person's words.

1 In groups of three, each talks in turn on a topic, for example 'if I could change one thing about myself'.

2 The two listeners listen intently and observe the body language of the speaker, trying to recognize the emotion behind the words.

Conveying the positive value of others

Conveying the positive value of others may be done using the following non-verbal signals:

- smiling
- eye contact
- listening skills
- calm movements
- open gestures

Both verbally and non-verbally the following values may be shown:

- empathy;
- acceptance and a non-judgemental attitude;
- respect for the individual;
- freedom from any type of stereotyping or discrimination;
- assurance of confidentiality, with its boundaries explained;
- encouragement of the client's self-determination, self-respect and dignity;
- conveying warmth, understanding and sincerity and beginning and ending the interview positively.

Factors which inhibit interpersonal interaction with individuals

DISTRACTIONS

A continuous noise outside an interview room is a distraction, but interaction between two people will be inhibited far more by interruptions. Suppose a client is telling his or her personal story to a care worker when the phone rings or there is a knock at the door. The worker takes his or her attention from the client and talks for some minutes to the person on the telephone, or the person at the door, about another matter entirely. The client will feel devalued, that his or her crucial communication is unimportant, and therefore that he or she is unimportant. The client will feel angry, and when the worker at last turns back, may have decided not to reveal any more about him or herself, and worker/client communication will have broken down. Any interruptions should therefore be dealt with briefly, with the worker making it clear that the client and his or her problems are the current priority.

DOMINATING THE CONVERSATION

Care workers are there to listen and should put their own concerns to one side. However, they may perhaps unintentionally dominate the conversation in any of three ways:

1 Making the client's story their own story: 'Oh, I'm sorry to hear that happened to you. My own sister/niece/uncle had a similar experience . . .'
2 By assuming responsibility for working out the problem and giving the client only a minor role. An extreme example would be to set out treatment/care plan, then impose it on the client.
3 By trying to scrutinize every area of the client's life, regardless of the actual service he or she requests.

MANIPULATION

The care worker or client can be manipulative if either one of them has a hidden agenda in the interaction. There are also specific ways in which each side may manipulate the other.

The care worker

This may be direct or indirect. Care workers may manipulate clients by manoeuvring them to choose modes of action in accordance with the care workers' judgement, in such a way that the clients are not aware of the process. If they are aware of it, they feel 'moved about' against their will.

Or care workers might use persuasion in a controlling way to urge clients to accept their decisions. This demotes the clients to playing a minor role in the play of their own lives, and denies them rights to personal choice and independence.

The client

This can happen when a client goes to several agencies for help and complains at each new agency about the lack of help received at the last agency. Such clients are often plausible and much time may be wasted.

BLOCKING THE OTHER'S CONTRIBUTION

In one-to-one, face-to-face interaction, communication can be blocked by one participant in a number of ways, verbal and non-verbal, some of which are subtle and minimal.

The care worker may block the communication of the client in many non-verbal ways, for example:

- a look of boredom;
- a yawn;
- the slightest expression of disgust;
- a smile at the wrong time;
- withdrawal of eye contact, turning away;
- drumming the fingers;
- fidgeting.

The care worker may block the communication of the client verbally by, for example:

- changing the subject;
- being critical;
- misunderstanding;
- joking at the client's expense.

ACTIVITY W

Practise interview skills by interviewing a friend about one of their interests. Try to get some in-depth information by preparing some questions in advance, and using open rather than closed questions.

Interview skills can be practised in role-plays with the case studies of Ivy Trent and Tracy Congdon (described at the beginning of this chapter).

On work experience, the supervisor at the day centre or hospital might suggest individuals who would enjoy being interviewed. Patients/clients would be assured that:

- they would not have to answer any questions they did not like;
- their names would not be used;
- they would be helping the students complete a project.

The content of the interview could be agreed in advance with the volunteer, for example to cover

- the client's childhood, or
- the client's employment history.

Students would:

- prepare questions in advance;
- study interview skills;
- tape-record the interview, with the knowledge of the volunteer.

Two willing volunteers should be found, with contrasting needs, and one with a communication disability.

PROMOTING COMMUNICATION WITHIN GROUPS

A group comes into being when a number of people share a common goal which they know cannot be achieved by any one of them alone.

Individuals in a small group are still communicating face-to-face, but everybody's behaviour is influenced by the larger number of participants. Many psychological experiments have been performed in the area of group pressure, obedience and collective responsibility, and readers are referred to the work of Asch (1951), Hofling (1966), Milgram (1963), Latane et al. (1968, 1969) and Piliavin et al. (1969) in *Psychology: The Science of Mind and Behaviour* by Gross.

Types of groups

In the health and social care settings there are many group formations. Two major types are:

- Multidisciplinary groups, for example a doctor, police officer, teacher, social worker and perhaps a parent at a conference on a child 'at risk'; or a doctor, physiotherapist, ward sister, occupational therapist, dietician and social worker at a ward meeting (see Case Study 1 on Mrs Ivy Trent at the beginning of the chapter).
- Groups of people in similar situations, for example, groups of people with similar diseases or disabilities, or people who have applied to be foster-parents awaiting their first child.

Each professional group has its own perception of a patient's problems and, if rigidly held, this can act as a barrier to communication with members of the other professions, to the detriment of the patient. It is important that the social worker, who often co-ordinates multidisciplinary assessments, is able to communicate clearly in speech and writing without the use of jargon, but is able to understand the jargon of each profession, in order, if necessary, to interpret it to other members of the team. Small details can have important consequences in these cases and should not be misunderstood.

ACTIVITY

M. Preston Shoot in 1987 identified the following types of groups:

- social or recreational groups
- group psychotherapy
- group counselling
- educational groups
- social treatment groups
- discussion groups
- self-help groups
- social action groups
- self-directed groups

Think of a group that would come under each of these headings.

The development of a group

A group which is assembled for a certain purpose and with regular meetings proposed develops through certain stages. Different theorists have named these stages differently, but all are agreed on what happens at each stage. Tuckman and Jensen 1977 called these stages of group development:

forming
storming
norming
performing
adjourning

THE GROUP LEADER

The role of the group leader will vary slightly according to the type of group, but always involves the difficult task of being sometimes central, sometimes motivating others, sometimes in the background, and then back in the centre again.

THE FORMING STAGE

In this stage members of the group move from finding out information about the group (orientation and exploration) in parallel communication directed at the leader, to increased communication with each other. The group and the leader are tested by each member to see if trust can be established.

Anyone joining a group will be aware that they will have to sacrifice individuality, and they will want to know whether the benefits of joining a group will compensate for this. The leader will take this and any similar opportunity to point out that the members of the group, by sharing their interests and problems, are in a position to understand and thereby help one another.

In the early meetings, a group leader will need to be able to perform the following tasks:

- give a short presentation of him or herself;
- ask each member to give a similar presentation;
- go over the information that was given to members before they joined the group;
- amend any aims and agreements;
- acknowledge initial uncertainties;
- get each person to say what they hope to gain from the group;
- summarize issues as they are presented;
- establish norms for listening and accepting;
- help the group interaction: 'does anyone else feel like this?';
- play the part of the absent member by putting into words what people may want to say but are not yet ready to risk;
- show concern for each individual;
- when asked questions, sometimes say: 'does anyone else know the answer to that?'.

THE STORMING STAGE

'Storming' is the period when people argue about how they see the group's function and structure. People reveal their differences and their personalities; some may be overbearing and disruptive. At this stage the question each group member is asking internally is no longer 'do I belong?' but 'do I have any influence here?'. Pairings and sub-groups might have formed among members of the group. Underlying the overt communications, a struggle for power and control is taking place, and there is a tendency to polarize around certain issues.

The leader and the group are tested out further. The group may break down at this stage if the leader does not provide enough security, while individual members query if they are going to get what they came for.

At this stage the group leader must:

- keep calm in the face of conflict between members of the group or towards the leader;
- not retaliate when his/her authority is challenged; the challenge may be due to ambivalence about membership or a transference reaction;
- model acceptance and openly recognize that people are different;
- not give particular attention to difficult or isolated members;
- try to choose the right time to intervene to encourage progress and the right time to keep quiet;
- start handing over responsibilities to the membership.

THE NORMING STAGE

When this stage is reached it means that group cohesion has been established. Intimate and personal opinions may be expressed by members to each other. People start to look for 'affection', that is, signs that they are accepted by the wider circle. Sharing information, co-operation and decision-making by consensus leads to action.

Members identify with the group and its future; there is a growing *esprit de corps* and 'we' talk develops.

At this stage rules for meetings are established. Norms are set up, specifying for example the kind of behaviour group members may expect from each other. Some groups opt for a business-like atmosphere, others find a more relaxed atmosphere appropriate. There will be some ritual ownership of seats, regular high attendance and a feeling of some exclusivity. Such norms are likely to make it difficult for new members to join the group. A lack of conformity to the group's norms can lead to scapegoating or group pressure to conform. New leadership may come from within the group and this may result in altering basic group norms.

The tasks for the group leader at this stage are to:

- retreat from a directing role into a listening, following one, therefore letting people help each other;
- facilitate the group by observing the group and commenting on what seems to be happening, offering ideas of his or her own and asking the group what their perceptions are;
- ask him or herself, and perhaps the group, what is going on here? What is this issue really all about? An apparently superficial and irrelevant topic, discussed heatedly, might hide a deeper issue.

THE PERFORMING STAGE

When performing occurs the group is working together to solve problems. It is no longer dependent on the leader, who moves into the background. The leader's tasks now are to:

- observe how the members of the group communicate with each other and deal with the tasks before them;
- show interest and express praise and appreciation of efforts (positive reinforcement);
- continue to model confidence, attitudes and problem solving.

THE ADJOURNING STAGE

This is the ending stage that follows the achievement of a task. All groups have to end at some time, or they may cease to be productive. Members will feel a sense of loss but also a sense of achievement. At this stage the leader becomes more active again. His or her tasks now are to:

- set goals for the time left in partnership with the group;
- review experiences, emphasizing gains as well as feelings of loss;
- mention and encourage interests outside the group;
- help the group return to the planning stage if they want to continue, but with some other purpose;
- evaluate the sessions and ask for feedback.

Different levels of participation in groups

Robert Bales in 1955 studied the performance of small, initially leaderless, discussion groups. He made the following observations:

- People do not participate to equal degrees. One or two members contribute much more than the others.
- The active members give information and offer opinions.
- The less active members confine themselves to agreeing or disagreeing, or asking for information.
- Group participants distinguish between the person they think the most influential and the person they like best.

Leadership styles

There has been much research into the leadership role in group performance, and four distinct styles have been described.

THE AUTOCRATIC STYLE

One member, usually the chairperson, holds the floor most of the time. He or she imposes his or her will on the others in the group, who may resent being 'steamrollered' and may lose interest in issues where their suggestions are not welcomed. A fair amount of work can, however, be achieved.

Example of this style in a health or social care setting: A ward meeting where time is limited and several patients' needs must be discussed. The meeting would be led by the consultant, senior doctor or ward sister.

THE LAISSEZ-FAIRE STYLE

Here a group does not have a leader, but may have a care worker who acts as a facilitator. Decisions are taken, but no one is chosen to carry them out. The meeting may be fun but little is achieved.

Example: a group meeting primarily for comparing notes and mutual social support – perhaps a group of first-time mothers with their babies.

THE DEMOCRATIC STYLE

This recognizes that everyone has a contribution to make. Leaders are elected for a term, or the leadership role rotates among all the members. A democratic group is one that takes the decision-making processes very seriously. Where unanimity is impossible, a vote is taken.

Example: Ongoing case conferences about children 'at risk', deciding whether they should be taken into care.

THE COLLECTIVE STYLE

A collective will avoid leadership roles altogether and work as a team of equals arriving at unanimity. In the health and social care context, a care worker might be present to act as a facilitator. This style entails long group discussions, but once decisions are taken, everyone feels committed to carry them out.

Example: A collective style might be chosen by a group of people with a certain disease or disability who feel the general public should be more aware of their needs.

Factors which inhibit interpersonal interaction in groups

DISTRACTIONS

Distractions which would interrupt the development of the group might include:

- outside intermittent noise (aircraft, pneumatic drill, chairs being pushed around in the floor above);
- constant knocking at the door – someone wanting to speak to a group member;
- telephone ringing – as above;
- group members coming and going all at different times;
- one group member leaning out of the window to talk to people outside;
- one group member distracting the others by silly behaviour.

Some of these potential pitfalls can be avoided by careful choice of venue. The leader can ask the group to solve the other problems itself.

IRRELEVANT TOPICS

Sometimes a group may heatedly and at length discuss a topic that seems irrelevant to the task in hand. Advanced group-work skills enable the leader to see the real meaning of the apparently irrelevant topic and explain to the group how this topic links to the main task.

DOMINATING MEMBER

One person may be aggressive and outspoken, with the rest hiding their feelings so as not to be different or unpopular.

The leader can point out that what the outspoken member is saying is felt by a lot of people, even though they may not admit it. The leader can explain that though some people may fear conflict, it does occur, and it is important to have the courage to confront it. If the leader does not handle the dominator in the group, members will start to be absent, or lose their tempers.

BLOCKING OTHER PEOPLE'S CONTRIBUTIONS

The problem with allowing someone to dominate a group is that this stops others with useful things to say from contributing. Intervention has to take place early on to prevent group structure hardening.

Stimulating silent members counteracts the dominance of the voluble member as well as making the group structure a more functional one. The leader should thank the monopolizer for all his or her contributions and state clearly that he or she would like to hear everyone's point of view.

MANIPULATION

At the other extreme from the dominator, a person may manipulate a group by remaining silent. Some groups resent this, believing that the person is quietly judging them or not sharing. The leader should ask pleasantly for a contribution from a silent member, thus modelling respect for each member. Conveying an interest in hearing from people can also be done non-verbally with a touch, gesture or eye contact.

The group may be manipulated by any of its members, including the leader, if they have a hidden agenda for the group.

Facilitating group work

ASSERTIVENESS

Assertive behaviour facilitates communications in groups and therefore it is useful if the leader explains the principles of assertion to certain groups at the outset.

Assertiveness in an individual or group situation may be defined as standing up for your basic rights and beliefs, without isolating those of others, and making your behaviour 'match' your feelings. It is distinct from both passive and aggressive behaviour.

Those who behave passively:

- allow others to make decisions for them;
- feel helpless, powerless, inhibited, nervous and anxious;

- rarely express feelings;
- have little self-confidence;
- do best when following others;
- are fearful of taking the initiative;
- feel sorry for themselves to the point of martyrdom.

Those who behave aggressively are:

- very expressive, to the point of humiliating and deprecating others;
- obnoxious, vicious, egocentric;
- able to make others feel devastated by an encounter with them;
- giving out the message that they are OK but the other person definitely is not.

If you are assertive in your behaviour, you:

- are expressive with your feelings, without being obnoxious;
- are able to state views and desires directly, spontaneously and honestly;
- feel good about yourself and others too;
- respect the feelings and rights of other people;
- can evaluate a situation, decide how to act, then act without reservation;
- are true to yourself;
- value winning or losing little compared to the value of expressing yourself and choosing for yourself;
- may not always achieve your goals, but the resolution isn't always as important as the actual process of asserting yourself;
- are able to say what you have to say, whether it is positive or negative, leaving the other person's dignity intact.

Most people are assertive at some times with some people, but it is possible to learn to be assertive in situations which cause stress.

ACTIVITY

Make an assertiveness self-assessment table. Each group member can make a hierarchy of the least and most anxiety-provoking situations for them.

Then make a daily log of successful assertive interactions.

Non-verbal techniques of assertion in the group situation include:

- good eye contact;
- confident posture, standing or sitting comfortably;
- talking in a strong, steady voice;
- not clenching one's fist and not pointing one's finger.

Assertive verbal behaviour includes:

- avoiding qualifying words (such as 'maybe', 'only', 'just');
- avoiding disqualifying phrases (such as 'I'm sure this isn't important but');
- avoiding attacking phrases (such as those that begin with 'you'; substitute assertive phrases that use 'I' language, e.g. 'I feel . . .'.

Other assertive behaviours to practise in the group situation are:

- the 'broken record' – calm repetition of the assertive message;
- 'fogging' – accept criticism comfortably without being defensive;
- 'negative enquiry': purposely invite criticism (this prevents manipulation);
- silence, and listening reflectively.

ADAPTING COMMUNICATION TO OTHER PHYSICAL AND COGNITIVE ABILITIES AND INDIVIDUALITY

As in the one-to-one situation (see the first part of this chapter), the care worker or leader assesses the abilities and needs of the group members and communicates appropriately.

For example, with a group of elderly people, some of whom are partially deaf and some of whom are visually impaired, communications might have to be both written and spoken, with non-verbal gesturing increased.

Children, those with a poor grasp of

English and the mentally handicapped are other examples of groups where the leader would specially adapt his or her methods of communication.

SUPPORTIVE SKILLS

Warmth, understanding and sincerity are supportive skills. These are conveyed by the leader in the group situation by modelling respect for each member of the group; assertiveness (verbal and non-verbal); confidence; attitudes; and problem-solving.

Humour can be used to relieve tension but must not involve teasing.

ACTIVITY

Practise group work in the classroom by using the case studies of Ivy Trent and Tracy Congdon (at the beginning of this chapter) for role-play.

In the course of study, you may do a project in groups, for example a video project. Each participant can analyse the development of this group.

On work experience, any meeting of professionals which the student attends could be used to analyse group communication.

Students should prepare in advance of their analysis:

- a record sheet
- a sociogram
- an analysis grid

to record who communicates with whom and what contribution each member makes.

ANALYSING THE CLIENT'S RIGHTS IN INTERPERSONAL SITUATIONS

This section examines the values which underpin social care work.

The charter of rights for someone receiving a service at home from social services

Most local authorities will draw up their own charter of rights for clients receiving social services, based on the general guidelines outlined in the citizen's charter. There are specific government recommendations for certain matters – for example, the document 'Working Together' deals with child abuse, and its guidelines will be adapted to the special circumstances of different localities. The following charter of rights is specific to Surrey Social Services, but may be considered as representative.

1 The right to remain living in your own home if that is what you want.
2 The right to maintain your chosen lifestyle.
3 The right to have your personal dignity respected irrespective of physical or mental disability.
4 The right to be treated as an individual, whatever your physical or mental disability.
5 The right to personal independence, personal choice, personal responsibilities and actions, including acceptance of risk.
6 The right to personal privacy for yourself, your belongings and your affairs.
7 The right to have cultural, religious, sexual and emotional needs accepted and respected.
8 The right to receive care appropriate to your needs from suitably trained and experienced workers.
9 The right to have, and participate in, regular reviews of your individual circumstances, and to have a friend and adviser present if you so wish.
10 The right to participate as fully as possible in the drawing up of your own care plan.
11 The right to be fully informed about the services provided by the Department, and of any decisions made by the Authority's staff that may affect your personal well-being.

12 The right of access to personal files.

13 The right of access to a formal complaints procedure and to be represented by a friend or adviser if you so wish.

14 The right to be represented by an advocate if you so wish, or are unable to make personal representation through mental incapacity.

BOUNDARIES ON THESE RIGHTS

1 **Rights**: In all situations it is Social Services' policy to respect people's dignity, individuality and confidentiality along with their rights to independence, choice and control over their own lifestyle. Therefore Surrey County Council has produced this Charter of Rights.

2 **Responsibilities**: Your personal choices and actions have consequences which may affect other people. Therefore, as a user of services at home, you are obliged to ensure that others are not disturbed or put at risk by your actions. For example, you have a responsibility to provide a safe working environment for those who enter your home to provide services.

3 **Risks**: It is important to realize that living at home independently brings an element of risk. Some degree of risk is a normal part of life for everyone. Avoidance of risk leads to an unhealthy way of life.

4 **Restrictions**: Some people with severe disabilities, learning disabilities, or mental health problems cannot exercise their rights in full. It is essential, though, not to take away their rights unnecessarily – and any restriction will be strictly limited and reviewed regularly.

Individualization

Individualization is the recognition and understanding of each client's unique qualities and the differential use of principles and methods in assisting each toward a better adjustment. Individualization is based upon the right of human beings to be individuals and to be treated not just as a human being but as *this* human being with his personal differences.

(Felix P. Biestek 1990)

This value incorporates the principle of freedom from any kind of discrimination.

THE ROLE OF THE SOCIAL WORKER

The skill of individualization requires the following attributes in the care worker:

- freedom from bias and prejudice;
- knowledge of human behaviour, from psychology and medicine – not just from personal experience;
- ability to move at the client's pace;
- empathy – the ability to enter into the feelings of other people;
- ability to keep perspective: the emotional involvement of the care worker should be controlled.

PRACTICAL WAYS OF INDIVIDUALIZING

The care worker may intend to individualize and not do so effectively; following these principles will demonstrate that he or she is doing so in a way the client cannot miss:

- thoughtfulness in details, such as timing appointments to help a mother with schoolchildren;
- privacy in interviews, ensuring that the care worker can give full and undivided attention and reassurance about confidentiality;
- care in keeping appointments;
- preparation for interviews – review the client's record before the interview starts;
- engaging the client – let clients make their own decisions, select their own goals, fill out their own forms, thus stimulating their self-confidence.

Purposeful expression of feelings

Purposeful expression of feelings is the

recognition of the client's need to express his feelings freely, especially his negative feelings. The care worker listens purposefully, neither discouraging nor condemning the expression of those feelings, sometimes even actively stimulating and encouraging them when they are therapeutically useful.

(Felix P. Biestek 1990)

BENEFITS TO CLIENT OF PURPOSEFUL EXPRESSION

- It relieves tensions and anxiety in the client who after 'letting off steam' will be able to see his or her problem more clearly.
- The care worker will understand more about the client.
- The client/worker relationship will be strengthened.

BOUNDARIES

Expression of feelings must be limited to those the agency can cope with. For example, deeply disturbed emotions need handling by a psychiatrist.

Controlled emotional involvement

The controlled emotional involvement is the care worker's sensitivity to the client's feelings, an understanding of their meaning, and a purposeful, appropriate response to those feelings.

Acceptance

Acceptance is a principle of action wherein the care worker perceives and deals with the client as he or she really is, including his or her strengths and weaknesses, congenial and uncongenial qualities, positive and negative feelings, constructive and destructive attitudes and behaviour, maintaining all the while a sense of the client's innate dignity and personal worth.

The purpose of acceptance is therapeutic: to aid care workers in understanding each client as they really are, thus making casework more effective; and to help each client free themselves from undesirable defences, so that they feel safe to look at and reveal themselves as they really are, and thus to deal with their problems in a more realistic way.

Client self-determination

The principle of client self-determination is the practical recognition that clients need, and have a right to, freedom in making their own choices and decisions. Care workers have a corresponding duty to respect that right, recognize that need, and stimulate and help to activate that potential for self-direction by helping the client to see and use the available and appropriate resources of the community and of his or her own personality.

The client's right to self-determination, however, is limited by the client's capacity for positive and constructive decision-making, by the framework of civil and moral law, and by the function of the agency.

It is this value which emphasizes the need for each individual to maintain his or her own identity, through exercising choice and independence.

The main reasons for enabling client self-determination are:

- to allow the client to regain self-confidence, which may have been lost in the present crisis;
- to allow the client to draw from that self-confidence a renewed ability to solve his or her own problems;
- to enable the client, through making his or her own choices and plans, with the support of the care worker, to experience personal growth and increased maturity.

FOUR PRACTICAL WAYS IN WHICH THE CARE WORKER MIGHT ENABLE CLIENT SELF-DETERMINATION

- Help the client to see his or her problem or need clearly and with perspective. This is done using listening and interview skills.
- Acquaint the client with the relevant

sources of help available in the community. The client should know precisely what help is available in the community. But it is up to him or her how far to use it.

- Introduce stimuli that will activate the client's own dormant resources. Through the care worker/client relationship, abilities in the client that had been crushed by the current crisis will be released.
- Create a client/care worker relationship in which the client can grow and work out his or her own problems.

It is unacceptable for care workers to impose plans on a client. A client will make progress in social responsibility, emotional adjustment and personality development only if he or she is allowed to exercise freedom of choice and decision.

THE LIMITATIONS ON CLIENT SELF-DETERMINATION

- Not all clients are equally capable of making their own decisions.
- A client cannot intrude on the rights of others without their consent.
- A client has the right to take some risks with his or her own safety but not with the safety of others.
- A client's plans and decisions should keep within the law.

The non-judgemental attitude

The non-judgemental attitude is based on a conviction that the function of the care worker excludes assigning guilt or innocence, or degree of client responsibility for causing the problems or needs, but does include making evaluative judgements about the attitudes, standards or actions of the client. The attitude, which involves elements of both thought and feeling, is transmitted to the client.

In helping clients it is important to understand their failures and weaknesses, but it is not the function of the care worker to judge.

The care worker provides the non-judgemental atmosphere and within this the client develops the strength to see him or herself objectively, and to do what is necessary for constructive change.

BOUNDARIES

The non-judgemental attitude does not mean indifference to value systems, or to social, legal or moral standards.

Confidentiality

Confidentiality is the preservation of secret information concerning the client which is disclosed in the professional relationship. Confidentiality is based upon a basic right of the client; it is an ethical obligation of the care worker and is necessary for an effective service. The client's right, however, is not absolute. Moreover, the client's secret is often shared with other professional persons within the agency and also in other agencies; the obligation then binds all equally.

One way in which 'confidentiality' could be described would be as having to do with people's rights over the property of their secrets. It is useful to make an analogy with material belongings, because this can help to highlight how much worth people attach to information concerning themselves and their lives, and the seriousness of the damage which can occur when their ownership rights in this area are infringed.

It therefore follows that 'to extract a person's secrets from him under false pretences, or to pass them on to others when they have been entrusted in confidence, might constitute a more serious violation of personal rights than the stealing of a material object' (Felix P. Biestek 1990).

Breach of confidentiality has been likened to theft, but it is more serious. The invasion of privacy resulting from a failure in confidentiality often leads to a greater and more fundamental loss than does theft.

Confidentiality relates directly to the principle of respect for other people.

A client wants to be reassured about confidentiality. But as the case will be recorded, his or her secrets will be known to the typist and the supervisor. The counsellor or care worker is not a freelance worker, but part of a social agency. The client should understand this.

How far this information should be communicated outside the agency is a different matter.

The client should be assured of the following rights:

- Other agencies and individuals should only be consulted with the client's consent (this may be overriden in extreme cases such as that of a child at risk).
- Records should only show information that is essential to provide the service, and in many instances should be available to the scrutiny of the client.

BOUNDARIES OF CONFIDENTIALITY

The client's right to confidentiality is limited by:

- the rights of other individuals;
- the rights of the care worker;
- the rights of the hospital/social agency;
- the rights of society as a whole.

ACTIVITY

The Code of Professional Conduct is issued by the United Kingdom Central Council for Nursing, Midwifery and Health Visiting. It states:

Each registered nurse, midwife and health visitor shall act, at all times, in such a manner as to justify public trust and confidence, to uphold and enhance the good standing and reputation of the profession, to serve the interests of society, and above all to safeguard the interests of individual patients and clients.

Write to the UKCC (for address see list at end of chapter) and ask for a copy of the Code. Read the section on confidentiality.

Anyone working in the health and social care fields is expected to understand and honour scrupulously the requirements of confidentiality. The following extract is an example of the formal commitment to do so that workers in a care institution may be expected to sign.

The following statement has been taken from the DHSS Steering Group on Health Service Information and should be adhered to by all hospital staff:

'In the course of your duties you may have access to confidential material about patients, members of staff or other health service business. On no account must information relating to identifiable patients be divulged to anyone other than authorised persons, for example medical, nursing or other professional staff, as appropriate, who are concerned directly with the care, diagnosis and/or treatment of the patient. If you are in any doubt whatsoever as to the authority of a person or body asking for information of this nature you must seek advice from your superior officer. Similarly, no information of a personal or confidential nature concerning individual members of staff should be divulged to anyone without the proper authority having first been given.'

The focal word in the definition of 'confidential' is TRUST. A patient must be able to have complete trust in the hospital and its staff with regards to private and personal information which they have given about themselves. A patient has a right to expect that information given in confidence will be used only for the purpose for which it was given and will not be released to others without their consent.

As a representative of the hospital, on a work placement programme, you are expected to ensure that you:

- Never discuss patients or hospital business with other persons either inside or outside the hospital.
- Never give out information regarding a patient to anyone.

- Always refer persons, who are requesting information, to your supervisor.

ACTIVITY

Read the following clinical profile and try to answer the questions at the end.

1 Mrs Irene McGregor is a 55-year-old married woman who lives on a housing estate in the suburbs of a large city. She has been admitted for a hysterectomy related to fibroids.

2 A routine chest radiograph shows evidence of previous tuberculosis. Other investigations are normal. In the past she has had no serious illness, but 10 years ago she was investigated for possible epilepsy.

3 She has three children, all of whom are well, but one has recently been suspected of drug-taking. She has told this only to the social worker. Her husband is a postman and she works part-time in a shop. There is an elderly mother-in-law who lives nearby and is visited daily by the family.

4 She is naturally anxious about the operation, and the fact that her eldest son may be involved with drugs has made her particularly anxious about the admission. She is otherwise well adjusted.

- This information, except for that associated with her son, has been obtained from the case-sheet. Who should have access to it?
- How much of each of the four points of information listed above should be shared with members of the professional staff?
- How much should be shared with other members of the team: e.g. porters, receptionists, etc.?

- Do all members of staff need to know all the information?
- During the weekly ward meeting, a member of the nursing staff feels that the patient is more anxious than she should be. How much information about the son should be divulged and openly discussed?

It is sometimes useful, when deciding on who should be given confidential information, to separate people into the following groups:

1 Those who must know
2 Those who should know
3 Those who could know
4 Those who shouldn't know

A typical team on a medical or surgical ward would include doctors, nurses, social workers, physiotherapists, dieticians, pharmacists and others. Related to this team are secretaries, receptionists, porters and ward maids. These individuals are vital to the working of the team. Look again at Mrs McGregor and the issues and questions which have been raised. Divide the professional groups, the supporting staff, and others into the categories listed above.

Confidentiality, outside the health care team: So far it has been assumed that information about an individual *might* be shared between members of the team. There are circumstances, however, when information about a particular patient is requested by other groups. Consider Mrs McGregor again. Information is requested by the following. Would you divulge it?

- The husband: He asks for information about the medical problems.
- A close friend: A neighbour (female) asks to see the ward sister and requests information about treatment.
- The social services: They are concerned about possible problems at home while the patient is recovering. They want details of the family background.

- The police: Questions are being asked about possible drug problems in the area and they suspect her son.
- The press: They have found out from the police that her son is a possible addict. They phone you for information.
- Your colleagues: You meet a colleague at a social event. He (or she) is very interested in family problems associated with drug-taking. He asks if you know anyone who might be able to help in this important research project.

These points raise important issues in confidentiality, and you should now be clearer about when, and to whom, you would divulge information.

Computers and records: The introduction of computers and data bases has introduced a new element in the maintenance of confidentiality. It has also introduced a new problem, that of access to records by patients. While it has always been possible (but rather difficult) to obtain access to case-sheets, the Data Protection Act makes the provision for this clear. While final decisions about access to computer-based medical information still remain to be made, there are fundamental moral questions which need to be answered.

- Should patients have a right of access to their own medical information?
- Will this prevent the writing down of sensitive information?
- Who else should have access to the information? Should all relatives be allowed to see it?
- What safeguards would you include to make the records confidential?

ACTIVITY

Consider the following dilemmas involving the values underpinning health and social care work. In each case, decide:

- Whose rights are being violated?
- Whose rights should take priority?

- What course of action should be taken?

1 A recently married man comes to see a social worker. He confesses that he recently on one occasion sexually abused his young step-daughter. He is desperate to get help so that this does not happen again. He was himself abused as a child; he has not told his new wife this, nor the fact that he has approached her daughter. He pleads that his wife should not know, fearing that she would have no more to do with him.

2 A teenager is benefiting from a series of counselling sessions in which she is discussing family problems. She reveals that a short while ago she stole something quite substantial from a shop, but swears that she will never steal again.

3 An elderly man is desperate to return from hospital to his own flat which is in a filthy state because of the numerous cats he keeps which have no access to outdoors. His health is frail following a heart attack and his movement limited. Hospital staff are pressing him to go to a residential home for his own well-being and safety, but he has lived in his flat for 50 years and feels that it is his home.

4 A mentally handicapped couple are considered fit to live in the community, and following discharge from hospital are housed in a ground-floor council flat. The woman is more severely handicapped than her husband. There have been complaints from neighbours about dirt and smells. The social worker visits and finds that the flat is very dirty and that the couple's standard of personal hygiene is very low (both have head lice and wear unwashed clothes). There is, however, a little food in the fridge and both husband and wife insist that they are managing. They do not want to move, or be parted.

REFERENCES AND RESOURCES

Atkinson, R.L. (1993), *Introduction to Psychology*, 11th ed. US: Harcourt Brace Jovanovich College Publishers.

Biestek, F.P. (1992), *The Casework Relationship*. London: Routledge.

Butrym, Zofia T. (1986), *The Nature of Social Work*. London: Macmillan.

Coulshed, V. (1990), *Social Work Practice: An Introduction*. London: Macmillan Education.

Eysenck, H. and Wilson, G. (1991), *Know Your Own Personality*. London: Penguin.

Gill, David and Adams, Bridget (1988), *The ABC of Communication Studies*. Walton-on-Thames: Nelson.

Gross, R. (1992), *Psychology: The Science of Mind and Behaviour*, 2nd ed. Sevenoaks: Hodder and Stoughton.

Hayes, N. and Orrell, S. (1993), *Psychology: An Introduction*, 2nd ed. London: Longman.

Mayer, John E. and Timms, Noel (1970), *The Client Speaks: Working Class Impressions of Casework*. London: Routledge and Kegan Paul.

Murgatroyd, Stephen (1985), *Counselling and Helping*. London: International Thomson Publishing Ltd.

Phelps, Stephen and Austin, Nancy (1989), *The Assertive Woman*. London: Arlington Books.

Preston-Shoot, M. (1987), *Effective Groupwork*. London: Macmillan Education.

Runciman, P. (1989), 'Health Assessment of the Elderly: A Multidisciplinary Perspective' in *Social Work and Health Care*, Taylor, R. and Ford, J. (eds). London: Jessica Kingsley.

USEFUL ADDRESS

United Kingdom Central Council for Nursing, Midwifery and Health Visiting
(PC Division)
23 Portland Place
London W1N 3AF

PHYSICAL ASPECTS OF HEALTH

HOW BODY SYSTEMS INTERRELATE

Body system organization

Most organs do not function independently but in groups called ORGAN SYSTEMS. These can also be called BODY SYSTEMS.

The following are the human body systems:

- digestive system
- cardiovascular system
- respiratory system
- reproductive system
- endocrine system
- nervous system
- sensory system
- urinary/renal system
- musculo-skeletal system

ACTIVITY

In order to complete the activities relating to body systems in this chapter, you will need to refer to specialist biology or human biology books.

1 Make a list of all the organs that make up each of the body systems listed here.

2 Take one organ of each system and make a list of the tissues that make up its structure. Note the contribution that each tissue makes to the function of the organ as a whole.

3 Consider the ways in which each of the organ systems are dependent on the other organ systems. For example, the cardiovascular system supplies each of the other systems with sugars and oxygen and removes waste.

The cardiovascular system

The cardiovascular system consists of the following tissues and organs:

- the heart
- the circulatory system
     arteries
     veins
     capillaries
- the blood
- the lymph
- the lymphatic system

THE HEART AND CIRCULATORY SYSTEM

The role of the heart and circulatory system is to carry blood between various parts of the body. Each organ has a major artery supplying it with blood from the heart and a major vein which returns it.

ACTIVITY

Copy Figure 3.1 and add the names of the vessels numbered 1–19. Use arrows to show the direction of blood flow. Shade the vessels containing oxygenated blood red, and those containing deoxygenated blood blue.

The flow of blood is maintained in three ways:

1 *The pumping action of the heart.*

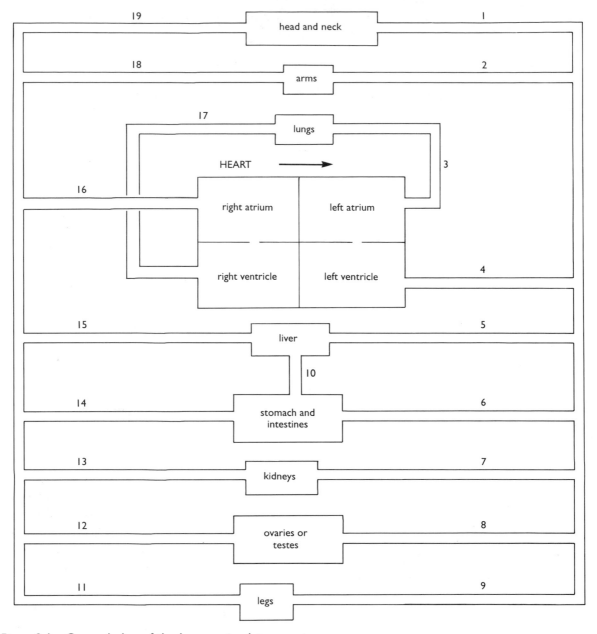

Figure 3.1 General plan of the human circulatory system

2 *The contraction of skeletal muscle.* The contraction of muscles during movement squeezes the veins and increases the pressure of blood within them. Pocket valves in the veins prevent backflow of blood and ensure that it flows back to the heart.

3 *Inspiratory movements.* The pressure in the thorax is reduced when breathing in, and this helps to draw blood back to the heart.

HEART STRUCTURE AND ACTION

ACTIVITY

1 Copy Figure 3.2 and label the parts A–Q. Indicate with arrows the direction of blood flow.

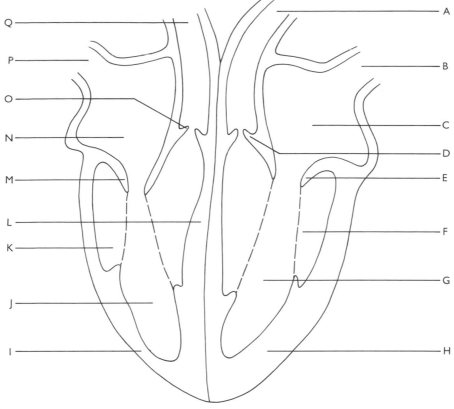

Figure 3.2   Structure of the heart

2 Note the function of each of the parts labelled A–Q.

3 Using a guide, dissect a heart (e.g. the heart of a sheep). Relate the diagram to the actual structure.

THE CARDIAC CYCLE

The following is the sequence of stages of a heartbeat:

1 *Diastole.* The atria and ventricles are relaxed. Deoxygenated blood under low pressure enters the right atrium and oxygenated blood enters the left atrium. The atria become distended as they become filled with blood. At first, the bicuspid and tricuspid valves are closed, but as the pressure in the atria increases the valves are pushed open, and some blood flows into the relaxed ventricles.

2 *Atrial systole.* When the diastole ends, the two atria contract simultaneously. This is called the atrial systole. This results in more blood being pushed into the ventricles.

3 *Ventricular systole.* As blood is pushed into the ventricles they contract almost immediately. This is called the ventricular systole. At this time, the bicuspid and tricuspid valves are closed. The ventricular pressure exceeds that of the aorta and the pulmonary artery, and the aortic and pulmonary valves are pushed open. Thus blood is expelled into these vessels. During ventricular systole the blood is forced against the closed atrio-ventricular valves and this produces the first sound of the heart beat ('lub').

4 *Diastole again.* The ventricular systole ends and the ventricles and atria relax again. The high pressure developed in the aorta and the pulmonary artery tends to force some blood back towards the ventricles, and the aortic and pulmonary pocket valves close rapidly. This causes the second heart sound ('dub').

One heartbeat consists of one systole and one diastole and lasts for about 0.8 seconds.

Figure 3.3 shows some of the changes that take place during one cardiac cycle.

ACTIVITY

From Figure 3.3:

1 Calculate the heart rate (beats/minute).

2 Explain what is happening in phases A, B and C.

3 Say what causes the first and second sounds of the heart beat?

HEART DISORDERS

There are many defects and disorders; some are acquired and some congenital.

A CONGENITAL condition is one that is recognized at birth or is believed to have been present since birth. Congenital malformations include all disorders present at birth, whether they are inherited or caused by an environmental factor. An example is the 'hole in the heart' condition.

ACQUIRED heart disorders are:

- *Coronary thrombosis.* A blood clot becomes lodged in the coronary arteries, which serve the heart muscle itself.
- *Atherosclerosis.* Narrowing of the arteries due to thickening of the artery wall caused by fat, fibrous tissue and salts being deposited on it. This is often called hardening of the arteries.
- *Spasm.* Repeated contractions of the muscle of the coronary artery wall.

Coronary heart disorders and heart attacks are often caused by a combination of these factors. If the main coronary artery is blocked, the whole heart muscle (the myocardium), or

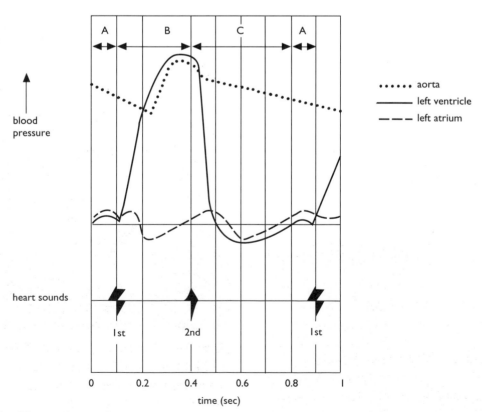

Figure 3.3 **The cardiac cycle**

part of it, may be deprived of blood, resulting in death. Sometimes only a portion of the myocardium is affected.

Angina is usually the result of reduced blood flow in the coronary arteries due to atherosclerosis, but sometimes it is due to thrombosis or spasm.

Factors causing heart disorders

- Smoking is a major cause of thrombosis and atherosclerosis.
- A raised level of fat, especially cholesterol, in the blood is a major cause of atherosclerosis. A high intake of saturated fat, found in meat and dairy products, is thought to be related to a high blood cholesterol level.
- High blood pressure, or hypertensive disease, contributes to atherosclerosis.
- A high level of salt in the diet contributes to coronary disease.
- Diabetes can be accompanied by coronary disease.
- Stress is thought to be a factor, and older individuals are more at risk than younger ones.
- Lack of exercise probably contributes to heart disorders and exercise can reduce the risk of heart problems.

ARTERIES, VEINS AND CAPILLARIES

ARTERIES carry blood away from the heart. VEINS carry blood to the heart. CAPILLARIES connect arteries and veins and form a network in the tissues.

ACTIVITY

1 Compare Figures 3.4 and 3.5. Can you see the structures labelled on the diagram in the photomicrographs?

2 Copy out the following table and complete it to compare the structures and functions of the three types of blood vessel.

	ARTERY	VEIN	CAPILLARY
1	Thick muscular wall	Thin muscular wall	No muscle
2			
3			
4			

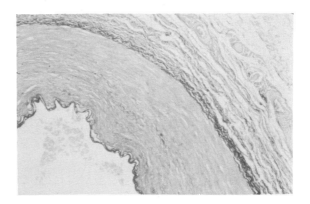

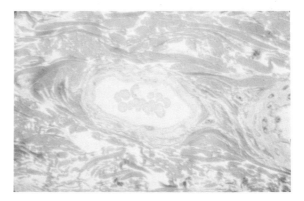

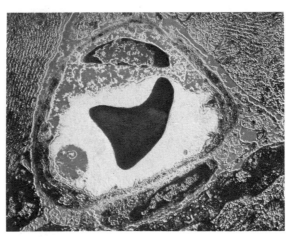

Figure 3.4 Photomicrographs of TS (a) artery, x 100 (b) vein, x 320 and (c) capillary, x 3,500
Photos: (a) Andrew Syred 1990, Microscopix;
(b) G.F. Gennard, Science Photo Library;
(c) CNRI, Science Photo Library.

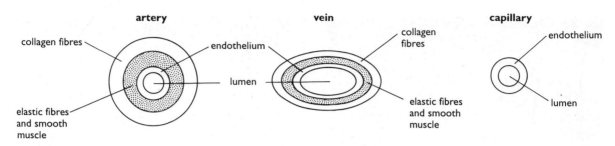

Figure 3.5 Diagram showing TS artery, vein and capillary

BLOOD

Blood is found circulating within the cardiovascular system, i.e. within the heart and blood vessels. Figure 3.6 shows the components of the blood in tabular form; Figure 3.7 is a photograph of a sample of blood.

Component	Appearance	Function	Nos. of cells mm⁻³
Plasma	straw-coloured liquid	Matrix in which a variety of substances are carried e.g. vitamins, products of digestion, execretory products, hormones	
Red blood cells or *erythrocytes*	Biconcave discs full of the red pigment haemoglobin. No nucleus. 7μm 2.5μm side view	Carriage of O_2 and some CO_2	500,000
White blood cells or *Leucoytes:*			
(a) *Granulocytes*	Granular cytoplasm. Lobed nuclei		
Neutrophils	12μm	Engulf bacteria	4,900
Eosinophils	12μm	Anti-histamine properties	105
Basophils	10μm	Produces histamine	35
(b) *Agranulocytes*	No granules seen under light microscope		
Monocytes	16μm	Engulf bacteria	280
Lymphocytes	10μm	Antibody production	1,680
Platelets	3μm	Clotting	250,000

Figure 3.6 The components of blood

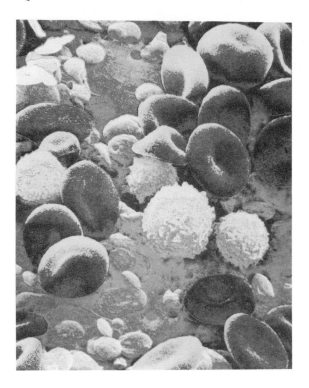

Figure 3.7 Photomicrograph of blood cells
Photo: Bill Longcore, Science Photo Library.

ACTIVITY

1 Figure 3.6 shows the components of blood. If possible examine a prepared slide of blood under the microscope and identify as many of the components as possible.

2 List three ways in which the structure of the red blood cells makes it efficient at carrying out its main function.

3 Red blood cells have a life span of about three months. How are the waste products from their breakdown excreted?

FUNCTIONS OF THE BLOOD

The functions of each type of cell in the blood are shown in Figure 3.6.

A major role of the blood is TRANSPORT.

ACTIVITY

Copy out the table and complete it.

Materials Transported	Examples	Transported to	Transported from	Transported in
Respiratory gases	Oxygen Carbon dioxide			Haemoglobin in red cells
Organic nutrients	Glucose Amino acids Vitamins			
Mineral salts	Calcium Iodine Iron			
Excretory products	Urea			
Hormones	Insulin Anti-diuretic hormone			
Heat	Metabolic heat			

Another major function of the blood is DEFENCE. There are three main ways in which blood defends the body against disease. These are by:

- clotting
- phagocytosis
- antibody production

Find answers to the following questions on CLOTTING:

- Which of the following are involved in clot formation: red blood cells, white blood cells, platelets?
- What do you think are the two main functions of a clot?
- What is thrombosis?

Some of the white blood cells engulf bacteria. This is known as PHAGOCYTOSIS. Once the bacteria are inside the cell, they are digested by enzymes contained in the LYSOSOMES. Pus formed at a site of infection is made up of dead bacteria and white blood cells.

ANTIBODIES are produced by white blood cells known as LYMPHOCYTES. They are produced in response to ANTIGENS – proteins or polysaccharides that coat foreign material such as bacteria. Antibodies are produced which are specific to a single antigen. The production of antibodies is not restricted to the blood; they are also produced by cells lining surfaces, for example in the respiratory system, and in the alimentary canal.

There are many different ways in which antibodies prevent the replication and harmful effects of micro-organisms.

Some of the ways in which they function are:

- They cause the foreign particles to stick together.
- They may neutralize the toxins produced by the pathogen.
- They may break down foreign material.
- They may stimulate phagocytosis (see above).

(Immunity will be explored in more detail later in this chapter.)

LYMPH

Lymph is a milky liquid which is rich in fats and contains lymphocytes. It is carried in lymph capillaries.

Lymph is derived from TISSUE FLUID, which bathes all the cells of the body. Tissue fluid is derived from blood, and is the means by which materials are exchanged between cells and blood. The lymph system drains into the circulatory system, so there is a constant flow of liquid from the blood to the tissue fluid, to the lymph and back into the blood (see Figure 3.8).

Formation of tissue fluid

The capillary walls are permeable to all components of the blood except red and some white blood cells and plasma proteins. When the blood enters the capillaries from the arteries it is under high pressure because of the decrease in diameter. This causes fluid to pass out of the capillary and into the spaces between cells, where it forms tissue fluid.

Drainage of tissue fluid

Obviously, as tissue fluid is continuously being formed it also has to be drained away. This occurs in two ways.

- By the time the blood reaches the vein end of the capillary, the pressure has dropped. This allows the osmotic effect of proteins in the plasma to cause the flow of tissue fluid back into the capillary. Osmosis involves the flow of water molecules from a region of high concentration of water molecules to a region of low concentration of water molecules, through a selectively permeable membrane. The tissue fluid has a high concentration of water molecules since the solute concentration is low. The plasma in the capillary has a low concentration of water molecules, chiefly because of the presence of the plasma proteins. The two solutions are separated by the selectively permeable plasma membranes of the epithelial cells lining the capillary. This situation therefore results in

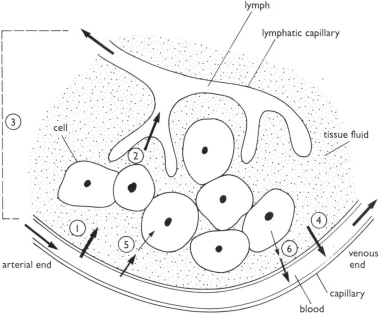

1 The high pressure at the arterial end of the capillary causes water to leave the plasma and pass through the capillary wall to the tissue fluid.

2 Water from the tissue fluid drains into the lymphatic capillary, by osmosis, to form lymph.

3 Lymph returns to the circulation system.

4 Water passes from the tissue fluid back into the capillary at the venous end. This occurs by osmosis.

5 Molecules, for example oxygen and nutrients, pass from the capillaries through the tissue fluid to the cells.

6 Waste materials, for example carbon dioxide and urea, pass from the cells through the tissue fluid and into the capillaries by diffusion.

Figure 3.8   Formation of tissue fluid and lymph

osmosis, and water from the tissue fluid passes into the plasma.

• Water from the tissue fluid enters the lymph capillaries, by osmosis, where it becomes lymph.

THE LYMPHATIC SYSTEM

The lymphatic system is a one-way system. Lymph capillaries drain the tissue spaces throughout the body. They eventually join up to form larger lymphatic vessels and join the blood system in two places:

1 On the left side via the thoracic vessel into the left subclavian vein.
2 On the right side via the right lymphatic duct into the right subclavian vein.

The larger lymphatic vessels have valves to prevent backflow. Lymph nodes are found as swellings on the larger lymphatic vessels; groups of lymph nodes are termed lymph glands.

Disorders connected with the lymphatic system

• Starving children may have grossly swollen abdomens from accumulation of fluid in and around the organ.

• Less seriously, if a person sits for a long time without moving their legs, their ankles may become swollen.

• A parasitic worm that blocks the lymph vessels causes a disease called *elephantiasis* (Figure 3.9). The most obvious symptom of this is the enormous enlargement of extremities, particularly legs, breast, or scrotum.

ACTIVITY

1 Construct a table to compare blood and lymph.

2 Draw a diagram to show the lymphatic system of a human.

3 At intervals along the lymphatic vessels are lymph nodes which produce lymphocytes and antibodies. Where in the body are the main sites of these lymph nodes?

4 Unlike the circulatory system, which has the heart, the lymph system has no

pump. Can you find out how the movement of lymph through the vessels is achieved?

5 What are the functions of lymph in addition to formation of tissue fluid?

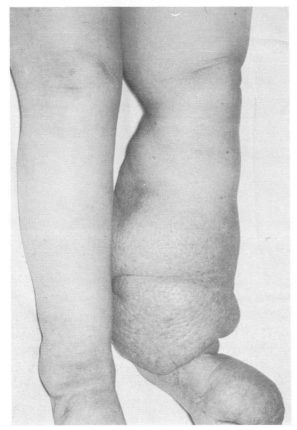

Figure 3.9 An example of the effects of elephantiasis
Photo: National Medical Slide Bank.

The respiratory system

The respiratory system consists of:

- Air passages connecting the respiratory surfaces with the outside air. These passages are found in the nose and nasal cavities, the mouth and throat, the trachea and the two bronchi. The passages are covered by mucus secreted by goblet cells in the ciliated epithelium which lines them. The mucus traps particles from the incoming air and also moistens it. The bronchi lead into further passages, the many bronchioles.

- The respiratory surface, which is formed by 350 million air sacs, the alveoli, in each lung. The total respiratory surface area is approximately 90 m^2. The surfaces of the alveoli are moist and form the site of gaseous exchange of oxygen and carbon dioxide. Each alveolus is surrounded by a capillary network, which conveys deoxygenated blood to the alveoli and oxygenated blood away from the alveoli.

- The structures which cause the breathing mechanism and ventilation of the lungs. Air is moved in and out of the air passages and the alveoli. The structures involved are the diaphragm, ribs, intercostal muscles and pleural membranes. The latter secrete pleural fluid into the pleural cavity; the function of the fluid is lubrication. Pressure in this cavity is always lower than that in the lungs, so that the lungs expand to fill the thorax.

ACTIVITY

1 Copy the diagram of the respiratory system (Figure 3.10).

2 Label the structures A–H.

3 Briefly note the function of each structure.

4 Inspect the photomicrograph of a bronchial tree (Figure 3.11). What structures can you identify?

ACTIVITY

1 Look at Figure 3.12. Why is it advantageous for the terminal chambers of the respiratory system to be divided into numerous small compartments rather than one larger spherical chamber?

2 What is the function of the capillary network covering the terminal group of alveoli?

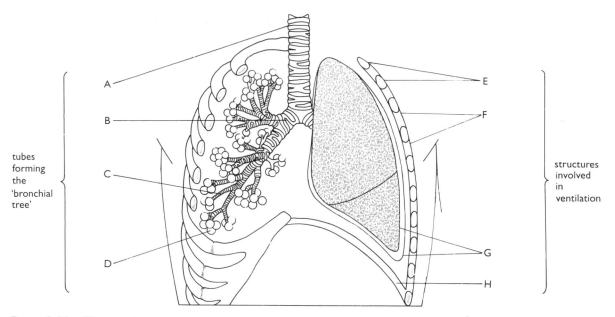

Figure 3.10 The respiratory system

tubes
forming
the
'bronchial
tree'

structures
involved
in
ventilation

GASEOUS EXCHANGE AT THE ALVEOLI

Each alveolus is made up of thin cells (squamous epithelium) and some elastic and collagen fibres. The network of capillaries that surrounds the group of alveoli brings blood from the pulmonary artery. The capillaries unite to form the pulmonary vein. The capillaries are also lined with squamous epithelium, and are very narrow so that the red cells within them are squeezed as they pass through. This slows down the flow of blood, allowing more time for diffusion, and increases the surface area of the red blood cell, thus giving a greater surface area for diffusion of oxygen into the cells. The oxygen from the inspired air dissolves in the moisture lining the alveoli and then diffuses across the alveolar and capillary walls into the plasma. From here it diffuses into the red cells and combines with the respiratory pigment, haemoglobin. Carbon dioxide diffuses from the blood into the alveolus to leave the lungs in the expired air.

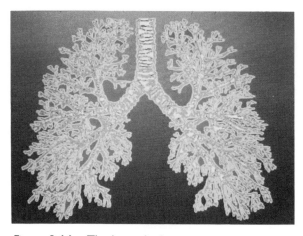

Figure 3.11 The bronchial tree
Photo: Alfred Pasieka, Science Photo Library.

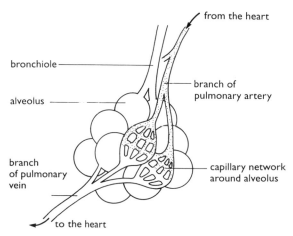

from the heart

bronchiole

branch of
pulmonary artery

alveolus

branch
of pulmonary
vein

capillary network
around alveolus

to the heart

Figure 3.12 A group of alveoli

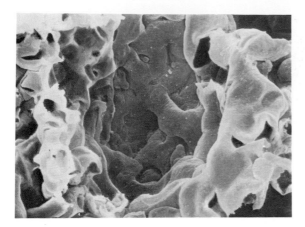

Figure 3.13   Photomicrograph of VS alveolus
Photo: Professor P. Motta, Department of Anatomy, University 'La Sapienza', Rome, Science Photo Library.

ACTIVITY

1 Inspect Figure 3.14. Why is the surface of the alveolus covered by a layer of water?

2 What properties are possessed by the squamous epithelial cells, which line both the alveolar and the capillary walls, that make them particularly suitable for their function here?

3 By which physical process do the oxygen and carbon dioxide molecules pass across the alveolar and capillary walls?

VENTILATION OF THE LUNGS

Ventilation of the lungs is brought about by changes in the volume of the thorax.

The rhythmical breathing movements occur 12 to 20 times a minute.

Inspiration (breathing in)

The volume of the thorax is increased by two movements:

1 The muscles round the edge of the diaphragm contract and pull it downwards so that it flattens.
2 The lower ribs are raised upwards and outwards by contraction of the external intercostal muscles which run obliquely from one rib to the next. The internal intercostal muscles are relaxed at this time.

The volume of the lungs increases as the volume of the thorax increases since they are thin and elastic. Thus air is drawn in (see Figure 3.15).

Expiration (breathing out)

The muscles of the diaphragm relax so that it resumes its dome shape. The external intercostal muscles relax and the internal

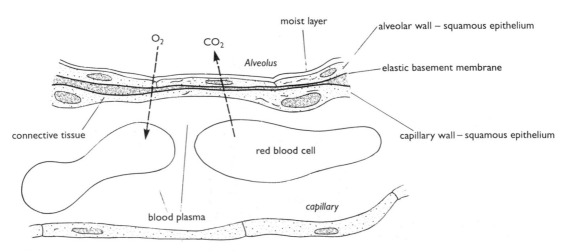

Figure 3.14   Gaseous exchange in an alveolus

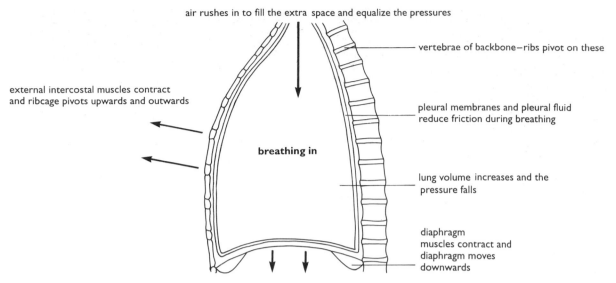

Figure 3.15 Breathing in

intercostal muscles contract. The volume of the thorax decreases and therefore the volume of lungs contract and air is expelled (see Figure 3.16). This is largely a passive process.

Changes to body systems as a consequence of lifestyle choices

Lifestyle choices, for example amount of exercise taken, diet, amount of stress (see Chapter 4) and smoking (see Chapter 5) can all cause changes to the body systems.

ACTIVITY

1 *Cardiovascular system*

- Investigate the evidence that could show that smoking is a major cause of coronary disease.
- Investigate the evidence that could show that a high cholesterol level in the blood is a cause of atherosclerosis.
- Investigate diabetes. Why should the risk of coronary heart disease sometimes accompany this disease?
- Why does exercise promote a healthy heart?

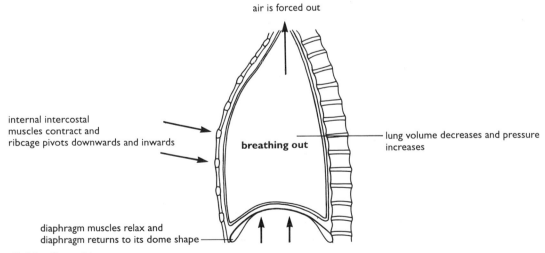

Figure 3.16 Breathing out

Design an investigation to show the effect of exercise on the heartbeat rate of five individuals. Record their pulse rate before exercise commences and then record the exercise undertaken. Record the heartbeat rate immediately after the exercise and find how long it takes for the rate to go back to normal.

What is 'fitness'? How do the results of your investigation relate to the 'fitness' of the individuals concerned?

• Investigate how a high level of stress may affect the heart. (See Chapter 4).

2 *Respiratory system*
Measure lung capacity using the equipment suggested in the diagram below. The subject being tested should breath in as far as possible, and then blow out as far as possible into the tube of the apparatus. The water displaced gives the *vital capacity*.

• Compare a group of 'fit' and 'unfit' individuals. How does exercise affect the respiratory system?
• Is there a difference between *breathing rate* of 'fit' and 'unfit' individuals?
• What else may affect vital capacity and breathing rate other than fitness?
• Compare a group of smokers' and non-smokers' vital capacities.

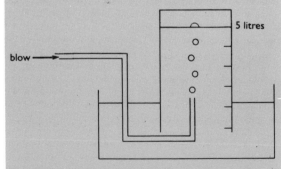

3 If the cardiovascular system and respiratory system are less effective, perhaps due to lifestyle choices, how will this affect other body systems?

What other effects will exercise, diet, stress and smoking have on these other body systems?

The effect of ageing on body systems

If we kept through life the same resistance to stress, injury and disease that we had at the age of ten, about half of us here today might expect to survive in 700 years time.

(Alex Comfort in The Biology of Senescence)

AGEING may be defined as the deteriorative changes taking place with the passage of time, eventually leading to the death of an organism. How fast a person ages depends on the following factors:

• environment;
• heredity or genetic programming;
• ethnic group;
• when the individual was born;
• level of wealth;
• gender.

Many physical changes occur with ageing, but the most common problems relate to poor mobility. However, 85% of elderly people can get around without assistance. Poor mobility may result from changes in more than one body system.

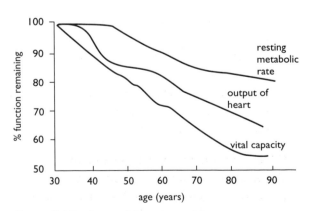

Figure 3.17 Loss of function with age

AN OUTLINE OF CHANGES CAUSED BY AGEING

- The hair thins and becomes grey due to pigment loss.
- The skin loses elasticity, causing wrinkling.
- *Bones* become lighter and more brittle. The discs of cartilage between the spinal vertebrae become thinner and harder, sometimes leading to hunching of the back.
- *Muscles* become weaker and less flexible.
- The nervous system becomes less efficient. Short-term memory is impaired along with the speed of reaction to changes in posture or position.

The cardiovascular system

- The heart becomes less efficient at pumping blood around the body. As a result, less blood flows through the kidneys and filtration is not as efficient.
- The tissue walls of the blood vessels lose elasticity and become rigid. Blood flow is impaired by this rigidity and by the build-up of fatty deposits on the vessel walls.

The respiratory system

- The muscles of the diaphragm become weaker resulting in shallower breathing.
- The walls of the alveoli lose elasticity and thicken, affecting gaseous exchange in the lungs.
- Certain disorders, e.g. bronchitis, may also affect the ability to inhale effectively.

The digestive system

- The muscles of the alimentary canal become weaker, which causes the digestive process to be less efficient.
- Peristalsis slows down, which may cause constipation.
- The breaking-down of food into small particles is less efficient, and as a result fewer valuable nutrients are absorbed.

The reproductive system

The menopause in women usually occurs between the ages of 45 and 55. The woman no longer ovulates and therefore can no longer have babies. Because of the drop in hormone levels of progesterone and oestrogen:

- the ovaries, uterus and cervix shrink;
- the Fallopian tubes shorten;
- the walls of the vagina lose elasticity;
- mucus production decreases and becomes alkaline.

While men can still father babies, certain natural changes occur in their reproductive system:

- sperm production decreases;
- sexual arousal takes longer;
- erections are less frequent and do not last as long;
- ejaculations are less powerful and less frequent.

The onset of all the changes in the male and female reproductive system is gradual and can be accommodated by the elderly couple as long as psychological factors do not interfere.

The endocrine system

Many of the body's metabolic functions are regulated by the production of thyroxine in the thyroid gland. In the elderly person:

- less thyroxine is produced, causing the metabolic rate to slow down, resulting in less energy and stamina;
- temperature control is also partly governed by thyroxine, which could account for an increasing inability to deal with temperature changes in old age.

The senses

Generally, the senses become less accurate as we get older.

- The lens of the eye loses elasticity. The eyes tend to become longsighted and focusing is difficult. The 'arcus senilis', an opaque ring at the outer edge of the iris, is of no significance.
- Hearing may be impaired, particularly for high-pitched sounds. The most common cause of hearing loss in the elderly is wax in the ear.

- Touch may become less sensitive. The receptors in the skin deteriorate and the skin becomes less elastic. These receptors are sensitive to pain, pressure and temperature and provide a measure of safety enabling a rapid response to avoid things which are too hot or cold.
- There is a marked reduction in the number of *taste buds* in the elderly and the sense of *smell* also deteriorates.

ACTIVITY

1 List the potential hazards resulting from:

- a raised pain threshold;
- failing eyesight and hearing;
- a reduced sense of smell and taste;
- weakening bones;
- wasting of the muscles.

2 The menopause is often called the 'change of life'. Research the causes, signs and possibe symptoms of the menopause. Use the following list as a guide:

- define the climacteric;
- possible emotional effects on the woman and her family;
- hormone replacement therapy;
- other available treatments.

HUMAN DISEASE

Classification of disease and illness

Diseases and illnesses may be divided into five main types.

PHYSICAL

Organ malfunction and injury

These diseases occur when there is a malfunction of an organ. There are various causes, which include injury. Examples are:

- diabetes
- goitre
- prostate enlargement
- heart disease
- malfunction of the cornea
- kidney disease

Environmental

These diseases are caused by a harmful environment. Some are deficiency diseases caused by malnutrition. Examples are:

- xeropthalmia (lack of Vitamin A)
- beri-beri (lack of Vitamin B)
- scurvy (lack of Vitamin C)
- rickets (lack of Vitamin D)
- kwashiorkor (lack of protein)
- goitre (lack of iodine)
- anaemia (lack of iron)
- pernicious anaemia (lack of Vitamin B12)

These diseases are discussed in the next part of the chapter, in 'a healthy diet'.

Others are occupational diseases, caused by a hazardous working environment. Many of these diseases are contracted through the respiratory system. Examples are:

- Pneumoconiosis, caused by inhalation of coal dust over a long period of time. The dust is engulfed and held by macrophages in fibrous nodules in the bronchioles. The flow of air to the alveoli is blocked and emphysema results.
- Asbestosis, caused by inhalation of particles of asbestos. The lower part of the lungs becomes fibrous. Lung cancer can result.
- Dermatitis. Skin infections can result from working with chemicals such as those used in hairdressing, or enzymic washing powders.
- Silicosis, caused by particles of silica from rock or stone. The inhaled particles are trapped in nodules in the alveoli and the lungs become fibrous and distorted. The surface area for gas exchange is reduced.
- Stress diseases. Ulcers of the stomach or duodenum and some coronary heart disease may be linked to stress.

Cancer tumours

The term cancer is applied to a group of *neoplastic* (literally meaning new growth) diseases in which normal body cells are changed into *malignant* ones.

Normally, the cells of tissues are regularly replaced by new growth which stops when old cells have been replaced. In cancer, this cell growth is *unregulated*. The cells continue to grow even after the repair of damaged tissue is complete. The malignant cells multiply and invade neighbouring tissues, thereby destroying the normal cells and taking their place. If the *lymphatic vessels* are invaded, the malignant cells are carried away in the lymph until their progress is halted by the filtering effect of the lymph glands. Here, they may be deposited and cause a *secondary* tumour (also called a *metastasis*).

Statistically, 1 in 4 of all infants born in the UK will develop cancer at some time in their lives and it is the second major cause of death.

There are over 150 types of cancer in humans, but they fall into two main groups.

- Sarcomas affect *connective* tissue, i.e. bones and muscles. They tend to grow very rapidly and are very destructive.
- Carcinomas affect *epithelial* tissue and make up the great majority of the *glandular* cancers, e.g. thyroid, pancreas and prostate. Also cancers of the breast, stomach, uterus, skin and tongue.

A *carcinogen* is any substance that causes cancer.

Biological factors and heredity play some part in the incidence of cancer, but, although it is known that there is permanent alteration in the DNA of the cell involved, it is not clear why some people succumb to a cancer and others do not. Research is still trying to discover the role of *viruses* in causing cancer. It is estimated that 70% of all cancers are caused by *environmental* factors:

- Cigarette smoking is directly related to approximately 90% of all cancers of the lung.
- Industrial pollutants such as asbestos,

benzene, solvents and insecticides.
- Radiation, prolonged exposure to the ultraviolet rays from the sun and the use of X-rays both in therapy and in diagnostic tests.

ACTIVITY

Find out the incidence of:

1 cancer of the lung and bronchus;

2 cancer of the breast;

3 cancer of the stomach;

4 cancer of the skin;

in

(a) UK,
(b) Japan,
(c) USA,
(d) Australia.

Prepare bar graphs or pie charts to display your findings and try to account for the variations found.

MENTAL

Some mental disorders are congenital. These are disorders that are recognized at birth and may be inherited or caused by an environmental factor. An example of a congenital condition is Down's Syndrome. Other mental disorders are described as neuroses or psychoses. A neurosis is a mental illness in which insight is retained but there is a particular way of behaving or thinking that causes suffering. The symptoms may include a severe emotional state such as an anxiety state or depression. Sometimes the symptoms involve distressing behaviour, as in phobias or obsessions. Other neuroses may be recognized by physical states, for example hysteria or hypochondria. A psychosis is a much more severe type of mental illness. The sufferer loses contact with reality and delusions and hallucinations often occur. Thought processes are usually altered. Manic depression and schizoprenia are the most commonly occuring psychoses.

INFECTIOUS

Infectious diseases are discussed in detail in this chapter. They are caused by parasites, which live and feed on another living organism, called the host. Ectoparasites live on the skin, while endoparasites are internal. Types of parasites are:

* bacteria
* viruses
* protozoa
* fungi
* worms (platyheliminthes, nematodes)

DEGENERATIVE

Examples are:

* Alzheimer's disease
* multiple sclerosis

INHERITED

These conditions arise from the genotype of the individual. They are hereditary conditions, and may be caused by dominant or recessive genes, or by chromosome abnormalities. Examples of hereditary disorders are:

* achondroplasia
* retinal aplasia
* phenylketouria
* haemophilia
* muscular dystrophy
* cretinism
* albinoism
* sickle-cell anaemia
* red/green colour blindness
* Down's Syndrome
* Klinefelter's Syndrome
* Turner's Syndrome

DEFINITION OF TERMS

1 *Congenital.* This term means 'present at birth'. A congenital abnormality may be inherited (i.e. passed down) from the parents; it may have occurred at the time of birth, or it may have occurred as the result of injury or infection in the womb. Congenital abnormalities are often called *birth defects*.

2 *Hereditary.* This term is used to describe the transmission of traits and disorders through *genetic* mechanisms. A disorder may be hereditary *and* congenital, but many hereditary diseases are not present at birth, e.g. Huntington's chorea and Friedreich's ataxia.

3 *Acquired.* Diseases and disorders which are neither congenital nor inherited are termed *acquired*. These are caused by external factors, e.g. infection, accidental injury or poisoning.

Infectious diseases

Infectious diseases are the leading cause of global mortality and debility, accounting for approximately one-third of all deaths and more than two-thirds of child deaths. Together with malnutrition, infectious diseases are largely responsible for the differential in infant mortality rates and life expectancies between developed and developing countries (UNEP 1987).

Infectious diseases are caused by *pathogens* (disease-causing organisms). These organisms are *parasites*, i.e. they are dependent on a live host for food and shelter. Parasites are found in many of the classification groups of diseases noted above.

VIRUSES

Viruses are, on average, about 50 times smaller than bacteria. They cannot be seen with a light microscope, and can only reproduce inside the living cell of a host. Viruses have a very simple, non-cellular structure. They contain a core of DNA or RNA surrounded by a protein coat.

ACTIVITY

1 The tapeworm and the liver fluke are parasites. What other examples can you think of?

2 Viruses are considered to be on the border between living and non-living. Which characteristics of living organisms do they possess, and which do they not possess?

3 List any viral diseases you can think of. How are these diseases spread?

The influenza virus

Four strains are known: A, B, C and D. Strains C and D are stable, whereas variants of strain A are very common, and strain B is rare. Epidemics break out frequently, affecting large numbers of people in a particular place. Sometimes the outbreaks are pandemic: they spread across continents. A serious pandemic outbreak occurred in 1918, when 20 million people died worldwide. This was caused by an A strain. Another strain of the A virus caused a pandemic in 1957–8; this was known as Asian 'flu. A similar outbreak happened in 1968, infecting about a quarter of the population in Britain, and killing 1,000 people. Nationwide epidemics of influenza caused by the A strain occur every two to three years, while B strains have a four- to six-year cycle.

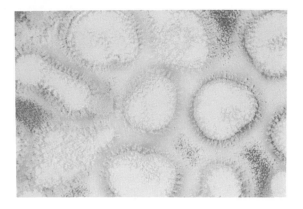

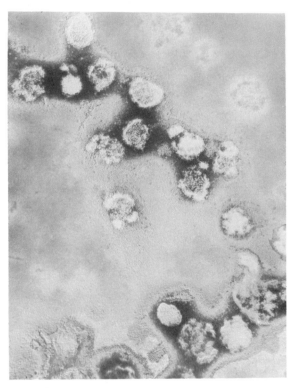

Figure 3.19 Photomicrographs of disease-causing viruses, (a) influenza, (b) rubella
Photo: (a) Omikron, Science Photo Library; (b) NIBSC, Science Photo Library.

The virus enters the respiratory tract in droplets, and attacks the epithelial cells lining the air passages. There is an incubation period of two to three days. Then the symptoms appear. The temperature rises to 40°C on the first day and this is accompanied by shivering, headache, sore throat and nasal congestion. Aches in limbs are common. After three to four days the temperature will fall, but a cough may develop due to damage of the trachea and bronchioles. Sometimes

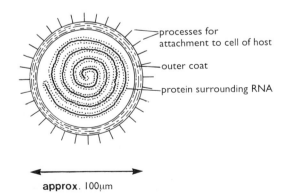

processes for attachment to cell of host

outer coat

protein surrounding RNA

approx. 100μm

Figure 3.18 Diagram of an influenza virus

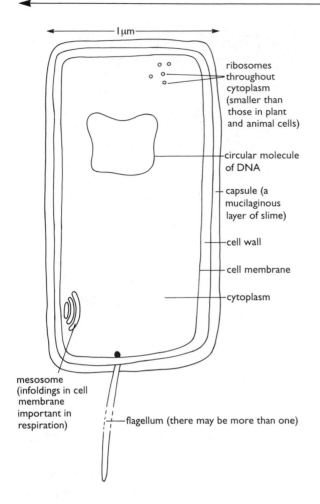

Figure 3.20 **Structure of a generalized bacterium**

pathogenic bacteria invade the damaged air passages and cause bronchitis or pneumonia.

BACTERIA

Bacteria are the smallest organisms which have a cellular structure (see Figure 3.20). They can be found in many environments, including in and on humans.

ACTIVITY

1 Study Figure 3.20. Construct a table to compare the structure of this cell with that of a generalized human cell.

2 If a single bacterium is placed into a fresh medium, and divisions take place every 20 minutes, how many bacteria will there be after 10 hours? You may be surprised by the answer!

Figure 3.21 shows the four main bacterial shapes.

If conditions (e.g. temperature, nutrient availability, pH (acidity) and oxygen availability) are suitable, bacteria reproduce by dividing into two identical daughter

Shape	Example	Disease caused	Shape	Example	Disease caused
spherical (cocci)			**rod-shaped (baccilli)**		
single			single	*Escherichia coli*	gut symbiont
chains	*Streptococcus pyrogens*	scarlet fever	chains	*Bacillus anthracis*	anthrax
clumps	*Staphylococcus aureus*	boils Pneumonia	flagellate	*Salmonella typhi*	typhoid fever
pairs in a capsule	*Diplococcus pneumoniae*	Pneumonia	**spiral-shaped (spirillum)**	*Treponemia pallidum*	syphilis
pairs	*Neisseria gonorrhoea*	gonorrhoea	**comma-shaped (vibro)**	*Vibrio cholerae*	cholera

Figure 3.21 Forms of bacteria

cells (*binary fission*). This may happen every 20 minutes which means huge numbers may be formed.

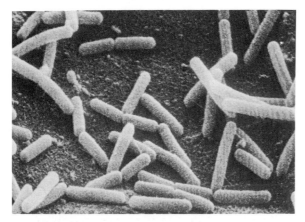

Figure 3.22 Photomicrograph of a disease-causing bacterium
Photo: Andrew Syred 1993, Microscopix.

ACTIVITY

Experiment to investigate the effect of temperature on bacterial growth

You will need five petri dishes of nutrient agar.

1 Leave the petri dishes uncovered in the laboratory for about 30 minutes.

2 Replace the lids and treat as follows:
   Plate 1: Leave at room temperature (20–25°C)
   Plate 2: Leave in a refrigerator (3–5°C)
   Plate 3: Leave in the freezing compartment of a refrigerator (below 0°C)
   Plate 4: Leave in an incubator (37°C)
   Plate 5: Heat in a hot oven or place in a pressure cooker for 15 minutes (121°C+) and then at room temperature (20–25°C)
   Label each plate.

3 After two to three days tape the two halves of each plate together for safety

reasons, and then examine. Make a table to show your observations.

4 To dispose of the plates safely, place in a disposable autoclave bag and autoclave for 15 minutes.

• At what temperature did bacteria grow quickest?
• What implications do your results have for food storage?

METHODS OF TRANSMISSION OF VIRAL AND BACTERIAL DISEASES

1 *Droplet infection*. Respiratory infections in particular are usually spread by droplet infection. Sneezing, coughing or even talking can result in a spray of droplets containing viruses or bacteria (see Figure 3.23). These can then be inhaled by other people.

2 *Direct physical contact (contagious)*. Relatively few diseases are spread through direct physical contact with an infected person. Examples include sexually transmitted diseases; the tropical disease yaws; trachoma (a common eye disease); the common wart; and herpes simplex, which causes 'cold sores'.

3 *Vectors*. An organism that transmits a pathogen is known as a *vector*. It may actually contain the pathogen which then

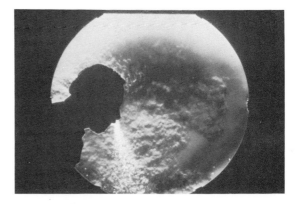

Figure 3.23 Photograph of a sneeze
Photo: Dr Gary Settles, Science Photo Library.

multiplies within it, for example, the flea as the vector of the endemic typhus bacteria; or it may carry the pathogen on the outside of its body, for example, a house fly might transfer cholera from faeces to food where it may be ingested.

4 *Contamination of food/water.* Salmonella and botulism are examples of true food-borne diseases. Pathogens found in faeces (e.g. cholera, typhoid and dysentery) may also be transmitted to another host via food or water.

5 *Contamination of wounds.* Disease can easily be caused through bacteria entering wounds, for example, tetanus.

ACTIVITY

1 Recommend precautions to prevent the transmission of viruses and bacteria by each of the methods outlined in the text.

2 Divide the following list into bacterial or viral diseases and, for each of them, find out by which of the methods listed in the text the pathogen is spread:

influenza; tetanus; common cold; diphtheria; mumps; tuberculosis (TB); whooping cough; measles; AIDS; gonorrhoea; syphilis; polio; typhus; German measles; yellow fever; rabies; chicken pox; yaws.

DIARRHOEAL DISEASES

Cholera affected many Latin American countries in 1991, the first such epidemic in the region this century. It had been assumed that improvements in water, sanitation, sewage treatment and food safety had eliminated this disease just as it had in Europe and North America in the late nineteenth and early twentieth century, when large-scale cholera epidemics in major cities had helped spur major investment in improving water supplies and installing sewers.

The epidemic first appeared in Peru in January 1991, and by the end of the year more than 276,000 cases and 2,664 deaths from cholera had been reported. At the same time, 39,154 cases and 606 deaths had been reported in Ecuador, and cases were also reported in other Latin American countries, plus 24 imported cases in the USA.

Cholera remains a serious problem in many African and Asian countries. It is endemic in India and Indonesia and has been reported in Iraq, although the number of cases and number of deaths at mid-July 1991 were relatively low; for all of Asia 6,700 cases were reported, with 68 deaths. Cholera was also reported in many African countries. In 1991 a total of 134,953 cases were reported in 19 of these countries, with 12,618 deaths. The actual numbers of cases of cholera will be substantially higher than the number reported in these countries, since no figures are available from other countries in the region known to have been hit by the epidemic.

(World Health Organization, provisional figures, 1991, in 'Our Planet, Our Health', WHO 1992)

Cholera is one of the more severe diarrhoeal diseases. Five million lives, mainly those of children, are lost each year through diarrhoea. Most of these deaths result from acute dehydration, and can be prevented by treatment with oral rehydration salts (ORS). In 1986 an estimated 59% of the population had access to ORS and it is estimated that this may have prevented some 700,000 diarrhoea-related deaths (UNEP 1991).

ACTIVITY

Study the extract from the WHO publication on cholera.

- What type of micro-organism causes cholera?
- How is it spread?
- What is meant by the terms *epidemic* and *endemic*?

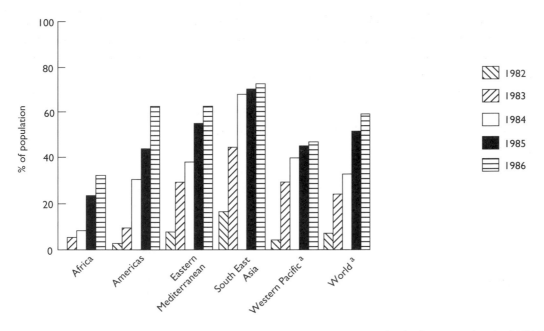

Figure 3.24 The proportion of world populations with access to oral rehydration salts, by WHO region, 1982–6
[a] excludes China.
Source: Martinez *et al.* 1988, 'Control of Diorrhoeal Diseases', *World Health Statistics Quarterly*, vol. 41, no. 2, pp. 74–81.

ACTIVITY

What can be concluded from Figure 3.24, which records the distribution of rehydration salts in 1982–86?

BACTERIAL FOOD POISONING

Serious diseases such as cholera, typhoid and dysentery may be caused by contaminated food or water. They have very specific symptoms, and a long incubation period. They are very dangerous, and can be described as food poisoning, but they are most commonly referred to by their names. The term 'food poisoning' is used to describe acute attacks of an explosive nature. Abdominal pain, diarrhoea and vomiting are associated with food poisoning episodes, and these symptoms usually arise between two and thirty-six hours after eating contaminated food.

Food poisoning bacteria divide very rapidly in conditions which are favourable to their growth. These include a warm temperature, humidity and a good food supply. Most bacteria usually require oxygen, but some can only multiply when oxygen is absent. These conditions are described as 'anaerobic'. The bacterium *Clostridium welchii* (*perfringens*) is a common cause of food poisoning. This is a bacterial organism which is the most common cause of *gas gangrene* (the breakdown of skin and muscle tissue by toxins and gas production). The organism is resistant to heat and may survive in pre-cooked foods, such as stews and pies, which are not correctly stored.

Some food poisoning bacteria produce heat-resistant spores. These form when conditions are unfavourable for growth. They survive heat treatment, then start to grow again when favourable conditions return. Some food poisoning organisms produce toxins, which can be very dangerous, for example *Clostridium botulinum*.

In order to investigate food poisoning, typhoid and cholera, carry out the class research exercise described overleaf.

ACTIVITY

Divide your class into five groups. Each group should investigate a different food poisoning organism(s) and will produce a display and a short presentation. Use the information provided and other sources obtained from the library or other centre.

Group 1   salmonella organisms
Group 2   *Staphylococci*
              Streptococci
Group 3   *Clostridium welchii (perfringens)*
Group 4   typhoid
              cholera
Group 5   listeria
              Bacillus cereus
              hepatitis A

You should consider the following aspects:

1   General characteristics of the organism. Different types.

2   Toxins produced? Spore-bearing?

3   How is the organism spread? Type of food involved?

4   What are the symptoms of the attack? How long do they take to appear? How long do they last?

5   Precautions and treatment.

6   Any other features of interest. How common? Recent outbreaks? Investigate these.

FOOD POISONING: CASE STUDIES

Study Table 3.1 and then read the following case studies. Answer the questions that relate to each case study.

Case Study 1: The steak and kidney pie

A person suffered from severe food poisoning for 24 hours, the symptoms arising 10 hours after eating a steak and kidney pie.

What organism caused the bout of illness?

Discuss the possible origin of the organism and factors which may have led to the contamination of the pie with enough bacteria to cause an infection.

Case Study 2: The duck egg mousse

Several people in a hotel suffered from food poisoning for a week after eating mousse made with duck eggs.

What was the likely cause of the illness?

Discuss factors which could have lead to the outbreak.

Table 3.1   Food poisoning organisms

Causative organism	Foods usually implicated	Incubation period	Duration of illness
Salmonella	Cooked meats, meat, poultry, eggs, warmed up meat pies, ice cream, shellfish	12–24 hours	1–8 days
Clostridium welchii (perfringens)	Joints and poultry reheated, large joints, gravy, stews, meat pies	8–18 hours	12–24 hours
Staphylococci	Custard, reheated meat, ice cream, poorly canned food	2–6 hours	6–24 days
Clostridium botulinum	Poorly processed food, meat paste, fish	24–72 hours	Death in 8 days, or a prolonged illness

Case Study 3: The shepherd's pie

An outbreak of food poisoning occurred among schoolchildren after eating shepherd's pie made in the school. A cook was later found to have a very septic finger.

What could have been the organism which caused the outbreak?

How could the bacteria have entered the pie?

Case Study 4: Scout camp

The following is an account of a food poisoning outbreak at a Scout camp.

Some meat pies were bought during the first day to be eaten that evening. By the next morning 21 of the 27 Scouts at the camp showed symptoms of headaches, fever, vomiting and abdominal pain. Many of these Scouts were ill for the first week of the camp.

Latrines were dug for sanitation but rain flooded them for several days. Water for the camp was obtained from a nearby stream. For the whole three-week period of the camp, there were always invalids suffering from the same symptoms as the first Scouts that were ill.

Identify the organism that caused the illness.

What conclusions can be drawn about the spread of the disease from one person to another from the evidence in the case history outlined above?

Why are meat pies more likely to cause food poisoning than lamb chops?

Case Study 5: School canteen

In a school canteen, large joints of beef (6–8 lb) were boiled for two hours in a large modern boiler. After removal from the boiler the joints remained covered in the kitchen overnight, left to cool down. This meat was served for lunch the next day (9–12 hours) later. Large numbers of children were subsequently ill with abdominal pain and diarrhoea. Some meat was left over; when tested it was found to contain the sporing bacterium *Clostridium welchii*.

Suggest how the meat became contaminated.

What factors in the treatment of the meat could have led to enough bacteria cells to cause an outbreak of food poisoning to be present in the meat?

Case Study 6: Salmonellosis from imitation cream

For many years, outbreaks of salmonellosis were traced to imitation cream. Yet when the cream arrived at the bakery in cans from the manufacturer it was quite clean and bacteriologically safe. All food in the bakery was tested and the only material found to be contaminated was imported bulk egg from China. This was found to contain salmonella organisms which were the same as those isolated from faeces of patients with salmonellosis. Yet this egg product was not used in the manufacture of imitation cream.

How do you account for the fact that the imitation cream contained salmonella?

Case Study 7: Typhoid outbreak – Aberdeen 1964

Over a three-week period, 400 people caught typhoid.

The investigation by the Public Health Inspector and his staff tracked down the origin of the outbreak as follows.

All typhoid sufferers had eaten cold cooked meat which had been purchased from the same small supermarket in Aberdeen. The investigation was hampered by the fact that typhoid has a two-week incubation period and that the sufferers had eaten two types of cold meat. There was not one type of meat which was immediately suspect. The origin of all cold meats was traced. Some corned beef from a certain cannery in the Argentine became suspect. This cannery had been traced as a source of contaminated ox-tongue which caused a smaller outbreak of typhoid in Britain in 1954. It was discovered then that the water from the river De La Plata was used for cooling cans of the tongue. The river had untreated sewage discharged into it and contained typhoid bacilli of the same type that caused the outbreak in Britain. It was postulated in 1954 that there must have been a tiny hole in the tongue can and that a few bacilli entered during the cooling process. After this event, the water was chlorinated before being used for cooling, but it was established that, in 1963, this chlorination plant had broken and again untreated water was used for cooling. So it was thought possible that the corned beef suspected of causing the 1964 outbreak in Aberdeen was canned during the period of using untreated water again. Typhoid bacilli caused no swelling of the can, no discolouration or bad odour, and no unfavourable taste.

However, this explanation did not account for the fact that not all typhoid sufferers had eaten corned beef. So, attention was turned to the hygiene of the supermarket. It was found that the can-opener, slicing machine, pedestals for window displays, price tickets and trays used for storage overnight were common to all cold meats. Although washing of these, and shelves, was carried out, no disinfectant was used and the clothes and scrubbing brushes were not thoroughly cleaned each day. So, for a matter of weeks, the typhoid organisms were lingering and were being spread around the shop. All cold meats became infected eventually, being contaminated by a single can of corned beef.

- Name two factors which hampered the investigation. Explain why.
- Why was the corned beef not immediately suspect?
- Why was it eventually suspect? Explain how experience of a previous typhoid outbreak contributed to an understanding of the 1964 outbreak.
- Draw a 'flow' diagram to show the passage of the typhoid bacillus from the river De La Plata to an Aberdeen resident.
- List four factors concerning the hygiene of the shop and show how they contributed to the outbreak.

FUNGI

Fungi are a third group of micro-organisms that can cause disease. However, unlike bacteria, they are far more likely to infect plants than animals, and few are human parasites.

ACTIVITY

Ringworm and athlete's foot are two common fungal skin infections. For each of these find out the symptoms, how it is treated and how it is spread. Suggest ways in which the spread can be prevented.

PROTOZOA

Protozoa are single-celled animals, some of which are parasitic. Many diseases are caused by these parasites, particularly in developing countries. The protozoan *Plasmodium*, which causes malaria, is probably responsible for more human deaths in the tropics than any other organism. It is estimated that about 100 million cases of malaria occur in the world each year (WHO 1987).

It has been estimated that in tropical Africa alone malaria accounts for approximately 750,000 deaths each year, mainly among young children. In some developing areas up to 5% of children under the age of five die from malaria each year (UNICEF 1986). In a number of areas the situation has been becoming worse since the late 1970s. This is largely due to the growing resistance of the mosquito vector to insecticides and of *Plasmodium* parasites to anti-malarial drugs.

Simplified life cycle of Plasmodium

When the *Plasmodium* first enters the human, it goes to the liver where it feeds and reproduces for about two weeks. During this time the person will start to feel ill, and there will be a rise in body temperature. A fever then develops as the parasite leaves the liver and enters the bloodstream. The fever subsides as each parasite enters a red blood cell. A few days later the fever returns as the red blood cells burst, releasing many more parasites, and their waste products, into the blood.

When the female mosquito feeds on the blood of an infected person, the protozoa enters her blood. The parasite undergoes sexual reproduction in the stomach of the mosquito, and the offspring make their way to the salivary glands. When the mosquito feeds again, the parasites are injected into the new host.

ACTIVITY

1 Draw a flow diagram to illustrate the life cycle of *Plasmodium* described in the text.

2 Can you suggest methods to help prevent malaria which could be used at different stages of the life cycle?

3 Find out what effect sickle-cell anaemia has on the susceptibility of the sufferer to malaria.

4 What other diseases are caused by protozoa?

5 What other parasites utilize an insect vector?

PLATYHELMINTHES

Two groups of platyhelminthes (flatworm) are parasitic: the tapeworms and the flukes.

The *pork tapeworm* and the organism that causes *bilharzia*, *Schistosoma*, are two well-known parasitic platyhelminthes. Their life cycles are shown in Figures 3.25 and 3.26.

ACTIVITY

1 Study the life cycles of the pork tapeworm and *Schistosoma* (Figures 3.25, 3.26). Suggest possible methods of disease control for each.

2 Bilharzia affects over a quarter of a million people in developing countries. It is often known as an *economic disease* as it makes people too weak to work. Can you find other examples of serious economic diseases?

NEMATODES

Nematodes are elongated, round 'worms' with pointed ends. They are found in very large numbers in a wide range of habitats. It is estimated that the 10,000 known species represent only about 2% of their full number.

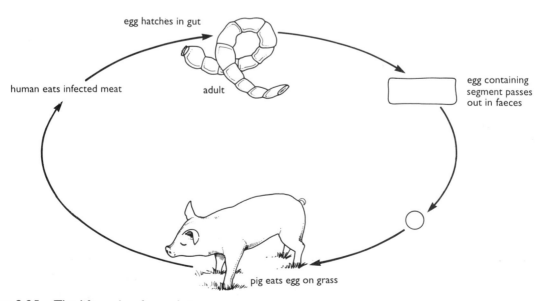

Figure 3.25 The life cycle of a pork tapeworm

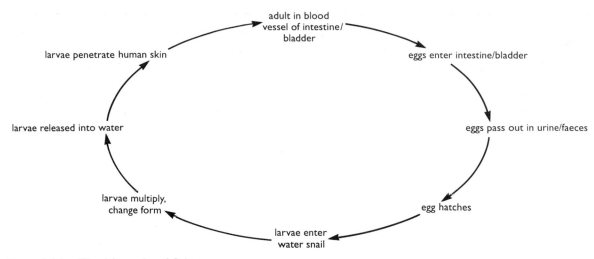

Figure 3.26   The life cycle of *Schistosoma*

Most are free-living, although the parasitic ones are the best known.

A well-known example of a disease caused by nematodes is *river blindness* or onchocerciasis. It is estimated that more than 17 million people are infected by this disease, mainly in west and central Africa. The severity of onchocerciasis is usually greatest in rural settlements located close to rapidly flowing rivers and streams which are the breeding sites of the blackfly, the vector of the disease.

Blindness rates as high as 10% have been reported in many endemic areas. Without sight, hundreds of thousands of people lose the ability to fend for themselves and die prematurely (see Figure 3.27).

In recent years, as a result of the control of the larvae of blackflies by the release of biodegradable insecticides into rivers, the disease has been eradicated in some areas. Remarkable achievements have also been achieved in the treatment of river blindness with drugs.

ACTIVITY

From Table 3.2, calculate the percentage of the total population:

(a)   at risk in onchocerciasis infected areas;
(b)   infected;
(c)   blind as a result of the disease.

NB: The figures in the table are likely to be an underestimate.

Table 3.2   Onchocerciasis morbidity: estimated number of persons at risk, infected and blind around 1983

Region	Total population (10^3)	Number at risk in onchocerciasis infected areas (10^3)	Number infected (10^3)	Number blind as a result of onchocerciasis (10^3)
Africa	293,750	78,273	17,121	366.6
Eastern Mediterranean (Sudan, Yemen)	26,590	2,060	540	8.4
Americas	265,850	5,251	97	1.4

Source: WHO 1987.

The bite spreads parasitic worms. They breed under your skin and produce hordes of microscopic worms called microfilariae which infest your body for years. You itch, you get skin problems, you become debilitated.

Then the microfilariae invade your eyes.

And you slowly become blind.

It's called River Blindness, "the disease at the end of the track". You'll find it in a host of fast-flowing rivers in West and Central Africa.

And there you will find most of the victims – the million or so who have already lost their sight and the seventeen million who have the symptoms and are at risk of blindness; their sight could be saved – quickly and easily.

The price of river blindness.

Consider what happens if you lose your sight in a poor African country. No disability benefit, no regular medical facilities, little prospect of remedial work.

There is just your family living at the harshest subsistence level. You

become a burden on them. You will need to be led from place to place. You can do little to contribute to their welfare.

For this is the particular agony of River Blindness. It takes years to gestate. When blindness strikes, you are likely to be in your thirties or forties. You are likely to be the family breadwinner. Without you, the family will lose their hard-won self-sufficiency and become dependent on the charity of neighbours.

And it is all avoidable.

THE BLACK SIMULIUM FLY

Ivermectin: it works, it's cheap, it's available.

Merck, Sharp and Dohme have developed a drug to halt River Blindness. It is a simple-to-take white tablet called ivermectin and it has been thoroughly tested in Africa. It not only prevents blindness but it tackles the painful symptoms as well. There are no serious side effects.

The manufacturers have generously agreed to supply ivermectin free. Sight Savers is committed to distributing it in Nigeria, Ghana, Mali, Uganda and Sierra Leone. We intend to expand the programme to include Guinea and Senegal.

If this sounds easy, it isn't. Sight Savers works worldwide and River Blindness is just one part of our work. So, a distribution programme on this scale will strain our resources to the utmost – we will need all the help we can get.

Then again, you have to allow for the reality of medical work in poor countries. In some of those countries there are village health workers or committees who we can train to distribute ivermectin. In others we are relying on nurses who go from village to village. We shall be very reliant on local people, village chiefs in particular, to guide much of this programme.

And there are transport problems. The dry flatlands of Mali make a 50cc motor cycle a reasonable means of travel; in the hilly, forest regions of Sierra Leone, we'll need a tougher 125cc machine. A lot of

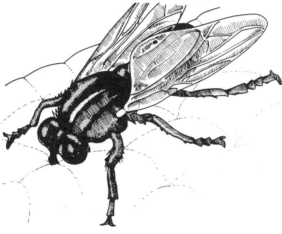

IT BITES YOU

ivermectin will be distributed by simple bicycle.

And the programme will go on for years. In each community at risk, ivermectin will have to be distributed annually for at least ten years to break the transmission cycle of the disease. Our aim worldwide is to ensure that, within twenty five years, nobody will lose their sight through River Blindness.

A massive campaign, then. But how can we look at that small white pill and at the terrifying statistics of River Blindness and at the harrowing stories of its effects... how can we know all these things and do nothing about it?

How much can you help us?

The whole world is full of claims on your generosity and the problems of the Third World will never go away in our lifetimes. But our River Blindness campaign is a hard-headed, practical and immediate chance to do something to prevent one evil once and for all.

It may help to think of your donation in very literal terms.

For it takes just £25 to protect twenty five people against River Blindness for a whole year.

£70 buys one of those bicycles for a medical assistant.

And £400 sponsors a training course for health workers.

But, whatever you can afford to send us, you will know of the scourge of River Blindness. There are not many things you can do that can achieve so much, so profoundly, so quickly.

Thank you for whatever you can do.

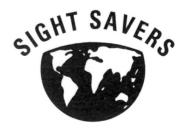

Sight Savers, FREEPOST,
Haywards Heath, West Sussex RH16 3ZA
Reg. Charity No. 207544

Figure 3.27   Advertisement publicizing treatment for river blindness
Source: Sight Savers.

Prevention of disease

Once the methods by which parasites spread have been understood, it is often possible to prevent disease. For example, *personal hygiene, food hygiene, clean water supply* and *efficient sewage disposal* are all important in the maintenance of a healthy population.

NATURAL DEFENCES AND IMMUNIZATION

The body's *natural defences* also play an important part in keeping the individual free from disease-causing organisms.

There are various mechanisms by which pathogens are prevented from entering the bloodstream:

- The *skin* has a dead, horny layer which is difficult for micro-organisms to penetrate.
- The cell layers which line the mouth, respiratory surfaces, alimentary canal and vagina contain antimicrobial enzymes and produce mucus to trap particles. In the respiratory tract, cilia can sweep these particles away.
- The *acid* in the stomach will kill many micro-organisms.
- If a wound occurs, *clotting* of the blood will help prevent the entry of micro-organisms.

If the mechanisms above fail and micro-organisms enter the bloodstream there are processes which may be able to eliminate the pathogens:

- phagocytosis (see earlier in this chapter)
- immune response

Immunity and vaccination

Earlier in this chapter the immune response (i.e. the production of antibodies in response to antigens) was described. This response can be artificially induced by VACCINATION. When the vaccine is introduced into the bloodstream, the antigens it contains stimulate the production of antibodies without causing the disease itself.

There are a number of different types of vaccine:

- *Living attenuated micro-organisms.* These are living pathogens which multiply, but they have been weakened, e.g. by heating, or by culturing them outside the human body, so that they are unable to cause the symptoms of the disease. Examples include the vaccines against measles, tuberculosis, poliomyelitis and rubella (German measles).
- *Dead micro-organisms.* Although harmless, they still induce antibody production. Examples include vaccines against typhoid, influenza and whooping cough.
- *Toxoids.* In some cases (e.g. diphtheria and tetanus) the toxin alone will cause antibody production. The toxin can be made harmless (e.g. with formaldehyde) and used as a vaccine.
- *Extracted antigens.* The antigens can be taken from the pathogens and used as a vaccine. For example, influenza vaccine can be prepared in this way.
- *Artificial antigens.* The genes responsible for antigen production in a pathogen can be transferred to a non-pathogen. This harmless organism can be grown in a fermenter where it will produce the antigen which can be harvested and used in a vaccine.

All the above methods produce what is known as *active* immunity because they cause the individual to synthesize his or her own antibodies. *Passive* immunity involves the acquisition or synthesis of antibodies. These can be acquired artificially. Antibodies from other mammals, e.g. horses, are injected in the form of a *serum*. For example, tetanus and diphtheria can be prevented in this way.

ACTIVITY

- Which type of immunity acts most immediately, active or passive?
- Which type of immunity would be the longest-lasting, active or passive?
- Suggest a situation in which passive immunization would be more useful than active immunization.

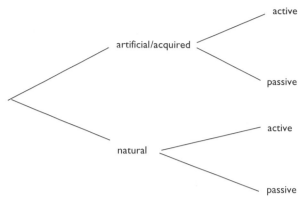

Figure 3.28 Summary of types of immunity

- These examples of active and passive immunity are *artificial* or *acquired*. The *natural* immunity described earlier in this chapter can also be *active* or *passive*. Natural active immunity is the synthesis of antibodies by an individual in response to antigens acquired by natural infection. In natural passive immunity the individual acquires antibodies. Where might these antibodies come from? (Clue: think about a baby.)

Immunization programmes

The progress made in the control and prevention of infectious diseases has been the result of a number of factors, including improvements in water supply and sanitation, personal hygiene and nutritional status. However, the development of vaccines and immunization programmes has been the most important factor in the prevention of many infectious diseases.

There is still a long way to go. Each year in developing countries almost four million children die and a similar number are permanently disabled from six of the most common childhood diseases: pertussis (whooping cough), diphtheria, measles, poliomyelitis, tuberculosis and tetanus. Of these deaths nearly two million are from measles, 800,000 from neonatal tetanus, 600,000 from pertussis and 30,000 from tuberculosis. It is estimated that 250,000 cases of poliomyelitis occur annually (UNEP 1990). There are effective vaccines against each of these diseases, but the immunization levels, although improving, are still not adequate in many parts of the world (see Figure 3.29).

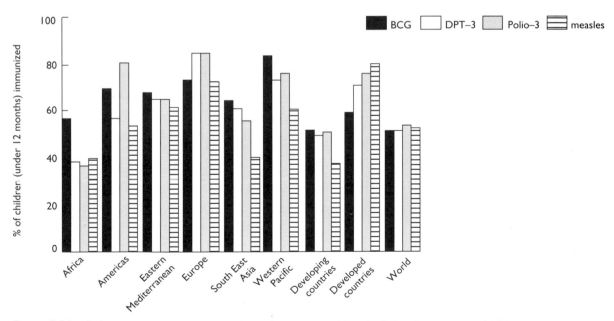

Figure 3.29 Immunization coverage, by WHO region and level of development, in 1987
BCG = vaccine for tuberculosis
DPT-3 = vaccine for diphtheria, pertussis and tetanus
Source: UNEP 1989, *Environmental Data Report 1989* (Blackwell, 1989).

In England, as in most countries, immunization coverage is continuing to rise (see Figure 3.30). The national target for childhood immunization is 90% and this has been reached for all infections except pertussis (whooping cough). It has been proposed that the targets should be increased to 95% by 1995.

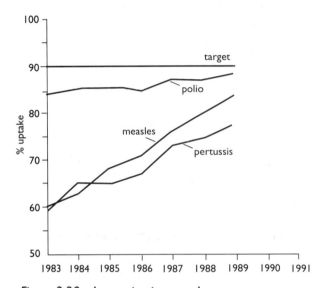

Figure 3.30   Immunization uptake rate, England, 1983–91
Source: Crown copyright. Reproduced with the permission of the Controller of Her Majesty's Stationery Office.

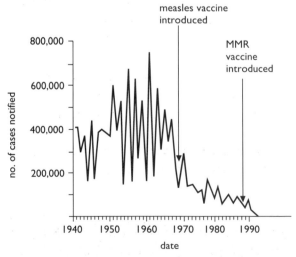

Figure 3.31   Notifications of measles, 1940–91
Source: Crown copyright. Reproduced with the permission of the Controller of Her Majesty's Stationery Office.

As the immunization uptake rate has increased, a corresponding fall in the relevant diseases has occurred. For example, in 1991 the lowest annual number of measles cases was reported since records began (see Figure 3.31). In October 1988 the MMR (mumps, measles and rubella) vaccine was introduced. Since then the number of cases of rubella has dropped, both for children and for pregnant women. There has been a corresponding drop in rubella-associated terminations of pregnancy and cases of congenital rubella.

The number of notifications of mumps has fallen to even lower levels than those for measles and rubella. It is likely that mumps will shortly disappear as a result of the very high uptake of MMR vaccine.

ACTIVITY

1   How does rubella harm the developing foetus?

2   Role play the following situation. In advance gather together and prepare appropriate materials to help you.

You are a health visitor in an antenatal clinic. A mother with a three-week-old baby comes to you for vaccination advice. Explain what the likely immunization schedule will be for her child. She tells you that she has heard that vaccines contain viruses and so is worried that they may endanger her baby. Spend about ten minutes responding to this, using simple visual aids to help you with your explanation.

3   Give an oral, visual or written presentation of an investigation into one named pathogen for which a vaccine is available. Your investigation should include the effect of the pathogen on the body, and the body's response. Investigate the effectiveness of the vaccine through the analysis of statistics, either globally or in one country.

CLEAN WATER

Often the answer to prevention of disease is the provision of a clean water supply to a community.

The first step in this process is the treatment of sewage.

The treatment of water by chlorination before it is taken to homes is a precaution against bacterial contamination.

ACTIVITY

1 Find out how a sewage-treatment works functions. Discover and explain the role of the following processes in sewage treatment:

- initial screens and disintegrator;
- grit tanks;
- sedimentation tank;
- biological filters;
- humus settling tanks.

Sometimes an 'activated sludge' process is employed. How does this work?

Draw a flow diagram to illustrate sewage treatment.

Visit your local sewage-treatment works if possible.

2 Water is treated before it is piped out to homes. Find out how it is purified. Consider the following processes, and draw a flow diagram to illustrate them:

- primary grid;
- settling reservoir;
- filter beds (primary and secondary);
- chlorination plant;
- pumping house.

3 Find out about water-borne diseases. Which of these have been eradicated in the UK by the treatment of sewage and the provision of a clean water supply? Which are still prevalent in other parts of the world?

Treatment of disease

Chemotherapy is the treatment of diseases with drugs. Chemotherapeutic substances are toxic to pathogenic microbes, but non-toxic to the host. Some chemotherapeutic substances are NARROW SPECTRUM, and affect only a few pathogens, whereas others are BROAD SPECTRUM, and attack a wider range.

The ways in which they are effective are as follows:

- inhibition of DNA synthesis, e.g. sulphonamides;
- inhibition of cell wall synthesis, e.g. penicillin;
- lysis of cell membranes, e.g. nystatin;
- inhibition of protein synthesis, e.g. streptomycin, chloramphenicol and tetracyclines.

Common chemotherapeutic drugs are:

- *Penicillin.* Broad spectrum and effective against most bacteria. Staphylococci are resistant to penicillin and erythromycin is used against these.
- *Cephalosporins.* Broad spectrum and used as an alternative to penicillin if resistance is encountered.
- *Chloramphenicol.* Used in the treatment of meningitis and typhoid.
- *Griseofulvin and Nystatin.* Used to treat fungal infections, the former for ringworm and athlete's foot, and the latter for oral and vaginal thrush.
- *Streptomycin.* A broad spectrum antibiotic used mainly to treat tuberculosis.
- *Tetracyclines.* Broad spectrum, used in the treatment of gonorrhoea.
- *Sulphonamides.* Used for treating infections of the urinary tract. Also useful in treating malaria.

ACTIVITY

Choose a common disease and then explain the basic principles relevant to its prevention. Refer to Chapter 4 and then investigate the socioeconomic factors (for example, level of wealth, housing, expenditure, diet) that affect the pattern of the disease.

THE COMPONENTS OF A HEALTHY DIET

Nutrients

The following elements (macronutrients) are important in the diet:

- proteins
- carbohydrates
- fats

Water is also required, as well as fibre and micronutrients.

PROTEINS

Proteins contain carbon, hydrogen and oxygen as well as nitrogen and sometimes sulphur. They are made up of AMINO ACIDS, ten of which cannot be made in the body and are therefore essential in the diet. There is a total of about 23 different amino acids. They are joined into peptide links which are broken down during digestion (see Figure 3.32). Polypeptides form proteins, which can contain hundreds of amino acids.

Table 3.8 on page 114 shows the protein content of many common foods. Proteins have many important functions and are major components in the structure of enzymes, haemoglobin and cell membranes.

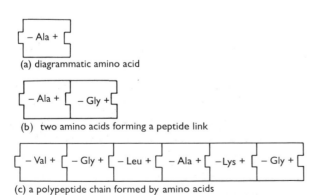

(a) diagrammatic amino acid

(b) two amino acids forming a peptide link

(c) a polypeptide chain formed by amino acids

(d) polypeptides form proteins, which have hundreds of amino acids

Figure 3.32   The formation of proteins

CARBOHYDRATES

Carbohydrates are the simplest carbon compounds, with a formula of $C_nN_{2n}O_n$. Their basic building molecule is a simple sugar or monosaccharide. This can be built up into more complex compounds:

- disaccharides – two monosaccharides, e.g. maltose and sucrose;
- polysaccharides – many monosaccharides, e.g. starch and glycogen.

Plants manufacture glucose, a mono-saccharide, in photosynthesis. The glucose is built up into more complex molecules; storage materials like sucrose and starch are synthesized. These substances are present in large quantities in:

- cereal crops – wheat, oats, maize;
- ground crops – potatoes, yams, carrots, turnips;
- Leguminous crops – beans, peas.

Carbohydrates are a primary source of energy.

FATS

Fats (lipids) contain carbon, hydrogen and oxygen. The proportion of oxygen to the other elements is very low. LIPIDS is the correct term to use for this group of compounds, although in dietary terms they are often called fats.

Plants tend to have liquid fats (oils) which contain mainly unsaturated fatty acids. Animal fats are solid at room temperature and contain mainly saturated fatty acids. There is thought to be a link between consumption of saturated fatty acids and cardiovascular disorder.

The terms SATURATED and UNSATURATED relate to the structure of the fatty acids which make up the fats. A typical unsaturated fatty acid is oleic acid. A typical saturated fatty acid is palmitic acid or stearic acid. Some fatty acids are essential in the diet since they cannot be synthesized in the body.

Fats are a secondary energy source in the diet. Sources of fat-containing foods will be found in Table 3.8 on page 114.

FIBRE (ROUGHAGE)

The diet should contain fibre as well as the food materials discussed above. Fibre consists of the various types of cellulose that are found in plant foods. Cellulose cannot be broken down in the intestinal tract since humans do not possess the enzyme that can carry out the breakdown. Cellulose therefore remains undigested and is eliminated in the faeces. Research strongly indicates that a diet low in fibre is linked to diseases of the bowel.

There are various theories put forward to account for this possibility. Some researchers think that cancer of the bowel is caused by fewer eliminations of faeces associated with a low-fibre diet. The cells of the bowel would be in contact with carcinogens in the food for a longer period. Other researchers think that a diet high in fibre decreases the pressure on the bowel wall, and it is this which helps to prevent bowel disease. A slow-moving bowel, because of lack of fibre, allows more water to be reabsorbed from the faeces and this causes constipation.

ACTIVITY

Read the section on 'Fibre' and answer the following questions:

- What is fibre?
- Why is it not digested?
- What can happen to people on low-fibre diets?
- What theories are there to explain the link between bowel disease and a low-fibre diet?
- Why is more water absorbed from faeces formed from a low-fibre diet?

MICRONUTRIENTS AND DEFICIENCY DISEASES

Vitamins

Vitamins are essential in small amounts in the diet. If they are missing from the diet illnesses develop. These are called vitamin deficiency diseases.

- *Vitamin A.* Keeps skin and bones healthy, helps prevent infection of the nose and throat, and is necessary for vision in dim light. Lack of Vitamin A causes poor night vision and increases the chances of infection of the nose and throat. Vitamin A is found in carrots, fish liver oils and green vegetables.
- *Vitamin B1.* Helps the body obtain energy from food. Lack of it reduces growth and causes beri-beri, when the limbs become paralysed. Vitamin B1 is found in yeast, wholemeal bread, nuts, peas and beans.
- *Vitamin B2.* Enables the body to obtain energy from food. Lack of it causes stunted growth, cracks in the skin around the mouth, an inflamed tongue, and damage to the cornea of the eye. Vitamin B2 is found in green vegetables, cheese, yeast, eggs, milk and liver.
- *Vitamin B12.* Enables the body to form protein and fat and to store carbohydrate. Lack of it causes pernicious anaemia, a disease in which haemoglobin is not produced for red blood cells. This vitamin is found in liver, meat, eggs, milk and fish.
- *Vitamin C.* Helps to heal wounds and is needed for healthy gums and teeth. A lack of it causes scurvy, a disease where gums become soft and the teeth loose, and wounds fail to heal properly. Vitamin C is found in oranges, lemons, blackcurrants, green vegetables, tomatoes and potatoes. It is destroyed by cooking food.
- *Vitamin D.* Enables the body to absorb calcium and phosphorus from food. These are needed to make bones and teeth. Lack of Vitamin D causes rickets, leading to soft bones, which bend under pressure. It is found in liver, butter, cheese, eggs and fish.
- *Vitamin K.* Needed for blood to clot in wounds. Lack of it causes haemorrhage when the skin is broken. It is found in cabbage and cereals, and is made by bacteria in the digestive system.

ACTIVITY

Experiment to investigate levels of Vitamin C in fruit juices

Collect five different fruit juices. Prepare six test tubes and a standard solution of Vitamin C which has a concentration of 1 mg Vitamin C/100 cm^3 water. Add 5 cm^3 of dichlorophenolindophenol (DCPIP) to each of the six test tubes. Add the standard solution of Vitamin C to the DCPIP in one test tube drop by drop from a syringe. Record how many drops it takes to cause the blue colour to disappear. Shake the test tube after the addition of each drop. Repeat for each of the fruit juices.

- Record all the results in a table.
- Calculate how much Vitamin C there is in each fruit juice by comparing the results for each juice with the standard Vitamin C solution.
- Comment on the conclusions that you draw from your experiment.
- Evaluate your experiment and comment on further investigations that could follow. Do your findings agree with the claims about Vitamin C content on the fruit juice containers?

Minerals

We need 15 minerals in our diets. Most of these are supplied by meat, eggs, milk, vegetables and fruit.

The following are some of these minerals:

	Daily requirement (mg)
Sodium chloride	5–10
Potassium	2
Magnesium	0.3
Phosphorus	1.5
Calcium	0.8
Iron	0.01
Iodine	0.00003

ACTIVITY

- What other minerals are required in the diet in addition to those listed in the text?
- Find out the functions of each of these minerals in the body.
- Find out what deficiency diseases are caused by a lack of each mineral in the diet.

Energy intake

Table 3.3 shows the different amounts of energy required throughout life, and in different occupations. Age, gender, occupation, pregnancy, and body weight all affect the amount of energy intake required.

A BALANCED BREAKFAST

ACTIVITY

Look at Table 3.4 and use the data to answer the following questions.

- Work out the total energy value of Breakfast A and Breakfast B.

Breakfast A	*Breakfast B*
Boiled egg (60 g)	Orange juice (100 g)
1 slice of toast (60 g)	Wholegrain cereal (30 g)
with butter (5 g)	with milk (100 g)
and marmalade (10 g)	and sugar (10 g)
Cup of tea (160 g)	Grilled bacon (30 g)
with milk (50 g)	Sausage (50 g)
	One slice of toast (60 g)

- Which breakfast forms a more balanced meal? Give two reasons for your answer. (You will need to refer to the section on 'Diet' later in this chapter.)

Table 3.3   Energy required daily and notes on diet

	Energy used in 1 day (kJ)*	Diet
Birth to one year		At least 2 g of protein are needed per kg of body weight from 0–6 months and 1.6 g per kg from 6–9 months, gradually reducing to 1 g per kg. Weaning usually begins at about 4 months
0–3 months	2,300	
3–6 months	3,200	
6–9 months	3,800	
9–12 months	4,200	
8 years (both sexes, active children)	8,800	At least 30 g of protein a day but 53 g are recommended
14–18 years		80–100 g of protein per day and 60% of this should be first-class protein
Males	12,600	
Females	9,600	About 300 g of carbohydrate per day except for those doing heavy work who should eat far more
Adult (light work)		
Males	11,550	Sugar should not be eaten in large quantities as it increases tooth decay
Females	9,450	
Adult (moderate work)		About 100 g of fat should be eaten per day
Males	12,100	
Females	10,500	
Adult (heavy work)		
Males	15,000–20,000	
Females	12,600	
Pregnant women	10,000	Pregnant women should eat about 85 g of protein per day increasing to 100 g during breast feeding, together with increased amounts of food containing calcium, iron, and all-vitamins
Nursing mothers	11,300	

*Books and magazines commonly use *calories* as the unit of measurement of energy, meaning kilocalories. 1 kC = 4.18 kJ.
Source: DHSS.

Table 3.4   Energy values and composition of foods

Food	Energy value (kJ per g)	Protein (g)	Fat (g)	Carbohydrate (g)
Bacon	18.5	0.24	0.38	0
Bread	10.0	0.07	0.01	0.4
Butter	30.5	0	0.85	0
Egg	6.0	0.12	0.11	0
Marmalade	11.0	0.001	0	0.7
Milk	2.5	0.03	0.04	0.47
Orange Juice	1.5	0.004	0	0.08
Sausage	15.0	0.11	0.24	0.11
Sugar	17.0	0	0	1.05
Tea	0	0	0	0
Wholegrain cereal	16.0	0.08	0.01	0.85

AN INDIVIDUAL DAILY DIET

ACTIVITY

Study Table 3.5 overleaf and use the data to answer the following questions:

- Given that 1 g carbohydrate yields 16 kJ energy and that 1 g fat yields 37 kJ energy, calculate the amount of energy that is provided in this diet by (a) fat and (b) carbohydrate.
- Comment on the relative contributions made by fat and carbohydrate to the doctor's daily energy requirement.
- Is this a balanced diet? Give reasons for your answer.
- Serena is overweight and decides to go on a diet by cutting out one meal. Which one should this be? Give reasons for your choice.

Table 3.5   The daily diet of Serena, a doctor

	Energy (kJ)	Protein (g)	Fat (g)	Carbo-hydrate (g)	Calcium (mg)	Iron (mg)	Vitamin A (mg)	Vitamin B complex (mg)	Vitamin C (mg)	Vitamin D (mg)
Breakfast	1,903	11.4	13.6	75.0	278	1.6	145	7.95	43.9	0.18
Snack	166	2.2	2.2	2.9	72	0.1	22	1.42	0.8	0.04
Lunch	3,049	25.0	46.1	57.5	310	4.2	525	9.86	13.6	3.34
Tea	979	5.0	8.9	35.3	112	0.9	57	2.21	2.3	0.07
Supper	3,332	40.2	38.6	76.6	221	3.3	2,349	18.52	30.8	0.49
Total dietary intake	9,429	83.8	109.4	247.3	993	10.1	3,098	39.96	91.4	4.12
Recommended intake	9,200	55.0	–	–	500	12.0	750	17.2	30.0	2.50

Table 3.6   Daily dietary energy allowances for boys and girls

	Age (years)	Mean body mass (kg)	kJ per day	Daily kJ/kg body mass
Boys	2	12	5,460	455
	5	18	7,120	393
	8	27	8,820	329
	11	36	10,500	288
	14	49	13,020	263
	17	63	15,120	238
Girls	2	12	5,460	455
	5	18	7,120	393
	8	27	8.820	329
	11	36	10,500	288
	14	49	10,720	222
	17	54	10,080	184

FOOD AND ENERGY REQUIREMENTS FOR DIFFERENT ACTIVITIES

Different activities use different amounts of energy. The following list gives examples of how much energy is used in one hour.

sleeping	200 kJ
sitting	300 kJ
light work, e.g. mending bike, housework	600 kJ
moderate work, e.g. woodwork	880 kJ
walking	1,000 kJ
cycling	1,600 kJ
swimming	1,800 kJ
energetic sports, e.g. hockey	2,200 kJ

DAILY ENERGY INTAKE FOR BOYS AND GIRLS

ACTIVITY

Using the data in Table 3.6:

- Draw graphs to show the relationship between the recommended daily kJ/kg of body mass and age for boys and girls.
- Suggest two reasons why 17-year-old girls require less energy per kg of body weight than boys.
- Express in words the relationship between 'mean body mass' and 'daily kJ' required per 'kg body mass' as boys and girls get older.

ACTIVITY

1 How does your body use energy when you are asleep?

2 Ranjit is 16 years old. He cycles to college, likes playing hockey and has a paper round. The following is a list of his activities for a typical day:

Sleeps 10 hours; sits at home 4 hours; sits at college 4 hours; household jobs 1 hour; woodwork 2 hours; walking 2 hours; cycling 0.5 hour; swimming 0.5 hour; hockey 0.5 hour.

Tabulate these activities together with energy used in each. What is his energy expenditure in 24 hours?

ENERGY USED BY A RANGE OF DIFFERENT INDIVIDUALS

Table 3.7   Energy used by children and adults

Age (yrs)	Energy used per day (kJ) David	Alison
2	5,500	5,500
5	7,000	7,000
8	8,800	8,800
11	10,000	9,200
14	12,500	10,500
18	14,200	9,600
25	12,100	8,800

A man weighing 70 kg uses the following amounts of energy in a day, depending on lifestyle/occupation:

Invalid	7,000 kJ
Senior citizen	9,000 kJ
Office worker	10,500 kJ
Factory worker	12,500 kJ
Coal miner	15,000 kJ

ACTIVITY

1 Explain why the different types of men listed above use up different amounts of energy.

2 Explain why some men in the same job use up different amounts of energy.

3 Using the information in Table 3.7, draw a line graph showing the energy used by David from birth to age 25. On the same graph draw a line to show Alison's energy use in the same way.

Use the graph you have drawn to answer the following questions:

- When does David use *most* energy in his life?
- When does Alison use *most* energy in her life?
- Between which ages did Alison and David use the same amount of energy?

4 Explain why:

- Alison and David used more energy as teenagers than as adults.
- David used up most energy per day at 18 whereas Alison did so at 14.
- David used up more than twice as much energy at 14 than when he was 2.

Diet

The components of a balanced diet are shown in Figure 3.33.

A balanced meal consists of about one part protein, one part fat and four or five parts carbohydrate. It should include mineral- and vitamin-rich foods.

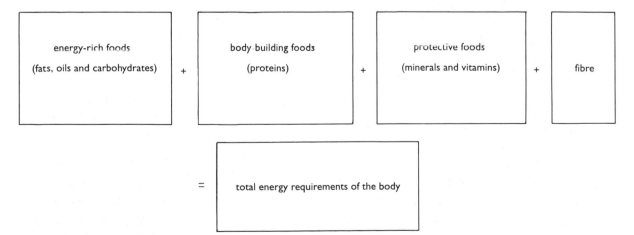

Figure 3.33   The components of a balanced diet

Normally 50–60% of protein would come from meat, and the rest from vegetable sources. In vegetarian diets a wide range of vegetables should be eaten to ensure that all essential amino acids are included.

A small amount of fat is required to supply the fat-soluble vitamins A, D and E and essential fatty acids. Fat can supply energy needs, but too much fat in the diet can cause atherosclerosis of the blood vessels.

Table 3.8 Composition of food per 100 g (percentage not accounted for is inedible waste, e.g. shell, bone, skin, water, etc.)

Type of food	kJ	Proteins (g)	Fats (g)	Carbohydrates (g)
Meat				
Bacon, grilled	1,852	24.5	38.8	0
Beef, roast	932	30.9	11.0	0
Chicken, roast	621	24.8	5.4	0
Liver, fried	1,020	24.9	13.7	5.6
Luncheon meat	1,298	12.6	26.9	5.5
Pork chop, grilled	1,380	28.5	24.2	0
Sausage, beef	1,242	9.6	24.1	11.7
Dairy produce				
Butter	3,006	0.5	81.0	0
Cheese	1,708	25.4	34.5	0
Eggs, raw, one	612	12.3	10.9	0
Ice-cream	805	4.1	11.3	19.8
Milk, liquid whole	274	3.3	3.8	4.8
Yoghurt, fruit	410	4.8	1.0	18.2
Fish				
Cod, fried in batter	834	19.6	10.3	7.5
Kipper	770	19.8	11.7	0
Sardines, canned	906	23.7	13.6	0
Cereals				
Bread, white	1,068	8.0	1.7	54.3
Bread, wholemeal	1,025	9.6	3.1	46.7
Rice, steamed	1,531	6.2	1.0	86.8
Vegetables				
Beans, canned	266	5.1	0.4	10.3
Brussel sprouts, cooked	75	2.8	0	1.7
Cabbage, cooked	66	1.7	0	2.3
Carrots, cooked	98	0.7	0	5.4
Lettuce	36	1.0	0	1.2
Peas, cooked	208	5.0	0	7.7
Potatoes, boiled	339	1.4	0	19.7
Potato chips, fried	1,028	3.8	9.0	37.3
Tomatoes	52	0.8	0	2.4
Fruit				
Apples	197	0.3	0	12.0
Bananas	326	1.1	0	19.2
Oranges, peeled	150	0.8	0	8.5
Plums	137	0.6	0	7.9
Strawberries	109	0.6	0	6.2
Miscellaneous				
Apple pie	1,179	3.2	14.4	40.4
Buns, currant	1,385	7.8	8.5	58.6
Coffee, white, 1 cup	84	0	0.5	0.5
Fruit cake, rich	1,546	4.6	15.9	55.0
Rice pudding	594	3.6	7.6	15.7
Sugar, white	1,654	0	0	100.0
Tea with milk, 1 cup	84	0	0.5	0.5

Source: Ministry of Agriculture, Fisheries and Food (1976).

ACTIVITY

Record your own diet for a week. Is it a balanced diet?

Use the information in Table 3.8 and elsewhere in this chapter to decide.

It is quite difficult to work out the actual mass of what you eat. You could weigh a few sample servings of food. Or you may have a computer program to help you.

ACTIVITY

This activity is designed to help you identify the nutrient content of common foods. Use the information in Table 3.8 and the section of the text on micronutrients.

carbohydrates (A)
fats (B)
proteins (C)
vitamin and minerals (D)
} Nutrients

Copy the following list of foods and add any others that you eat. Put letters A, B, C and D by each food as appropriate to indicate the nutrient content.

chocolate
baked potato
fried potato
rice
brown bread and butter
white bread and butter
fried cod
beans
apples
pork
cheese
orange juice

raw egg
egg, lettuce and tomato salad
fried bacon and egg
milk
fried fish, chips and peas
cod liver oil
roast chicken

CULTURAL FACTORS AFFECTING DIET

Hindu

Orthodox Hindus will be vegetarian and beef is especially strongly prohibited. Milk and its products may be eaten, but fish and eggs are rarely eaten.

Moslem

No pork or any pig products may be eaten. The only meat permitted is that from cloven-hooved animals that chew the cud and it must be *halal*, i.e. ritually slaughtered. Only fish that have fins and scales may be eaten; shellfish and eels are therefore forbidden. Dairy products and cheese are permitted, but this must be vegetarian cheese made without rennet.

Moslems may find kosher meals acceptable if these are available. They may be wary of many foods in case they contain pork or other animal products which may not be *halal*. Alcohol is forbidden.

Sikh

Many Sikhs, particularly women, will be vegetarian. Beef will be strictly forbidden. Any meat has to be ritually slaughtered.

Jewish

All pork and pig products are forbidden, as are fish without fins or scales. Only animals which have cloven hooves and chew the cud and have been ritually slaughtered may be eaten. Meat and milk dishes are never mixed within the same meal. Food must be prepared in a special way so that it is kosher ('fit') according to Jewish law.

Rastafarian

Some Rastafarians are vegan or vegetarian. The diet will often be called I-tal. Products of the vine, such as wine, currants, grapes are forbidden by some Rastafarians. Food must only be cooked in vegetable oil. (Rastafarians want food to be pure and prefer whole foods to processed foods.) For strict Rastafarians, diet is of the utmost importance.

The techniques of western medicine may be treated with suspicion as the movement advocates herbal and natural medicines.

Alcohol is forbidden.

SPECIAL DIETS

Sometimes a special diet is needed for a particular purpose, such as controlling weight, or a disease. You could do a project on special diets.

Two articles on diet are included at the end of this chapter to provide information: one is about a special diet to help control diabetes, and one is about low-cholesterol diets to help people with cardiovascular problems.

ACTIVITY

Research and compile diets of the following types:

- weight-controlling
- vegetarian
- vegan
- diabetic
- low-cholesterol
- low-salt

SOCIOECONOMIC FACTORS THAT AFFECT DIET

ACTIVITY

1 Go round a supermarket and find out how much it would cost to feed a family of four on a healthy diet for a week. Using half this amount, go round the

supermarket again. How would you feed this family on this amount?

Relate your findings to research that you could do to find out about dietary deficiencies in Britain today.

2 Read the article 'Food, Diet and Health' at the end of this chapter to give you a worldwide perspective on the relationship between poverty and disease. Choose one aspect and investigate it further.

EXTRACT 1: THE FACTS ON DIABETES

Diabetes mellitus, a growing public health concern worldwide, is quite common in the United Kingdom. Today, up to 2% of the population is affected, and the problem is increasing. The following information, extracted and adapted from literature provided by the British Diabetic Association, offers an overview of the disease, its symptoms, causes and treatments.

What is diabetes?

Diabetes is a disorder in which the body is unable to control the amount of sugar in the blood, because the mechanism which converts sugar to energy is no longer functioning properly. This leads to an abnormally high level of sugar in the blood, which gives rise to a variety of symptoms initially. If uncontrolled over several years, it may damage various tissues of the body. Therefore the treatment of diabetes is designed not only to reverse symptoms which manifest themselves at the beginning, but also to prevent any serious problems from developing later.

Some healthy eating tips

- Eat more wholemeal or high fibre bread, wholegrain breakfast cereals (or those which contain bran or oats), brown rice, wholemeal pasta, fruit and vegetables.
- Use wholemeal or whole-wheat flour for

baking, or try half wholemeal and half white flour.
- Try to include more peas, beans and lentils in your diet. In many meals you can replace some of the meat with beans. This is less expensive and very nutritious.
- Use skimmed or semi-skimmed milk instead of whole milk in cooking, on cereals and in drinks.
- Use low-fat spread or no spread instead of butter or margarine.
- Use cheese sparingly or look for the low-fat varieties.
- Try saving cream for special occasions and use low-fat yogurt as a routine.
- Try to limit pies, cakes and pastries as they tend to be high in fat.
- Choose low calorie soft drinks, e.g. low calorie squash.
- Choose fish, poultry (remove the skin) and lean cuts of meat.
- Buy fruit tinned in natural juice rather than in syrup.
- Try halving the sugar you use in recipes.
- Use reduced sugar or pure fruit spreads, jams and marmalades.
- Try using an intense sweetener such as saccharin or aspartame if you normally sugar your drinks or cereals.
- Try diet yogurts which have a lower sugar content than normal low-fat yogurts.
- Don't put salt on the table.
- Cut down on snacks and convenience foods with high salt content.
- Cut down on salted meats and fish such as bacon, gammon and mackerel.

Source: British Diabetic Association.

EXTRACT 2: CHOLESTEROL: THE 'VILLAIN' REVISITED

Cholesterol has been high on the list of dietary villains for years. Indicated as a serious contributor to the development of coronary heart disease – the leading cause of death in the UK – cholesterol's strong presence in the national diet has spurred widespread education efforts aimed at limiting the public's intake of harmful fats.

But a new wave of research, some of it highly controversial, is focusing some of the blame elsewhere. According to recent studies, the problem may not lie with the cholesterol itself, but the way in which it reacts with oxygen (or oxidizes) in the bloodstream. In other words, high cholesterol alone is not the problem, high oxidation of cholesterol is.

When there are enough antioxidants circulating in the blood, cholesterol is prevented from oxidizing. Without enough, the opposite is true. And then the damage to arteries begins.

The process involves the macrophage, an immune cell that serves as a kind of micro-scopic vacuum cleaner in the bloodstream. Globules of fatty, oxidized cholesterol are devoured by roaming microphages. But because the oxidized cholesterol is so fat and greasy, macrophages become bloated and end up lodged in the walls of the arteries, roughing them up and impeding the passage of blood. This is the beginning of atherosclerotic plaque – a direct precursor of heart disease.

Because this cholesterol-laden plaque was always found in the arteries of people who had died from coronary heart disease, researchers naturally assumed that cholesterol was the main causative factor.

If what many researchers around the world are beginning to believe is true, then it could be possible to develop a method of introducing high-impact natural antioxidants into the diets of people who are under significant oxidative stress – for instance, the elderly, smokers and athletes – and thus help them combat cholesterol's transformation into atherosclerotic plaque.

To guard against oxidized cholesterol: an antioxidant shopping list (selected foods)

Vitamin C

peppers, red/green	grapefruit*	Brussels sprouts
strawberries	oranges*	broccoli
lemons	blackcurrant*	cabbage
tangerines	raspberries	cauliflower

*natural juice or whole fruit

Vitamin E

wheat germ	soya beans	hazelnuts
oatmeal	chick peas	sunflower seeds
rye flour	olives	peanuts
muesli	almonds	margarine

Carotenoids

carrots	tomatoes	broccoli
apricots	cabbage	leeks
mango	spinach	peas
cantaloupe melon	green beans	courgettes

Mixed antioxidants

curry powders: chilli powder, paprika

herbs: parsley, mint, sage, rosemary, oregano, thyme

spices: nutmeg, cloves, pepper

wheat bran, sesame, rice, green tea, wine

Source: Nestlé Dietetic Information Services, UK.

EXTRACT 3: FOOD, DIET, AND HEALTH

The existence of hunger and malnutrition and the persistence of diseases for which medical science has found the cure reveal the inequalities in the modern world. While food supplies are sufficient to meet the world's aggregate minimum requirements, they are so inequitably distributed among the different countries and among the people of each country because of income disparities that the lives of hundreds of millions are affected.

Interactions between nutrition and infec-tion to produce the 'malnutrition/infection complex' create the greatest public health problem in the world. Infection influences nutritional status through its effects on the intake, absorption, and utilization of nutrients and in some cases on the body's requirement for them. A child's rate of growth may be retarded by too little food and/or too many infections or parasites. Malnutrition may result in lowered immunity. Infection can lead to loss of appetite, decreased efficiency of food and nutrient utilization, increased energy requirements, and decreased growth. The relationship between diarrhoeal diseases and physical growth has been clearly shown. These interrelationships produce the malnutrition and infection cycle so prevalent in many developing countries. The vulnerability of malnourished people to environmental health risks has been widely documented. Hence the importance of improved water supplies, sanitation, and safe food to reduce water-related and foodborne diseases and of programmes to control disease vectors supported by education and health care.

It is now widely accepted that chronic hunger is due more to lack of purchasing power or of land on which to produce food than to the non-availability of food. Alleviation of poverty is at the forefront of the development agenda, but waiting for its decline to alleviate malnutrition may take decades. The results of poverty – hunger, sickness, debility, early death – are centred on nutrition. Malnutrition results, and preventing malnutrition is an aim that can be monitored.

Nutrient deficiency diseases
Iodine
Goitre and cretinism are clinically obvious and easily recognizable forms of this deficiency. But the more pervasive effects of milder deficiency on the survival and physical and mental development of children and the intellectual ability and work capacity of adults are now being recognized. About 1,000 million people are affected in more than 80 countries; the Andes, Alps, Great Lakes basin of North America, and Himalayas are particularly iodine-deficient areas, but coastal areas and plains may also be deficient. Excessive intake of goitrogens (for example through eating cassava) interferes with the normal intake and metabolism of iodine and may amplify the effects of iodine deficiency.

Vitamin A
Vitamin A deficiency, leading to xerophthalmia and sometimes blindness, continues to be a widespread problem among children. This deficiency also decreases resistance to infections and thus increases mortality. Analyses of food supplies from different regions show that the availability of vitamin A is limited and the problem exacerbated by any tendency to withhold vegetables from children for cultural or other reasons. The problem is most pronounced in Asia because the overall availability of vitamin A is less than that required and any maldistribution of foods high in vitamin A within a population worsens the problem. Xerophthalmia continues to be a major problem in about 40 countries.

Iron
Anaemia, whose dominant cause is iron deficiency, remains a major problem. Estimates made in 1980 suggest that it affects close to 200 million children between 0 and 4 years of age, 217 million between 5 and 12 years, 174 million men, and 288 million women (including 54 million pregnant women). Most are in Southern Asia, although the proportion of those affected is high in Africa; in both these regions half or more of all children in both age groups and close to half of all women are affected. More than three-fifths of all pregnant women are affected in these two regions. Anaemia also affects significant proportions in each of the above groups in other developing countries. In many areas of the tropics or subtropics, dietary iron deficiency due to low intake and/or poor absorption may be complicated by hookworm infection, which causes intestinal blood loss and may lead to profound iron deficiency anaemia.

Others
Fluoride deficiency increases the incidence of dental caries. (On the other hand, excess of fluoride leads to mottling of teeth and in severe cases to bone damage.) Rickets, which is still widespread in parts of Northern Africa and the Eastern Mediterranean and is reported to be increasing in Mexico, is attributable to insufficient exposure to sunlight and lack of vitamin D in the diet. Ascorbic acid deficiency is a problem in some drought-affected populations, especially in Africa. Vitamin B12 deficiency, which causes anaemia and, if

severe, neurological disorders, may occur in those consuming exclusively vegetarian diets.

Unlinking drought and malnutrition: the example of Botswana

Botswana suffered from six consecutive years of severe drought between 1982 and 1988 and yet managed to contain hunger and malnutrition in many of the rural areas.

The figures below show the food production index, the kilocalories available per day, and the prevalence of underweight children aged under five years for the period 1980–87.

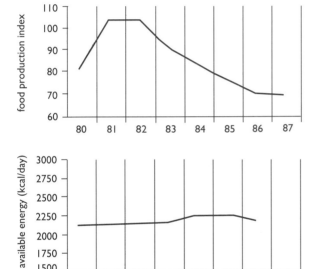

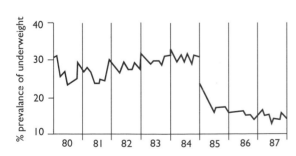

The drought began in 1982. Cereal production declined from nearly 50,000 tonnes in 1982 to only 6,000 tonnes in 1984. The number of head of cattle was reported to have fallen by about a quarter between 1982 and 1987. Cereal imports and food aid

increased in the early years of the drought so that, by 1984, total cereal availability and calorie availability were higher than before the drought. The relative cost of food increased from 1980 but was largely stabilized by 1984.

Restoring the overall availability of food was only part of the strategy; access to food in rural areas was also tackled through compensating for income loss by labour-based relief programmes and food distribution. An estimate in 1985–86 suggested that nearly 700,000 people out of a national population of 1.2 million benefited from the drought food programme and some 74,000 workers participated in labour-based relief. The cost of the 1985–86 drought relief programmes was the equivalent of around US$40 per beneficiary – the amount split between governments and donors. The experience demonstrates that well organized rural programmes to provide income and food linked to a widespread system of nutritional surveillance can minimize the hunger and malnutrition that usually accompany drought.

Source: WHO (1992).

REFERENCES AND RESOURCES

Comfort, Alex (1979), *The Biology of Senescence*, 3rd ed. Edinburgh: Churchill Livingstone.

Martinez, C.A., Barua, D. and Merson, M.H. (1988), 'Control of Diarrhoeal Diseases', *World Health Statistics Quarterly*, vol. 41, no. 2, pp. 74–81.

Ministry of Agriculture, Fisheries and Food (1976), *Manual of Nutrition*. London: HMSO.

UNEP (1989), *Environmental Data Report 1989*. Oxford: Blackwell.

UNEP (1992), *The World Environment 1972–1992*. London: Chapman and Hall.

UNICEF (1986), *The State of the World's Children 1986*. Oxford: OUP.

World Health Organization (1987), *WHO Expert Committee on Onchoceriasis – 3rd Report*, Technical Report Series 752. Geneva: WHO.

World Health Organization (1992), *Our Planet, Our Health*, Report of the WHO Commission on Health and Environment. Geneva: WHO, HMSO.

USEFUL ADDRESSES

British Diabetic Association
10 Queen Anne Street
London W1M 0BD
Tel.: 071 323 1531

Save the Children Fund
17 Grove Lane
Camberwell
London SE5 8RD

PSYCHOLOGICAL AND SOCIAL ASPECTS OF HEALTH AND SOCIAL CARE

THE DEVELOPMENT OF INDIVIDUAL IDENTITY

The role of social factors in the development of individual identity

SOCIALIZATION refers to the many processes that mould the human being into an active member of society.

The agents of socialization are parents, other members of the family, peers, workmates, schools, churches and the mass media. They all present the values, beliefs and conventions of society by means of communication.

THE ROLE OF LEARNING PROCESSES IN THE DEVELOPMENT OF IDENTITY

From a psychological point of view, two theories of learning are relevant to the socialization process: first, the theory of classical and operant conditioning, whereby behaviour is learnt for a reward (see page 131), and second, social learning theory. Social learning theorists believe that a child's personality and behaviour develop through social interaction. Operant conditioning plays its part here, in the form of rewards and punishments, but behaviour is also learnt through imitation, identifying with particular role models and conforming to expectations. MODELLING, in this context, means providing an example which a child can imitate in order to learn styles of behaviour.

Socialization starts at birth. A mother responds to her baby's needs for food and warmth, giving security and affection (see 'Attachments' on page 124); when the time comes for weaning she begins to control the baby's behaviour. Conforming behaviour will be rewarded with smiles, approving sounds and appropriate words (positive reinforcement). This process of rewarding acceptable behaviour and controlling unacceptable behaviour continues through a child's life. Parents are later joined by teachers in this role.

THE ROLE OF CULTURALLY AVAILABLE CONCEPTS IN THE FORMATION OF INDIVIDUAL IDENTITY

Culturally available concepts include stereotypes and labels, and the self-fulfilling prophecy (see page 134) ensures that the inner self-concept can be permanently affected by these.

At school, language is often the key to success: see Labov's concept of Black English, discussed in Chapter 2. Total failure to cope with formal education has led some, mainly working-class young males, into crime. The education system for them fails as a socializing agent and they may be labelled as deviants. This is a sociological explanation of deviance; psychologists would put forward different reasons for deviant/delinquent behaviour, for example, long-standing family discord.

Some comprehensive schools in inner-city areas, with a high proportion of pupils from minority racial groups and many pupils from disadvantaged homes, nevertheless succeed in compensating for problems at home and reaching minority groups. The following extract from a report in *The Times* describes one such school:

Mulberry school is typical of the 'little beacons of excellence' in the inner cities that John Patten, the education secretary, wants other schools to learn from. Even though 97% of the girls in the fifth year were classed as having English as a second language, more than three-quarters achieved at least one GCSE at grades A to C. Nearly one in six (16.4%) gained at least eight top grades.

Its success is, in fact, a tribute to a truism now gaining ground even in the education establishment: people matter. For two decades it had a remarkable headteacher, Daphne Gould, who established a reputation for firm leadership, improving academic standards, good discipline and strong links with parents in the Bangladeshi community.

(The Times, 22 November 1992)

PSYCHOLOGICAL AND SOCIAL CAUSES OF THE INCREASING CRIME RATE AMONG JUVENILES

There has been recent national concern at and a heated debate about possible causes of juvenile crime. Proposed causes for this, based on research over the years, have included separation from the mother at an early age, a failure to form any strong attachment bonds in infancy (affectionless psychopathy), and long-standing marital discord, as well as social factors such as high unemployment, alienation from school and truancy. Now, controversially, the lack of a socially responsible father in many families is also seen as a contributory cause.

The importance of the father

In the past the father has been seen as having mainly indirect value as an emotional and economic support for the mother. The notion of 'paternal deprivation' has hardly been considered until the present day. While the importance of a father's secondary role as provider of emotional and economic support for the mother has changed but not diminished, research is now showing that children raised without fathers are more likely to be poor, do badly at school, have a drink or drug problem and end up in jail.

The role of the father does not supplant that of the mother and should be viewed as providing increased involvement with his children and concern for their social and emotional welfare, both directly in partnership with the mother and through support for the mother.

The father is now considered to be of direct emotional and social significance to the developing child in the following ways:

- A father is an important attachment figure for small children, who form a different quality of attachment with their mother and father and choose one or other according to the circumstances. For example, the mother might be preferred as a source of comfort, the father as a playmate.
- A father provides an adult male role model which is important for girls, but seems to be particularly necessary for boys.
- Affection and discipline from two parents protects against acquiring a criminal record. Past research has established that children from homes where there is long-standing marital discord are more likely to acquire a police record. But recent research has shown that children from fatherless families are at similar risk.

One of the factors must be that where there are several children, two parents can provide more affection, supervision and discipline than one parent trying to do everything alone.

There is now a large body of American and British data to demonstrate the disastrous effects of raising children without fathers. In the USA, more than 70 per cent of all juveniles in state reform institutions are from fatherless homes. Studies suggest that the most damaging lack in lone-parent families is the example of two adults engaging in negotiation and concession, a model of behaviour that may be sometimes irreplaceable in a child's development. Easier divorce, while improving the happiness of adults, can thus reduce children's experience of give-and-take.

(The Times, leading article, 6 July 1993)

The underclass

Several years ago, a right-wing American political scientist, Charles Murray, claimed to have discovered the existence in Britain of a section of society he called the underclass, characterized by high levels of illegitimacy, a propensity to crime and chronic unemployment.

The recent concern about the growth of single-parent families is not so much about the more mature single parent who has become homeless as a result of marital breakdown but wishes to be independent and work; the most vulnerable to the underclass growth are teenagers, and women between 20 and 24 years, the traditional child-bearing age. The young single mothers of the underclass may talk of having a baby without a husband as utterly normal. The mother receives from the baby the unquestioning love she finds nowhere else, and she may believe that having a baby may give her priority on the council housing list, and access to a range of benefits.

On some housing estates today there is a lack of men.

Something is missing on the Meadow Well estate on North Tyneside. There are women and children aplenty, and scores of youths. But where have all the fathers gone? Most of them seem to have vanished: to the pub, the betting shop, prison, or points unknown.

That men should get and hold a job, live with their children, plant the garden, keep an eye out for the local villains or organise a Scout troop is an idea so detached from the reality of life at Meadow Well as to be farcical.

Meadow Well has become a classic sink estate of impoverished women, deprived children, loutish adolescents and a prevailing nihilism, underwritten by the state: in short, the 'underclass'.

(Sunday Times, 11 July 1993)

The problems on this estate are not its design (the houses are well spaced) or a lack of community initiatives (many programmes have been started here); they reflect deeper problems – of 'growing illegitimacy and family breakdown, the reduction in the work ethic and rising crime which are part of a general malaise threatening the whole of British culture' (*Sunday Times*, 11 July 1993).

What problems or benefits might occur for a child raised in a single-parent family, on an estate surrounded by similar families, without the back-up of relatives?

A recent report carried out by Family Policy Studies Centre and Crime Concern 1993 states that more emphasis needs to be placed on the roles played by men in bringing up children and their influence on the raising of socially responsible adults. The report states: 'This is not merely because men so heavily outnumber women as known offenders, but because the role of fathers in raising pro-social responsible children has been unjustly neglected.'

There is now a national campaign to prevent youngsters turning to crime and courses on parental skills will be offered in areas across the country. The following extract from *The Times*, July 1993, describes examples.

A block of flats and the lives of its residents have been transformed by the provision of a neighbourhood centre offering a range of support facilities for young mothers and fathers.

The flats on the ground floor of one of three tower blocks at Hockwell Ring, Luton, Bed-fordshire, have been converted to provide a community room, nursery, toilets and reception areas. A nursery school and 'mums and tots' club operates five days a week and, once a week, there is a drop-in club for mothers and children and a lunch club. A six-week basic child-care course has been held and a ten-week course for those who want a certificate is planned.

Inside Lancaster Farms young offenders' institution, Lancashire, staff are also running a parentcraft course for young men aged 17 to 21. The course includes talks on sexual behaviour, contraception and how to feed, bath and look after a baby.

ACTIVITY

Discuss the following questions in your class, or in smaller groups.

- The concept of an underclass is highly contentious. To what extent does other sociological and psychological research support these ideas?
- The growth of the idea, starting in the 1960s, that people should not have limits on their happiness or rights – including the rights both to have children and to get divorced – has been blamed for the breakdown of the traditional family. Do you agree with this?
- In some cultures the extended family (grandparents, uncles, aunts, etc.) all help each other in raising children, so that there is less pressure on the 'nuclear' family. Could anything be done in this country to encourage the extended family? Or do you think this would be a backward step?
- If everyone watches TV soaps, should more effort be made to give good parenting models in these shows? Do you think this is already being done?
- If the father's role in the family is important, what qualities should he possess? What behaviour should he show? What behaviour should he not show?
- Find out what parenting courses and other types of support are offered to young mothers and fathers in the area where you live.

Attachments

DEPRIVATION AND PRIVATION

Psychologists since Bowlby have been divided about how important the mother is to the child's emotional development. There is agreement, however, that the formation of strong attachment bonds (not necessarily with the biological mother) before the age of three years, is vital to the emotional health of the growing child.

If these bonds have been made, and are then for some reason disrupted, perhaps by divorce, death, moving house or hospitalization, the child will be distressed, the distress typically showing three phases: protest, despair and detachment. This distress can with time and care be overcome, more quickly if an infant can be with someone else to whom he or she is attached.

What is far more serious for the long term is if an infant fails to make any bonds at all (privation). This may happen if a baby has multiple changes of carer, or if he or she is in the kind of institution where staff change regularly and 'favouritism' is discouraged, or if the child has emotionally neglecting parents (see section on emotional abuse on page 141). A child may then suffer from 'affectionless psychopathy' (Bowlby) which is characterized by:

- a phase of very clingy, dependent behaviour, followed by
- attention-seeking behaviour and indiscriminate friendliness, and finally
- a personality which shows no feelings of guilt, is unable to keep rules and is unable to form lasting relationships.

A life on the fringes of society, or involvement in crime, is a strong possibility for such people. Psychopathy is rare, but behaviour that tends towards it is quite commonly observed.

For an infant it is certainly better to have loved and lost (deprivation) than never to have loved at all (privation).

WHAT IS AN ATTACHMENT?

Maccoby (1980) defined an attachment as 'a relatively enduring emotional tie to a specific other person'.

In infancy and early childhood, attachment is demonstrated by:

- trying to be near the other person;
- being distressed if separated from that person;
- showing joy and relief when the person reappears;
- being generally oriented towards that person, even when they are not close by, through, for example, listening to their voice and watching what they do.

HOW DO ATTACHMENTS DEVELOP?

Attachment bonds build up slowly from birth between a baby and his or her adult carers, through:

- touch, skin contact, comfort;
- vocal interaction;
- feeding and handling;
- eye contact;
- stimulation.

A small baby will usually allow anyone to handle him or her but at about six months will protest if a stranger does this, thus demonstrating that attachments to special people have been established.

CASE STUDY 1: PETER

At the Tavistock Clinic with Dr Bowlby were James and Joyce Robertson, who specialized in the emotional needs of young children. Joyce Robertson worked with mothers attending the clinic and found an interrelation between deficient mothering and disturbed infant development. One of her case studies follows:

When first seen at a few weeks old, Peter was a picture-book baby, contented and round, delicately coloured and presenting no problems. His mother handled him competently but appeared harassed and depressed. She was conscientious, devoted to her son and pleased with his development. But she was an unhappy woman, seriously inhibited in her ability to express feeling or to witness it in others.

Peter first smiled at about six weeks, but did not progress to the free smiling which is typical of babies between two and three months. When talked to he would listen and look, move his limbs and head and lips, but only rarely would the expected smile appear. His mother did not try to elicit smiles from him and she became uneasy when I tried to do so. When he wriggled in response to my talking to him, she said, 'He is embarrassed', and thereby gave the first clue to her inhibition. We were to become very familiar with this inability to elicit or to answer to an emotional response.

She did not talk to her baby or play with him. In the waiting-room mother and child would sit silent and still like two wooden figures. By the time Peter was seven months old his lack of facial expression, lack of bodily movement and lack of expression of feeling were conspicuous.

When he cried she would hold his shoulder as one might do a strange schoolchild crying in the street. Inadequate comforting led in his case to the gradual development of an exceptional ability to control his tears when in pain. He would tremble, flush, screw up his eyes and swallow his tears. By the time he was a year old this meagre response had gone; even injections did not make him cry.

He was slow in attaining the usual developmental steps: he sat up, crawled and pulled himself into a standing position just before his first birthday. He walked at sixteen months and said his first words at two years.

It became clear that this subdued unresponsiveness was what his mother wanted. The attention and stimulation that came his way during illness, or on one of the frequent holidays spent in hotels, brought about more demanding behaviour. In our judgement, this behaviour was more normal, but it invariably caused his mother to complain.

Peter always looked healthy, but there was no animation or pleasure in his body movements or in his facial expression. In the consulting-room he sat silently on his mother's knee, intently watching whatever was going on but rarely responding. His watching sometimes had a self-protective quality, like that of a petrified animal – eyes staring, body tense and stiff – waiting and watching for danger. When a therapist first observed him at eighteen months of age his unwillingness to respond to stimuli made her ask: 'Is he psychotic?'

At three years he sucks his thumb a great deal, and his play is hindered by it. He is passive – watching rather than doing or responding. When he is excited he has a disturbing habit of standing rigid, trembling and making unusual hand and finger movements.

ACTIVITY

1 Read the case study of Peter.

2 Observe for 15 minutes a mother and baby. (If a live mother and baby cannot be arranged, the students could watch a video.)

3 Note:
  • age of baby,
  • relationship of carer to baby.

4 Note what the carer does with body, voice, eye contact.

5 Note how the baby responds.

6 Write down a case study of this mother and baby from your notes.

7 How does the behaviour of this mother and baby differ from the behaviour of Peter and his mother?

8 How much do you think your presence affected the behaviour of the mother?

9 Discuss which factors favour attachments and which inhibit them, using books from the library for your research.

ATTACHMENTS: SUMMARY

• There is no foundation for the belief that the biological mother is uniquely capable of caring for her child.
• The 'mother' does not even have to be female.
• Multiple attachments rather than a distinct preference for a mother-figure is the rule rather than the exception for even young infants.
• Attachment is unrelated to the amount of physical caretaking the baby receives from the attachment figure.

Attachments are determined by:

• *Intensity of interaction*: quality of time is more important than quantity of time.
• *Sensitive responsiveness* to the baby's needs by the carer.
• *Consistency*: people must be a predictable part of the child's environment.

Eight psychosocial stages in the life cycle

Erik Erikson (b. 1902), accepting some parts of Freud's theory of the personality and the psychosexual stages, believed that development continues throughout the life cycle. He identified eight psychosocial stages. Each one centres on a developmental crisis where a choice must be made between two conflicting personality characteristics.

These eight stages, summarized in Table 4.1, may be used as a basis for exploring the changing needs of the person and the way in which personal identity is established.

Table 4.1   Erikson's eight psychosocial stages

Number of stage	Name of stage (psychosocial crisis)	Radius of significant relationships	Human virtues ('qualities of strength')	Approximate ages
1	Basic trust versus Basic mistrust	Mother or mother-figure	Hope	0–1
2	Autonomy versus Shame and doubt	Parents	Willpower	1–3
3	Initiative versus Guilt	Basic family	Purpose	3–6
4	Industry versus Inferiority	Neighbourhood and school	Competence	7–12
5	Identity versus Role confusion	Peer groups and outgroups, models of leadership	Fidelity	12–18
6	Intimacy versus Isolation	Partners in friendship, sex, competition, co-operation	Love	20s
7	Generativity versus Stagnation	Divided labour and Shared household	Care	Late 20s–50s
8	Ego integrity versus Despair	'Humankind', 'my kind'	Wisdom	50s and beyond

STAGE 1: BASIC TRUST v. BASIC MISTRUST (0–1 yr)

The quality of care that a small baby receives is important if the baby is to develop a sense of the world as a safe and comfortable place to be, as opposed to a place full of hazards.

If the baby is cuddled, played with and talked to, and his or her needs met as they arise, the baby will sense that people are dependable and helpful and that the world is safe. This sense of trust allows the baby to accept new experiences and to learn gradually to tolerate fear of the unknown.

However, if there are frequent changes of carer, if no effort is made to relate to the baby, or if care is inconsistent, the baby will develop a sense of mistrust, fear and suspicion. This shows itself as apathetic or withdrawn behaviour, where the baby has a sense of being controlled rather than being in control.

This is clearly shown in videos recording parents interacting with their babies. Very often the baby initiates the interaction, perhaps by eye contact, a vocal sound, or moving a limb. If the parent responds the movements increase and the baby smiles (if old enough). But if the parent does not respond the baby gives up, withdraws and turns his or her head away.

STAGE 2: AUTONOMY v. SHAME AND DOUBT (1–3 yrs)

The child's cognitive and muscle systems are developing and he or she is becoming more mobile. The child's range of experiences and choices is also expanding. The child is just beginning to see him or herself as a person in its own right and is beginning to sense independence.

This stage has sometimes been called the 'adolescence of childhood', as the child, though in many ways still a baby with a baby's needs, also wants to do everything him or herself. This can be a demanding time for parents who are often caring for a small baby as well. In this age group there are wide cultural/family/class differences on matters such as weaning and toilet training. Some psychologists of the Freudian school would say that attitudes to these matters have lasting effects on the personality. Others would discount this, saying that the important thing is that the child is allowed to do things in his or her own time, encouraging a sense of autonomy and self-esteem, and not criticized or ridiculed for slowness, mistakes or failures, which could lead to a sense of shame and doubt.

Most experts would recommend individual care in the home for younger children (up to age 2 or 3) whose mothers work, rather than a large day-care centre or nursery, as they need security and one-to-one care.

STAGE 3: INITIATIVE v. GUILT (3–5/6 yrs)

Rapid development takes place at this stage, physically, intellectually and socially, and the child is eager to try out growing skills and abilities to achieve all sorts of new goals.

The child wants to ask questions, indulge in fantasy play, play alone and be with other children, run and jump, climb and ride a bike.

If encouraged to do these things, the child's sense of initiative will be reinforced. But if parents or carers ridicule the child's fantasy play, find the artistic play too messy or inaccurate, the physical activity too dangerous, the questions embarrassing or a nuisance or too difficult to answer, then the child might come to feel guilty about expressing him or herself and inhibit natural initiative and curiosity.

At this age a child's physical and intellectual development will be affected by DEPRIVATION (see Table 4.2), especially sensory and intellectual deprivation. A home without space to play, toys to play with, books to look at, things to see, hear or touch will have detrimental effects on the child's development. Many children do not have access to a safe place outdoors where they can play with others.

Many people believe that free nursery education, where children have space to run around in a safe environment and freedom to express themselves with paint, sand and fantasy play, should be available to all pre-

school children. For those from deprived homes it is a necessity, while those from the most stimulating homes benefit from the social contact of nursery school.

Ramey 1981 found that, for children aged 2–5 yrs, social and intellectual development can be greater for those who attend day-care centres than those who stay at home. This applies especially to those children from deprived homes with poorly educated parents, who typically experience a decline in intellectual performance after the age of 2 years if they stay at home.

Poverty contributes to deprivation and family stress, but of course many children from poor homes are not deprived. A child from a wealthy home may be deprived by frequent changes of nanny, or by being given material goods in place of personal attention.

John Bowlby said at first that the family home is always a better place for a child than an institution.

Later he revised this, saying that some family homes are just awful.

The policy of Social Services Departments today is to promote the welfare of children in need by providing services to help them to be brought up within their own families as far as possible. If a child has to be taken into care, foster family homes are used in preference to institutions. When choosing a foster home the child's race, religion, culture and language will be taken into account, as well as his or her particular personality and needs. Foster-parents have to be visited and approved by Social Services before they are registered and allowed to take a child.

Foster-parents receive support and counselling from social workers and they receive a professional wage. The support is particularly necessary in the early weeks of a fostering when a child, who may have had many previous disappointments, will be testing them to the limit.

Regular support and advice is especially important to families who foster children who have previously been abused, for the foster-parents will find that here, the best of

Table 4.2 The various forms of deprivation that can affect small chiildren

Age group particularly affected	Type of deprivation	Effects
0–3 years (also 3–5 years)	Lack of basic care: warmth, food and clothing	Lack of food can lead to 'deprivation dwarfism'
	Lack of mother or other sensitive, caring adult to become attached to	Failure to make attachment bonds can lead through retarded development to maladjustment
2–5 years	Lack of sensory stimulation – colour, taste, sound, things to feel, e.g. in a flat with no access to outdoors	Will hamper intellectual development
2–5 years	Lack of intellectual stimulation – books, toys, conversation	Will retard speech and otherwise hamper intellectual development, as above. Boredom has also been related to behaviour disturbance
3 years–adolescence	Stressed relationships between adults	May lead to neglect of child Also, family discord has been related to behaviour problems and acquiring a criminal record
	(controversially) Lack of father or father figure Illegitimacy Underclass environment	Increased likelihood of: poor attainment at school substance abuse acquiring a criminal record

intentions are not enough. Such children may show very odd and disturbing behaviour, and foster-parents need to be told what to expect and how to handle the behaviour over a long period.

Typically now about 60% of children in care are placed in foster-homes, and a residential community home will be available to look after those with more serious difficulties and behaviour problems. There are also smaller community homes, especially for teenagers.

The case for adoption

If a child has failed to make attachments as an infant, and is 'affectionless' or 'maladjusted', is this effect permanent?

Tizard and Hodges investigated this. They looked at children who had spent their whole lives in institutional care, and who weren't adopted till late on in their childhoods.

They found that, given time, even the children who had seemed 'affectionless' could develop a deep and loving relationship with the right adoptive parents.

The early stages in the relationship were difficult. But if the adoptive parents received support and help, and if they were patient with the child, then they could overcome this problem, and the child would eventually learn to trust them. But since it was so hard at the beginning, a lot of people gave up.

It does seem from this, though, that even early privation can be successfully overcome in the right kind of environment.

ACTIVITY

Find out about the care of children in need in the area you live in.

- Are there many community homes?
- Are children placed with foster-parents where possible?
- Are family aides available to help during a temporary crisis (if, for example, a mother has to go into hospital and the father cannot take time off work to look after young children)?
- Are free day care places available?

CASE STUDY 2: ANTHONY

The following description of Anthony's case is taken from 'The Lost Boys', *Sunday Times*, 22 September 1991.

The police started calling for Anthony when he was 4. He got into trouble from the moment he was allowed to play outside his home on a big pre-war housing estate in west London. First he abused bigger boys with racial taunts until they beat up his eldest sister. (Anthony, they felt, was too small to hit.)

Then he smashed a neighbour's windows and discovered vandalism. At the age of 5 he learnt about theft, breaking into a BT van and stealing the equipment.

'He always denies everything. It's never him,' his mother says. 'He's done so many things I can't remember half of them. I've done everything they've told me to, like keep him in and stop his treats and put him in his room and leave him. But he just climbs out of the window.'

Home is a clean but sparsely furnished ground-floor flat. There are no books; the only wall fitting is an electric clock. There used to be a telephone, but it melted when one of Anthony's younger sisters burnt the flat down.

Trying to alter Anthony means tackling emotional damage that goes back to birth. He was sick with lung trouble from the age of three months, passed much of his infancy in hospital, and from the age of 18 months spent his days in a nursery because another baby, Frances, had come along. His mother adored the new child, regarding Anthony, by contrast, as spoilt.

At the nursery, Anthony hit other children as soon as he could walk. 'I thought it was normal because he was only two. All kids are spiteful at that age. He was just very active,' Bridget says. But his violence continued. Bridget stopped his medication, believing it was the cause, but it made no difference.

Anthony's teachers arranged child guidance and mother-and-son counselling with a psychologist. Nothing changed.

At infants' school the teachers kept a book in the playground for the names of misbehaving children. If a child featured twice in one week, a letter was sent to parents. Anthony was named twice a day; the school wrote only if he did *not* appear. That happened once, and his mother rewarded him with a budgie, christened Gazza. Within days Gazza was forgotten and Anthony was back in the book.

In some ways, he is a bright and endearing child, who climbs trees and loves pigeons, often bringing them home. When he grows up, he says, he wants to be a policeman.

But wherever he goes, his behaviour is the same. When he and his sister were given summer holidays with host families outside London this year, Frances returned with a present and a promise that she would be welcomed again. Anthony's hosts said the family was glad to see the back of him.

Asked about the holiday last week, Anthony said: 'I don't know. I forget now. I forget everything.'

His mother, living a cycle of boredom during the day, and 'murderous' weekends with all the children home, sees her only hope in a move from their estate. Unless this happens, she believes, Anthony is doomed.

'If he carries on the way he's going now, he will end up in prison. I know it's horrible to say. But I don't see any future for him.'

ACTIVITY

Read Anthony's story. Then use the following questions as the basis for discussion or a written essay.

- Is Anthony an 'affectionless' child?
- What stresses did he experience in infancy which might have contributed to his present behaviour?
- In what ways is his home deprived?
- What positive signs are there? Does Anthony demonstrate any attachments at all?
- What help would you suggest for Anthony and children like him?

LEARNING

Children who have learned the benefit of behaving acceptably at home and conforming to the culture of their parents will take this knowledge with them to playgroup, nursery school and infant school.

Learning is a relatively permanent change in behaviour which occurs as a result of experience. It is dependent on other cognitive abilities, particularly memory and perception.

Behaviourist psychologists have identified two levels of learning known as classical conditioning and operant conditioning. Both processes were studied originally using laboratory animals, but the principles of each type may be applied to human learning.

Classical conditioning

In the early part of this century, Ivan Pavlov, a Russian physiologist, was studying the digestive system of dogs.

Pavlov had a tube inserted into the cheek of a dog to measure salivation, which occurred when food was brought. He noticed that the dog salivated when it saw just the assistant with a bucket. Pavlov then experimented with a buzzer and a shining light. He sounded the buzzer or shone the light every time the food was presented. After a while he found that the buzzer or the light on its own, without the food, would cause salivation.

Salivating is a REFLEX. The unconscious conditioning of involuntary reflexes in this way is called classical CONDITIONING.

Classical conditioning (learning by association) is involved, largely unconsciously, in the socialization of young children, and it also plays a part in the development of phobias. The principles of classical conditioning are behind the methods of treatment used for phobias. Classical conditioning is used in the treatment of alcoholics, by creating a phobia. This is known as AVERSION THERAPY. A drug called antabuse can be implanted under the skin, so it remains active in the body over a long period of time. If the alcoholic person has a drink during that time, they instantly fall sick, and often actually are sick. The alcohol becomes linked with nausea, and so the patient comes to avoid it.

Operant conditioning

Some responses are learned, not just because of a simple stimulus response connection but because they produce pleasant consequences.

In the 1930s B.F. Skinner, a psychologist, developed the Skinner Box. This contains:

* a metal grid floor;
* a food delivery chute;
* a lever or some kind of easily operated switch;
* a light.

It is used as follows:

* A hungry animal (a lab rat or hamster) is put into the box.
* Because it is hungry it is very active and explores the box.
* As it wanders it will accidentally press the lever, and a pellet of food is delivered into the chute.
* Gradually the rat builds up a connection between pressing the lever and getting the food reward.

When the animal is pressing the lever frequently and then looking in the chute it has 'learned' the activity.

* The food reward is called reinforcement.
* It strengthens the response.
* There is no thinking involved. This is learning by trial and error. Rats, pigeons, even worms can do it.

Operant conditioning can be used in two ways:

* positive reinforcement, where a behaviour is learned for a reward;
* negative reinforcement, where a behaviour is learned to avoid a punishment.

In operant conditioning, responses that bring about satisfaction or pleasure are likely to be repeated (this is positive reinforcement), while those which bring about discomfort are likely not to be repeated (negative reinforcement). Behaviour shaping (in which approved behaviour is gradually produced by the rewarding of actions which build up to the desired response) is used consciously to promote socially acceptable behaviour. Behaviour shaping may be used, for example, in the management of misbehaving children at school; to help those with learning disabilities; or to help the long term mentally ill who have lost their social skills.

Primary reinforcers are those which satisfy a basic need or drive, for example food or water or praise. Secondary reinforcers acquire their reinforcing properties through the association with primary reinforcers, for example money, tokens, stars.

In psychotherapy, the therapist may reward good or positive behaviours that the client is describing with signs of approval, e.g. a smile or a nod, therefore reinforcing them. Praise and approval appear to be deeply necessary to humans, and can similarly be used in any counselling or helping interview.

A common error in dealing with difficult children is to ignore them when they are being 'good' and to pay them attention only when they are misbehaving. But for some children even cross attention is better than none, and so the bad behaviour is reinforced.

CASE STUDY 3: NICKY

Nicky causes problems in her class because she leaves her chair all the time to talk to other children. Every time she does this the teacher walks over to her and tells her to sit down. After advice from a psychologist, the teacher ignores Nicky when she wanders around the room and only gives her attention as soon as Nicky sits at her desk. The table shows the results of this action.

ACTIVITY

Read the case study about Nicky, then answer the following questions.

- What is the unacceptable behaviour?
- What is the acceptable behaviour?
- What happened to Nicky's behaviour over the five-week period?
- Why did the psychologist advise the teacher to ignore Nicky's unacceptable behaviour?
- What positive reinforcers did the teacher use? Explain your answer.
- State what is meant by 'shaping' and explain how the teacher could have shaped Nicky's behaviour.
- Using secondary reinforcement, such as tokens, how could you change children's behaviour in the classroom?

STAGE 4: INDUSTRY v. INFERIORITY (7–12 yrs)

Industry refers to the child's concern with how things work, how they are made and their own efforts to make things.

This is reinforced when the child is encouraged by adults, who now are no longer confined to the parents. Teachers begin to be very significant in the child's life, and the child, helped by teachers and parents, begins to develop all sorts of new skills valued by society.

The peer group becomes increasingly important, relative to adults, and plays an important part in the development of self-esteem. Children begin to compare themselves with other children as a way of assessing their own achievement.

Self-esteem and the esteem of others stem largely from completing tasks successfully, being allowed to make things and being given guidance and encouragement by adults.

A child may have potential abilities which

	Behaviour during a 40-minute lesson	
	Acceptable to teacher	Not acceptable to teacher
Week 1	2 mins	38 mins
Week 2	10 mins	30 mins
Week 3	35 mins	15 mins
Week 4	39 mins	1 min
Week 5	39 mins	1 min

if not nurtured during this period may develop 'late or never'. A lack of encouragement, and cold, uninterested or critical parents, may lead to a failure to achieve new skills and a sense of failure and low self-esteem.

Language and cultural differences

At this age children may begin to fall behind seriously at school if they have not mastered the middle-class 'elaborated' code of English used in school, perhaps because they come from immigrant communities or if their parents only use a 'restricted' code. See the sections on 'Bernstein's theory' and Laov's work on 'black English' in Chapter 2.

It is at this age that children become aware of the implications of belonging to a particular cultural or religious group. They realize that this affects their family rules, family activities and diet, which may be different from those of the majority. If they belong to a sect or racial minority group which is subject to prejudice in the area, they will become aware at this age of stereotypes and may absorb the stereotype of their own particular group into their own self-concept (see the section on stereotypes and self-fulfilling prophecy on page 134).

A good school, which believes in the value of each individual, can help substantially in overcoming these difficulties.

PARENTING

Styles of parenting differ, and psychologists have tried to categorize these many differences. Figure 4.1 shows one method of characterizing the various styles.

Authoritative parents combine control with acceptance and child-centred involvement. Their control and demands are combined with warmth, nurturance and two-way communication. Children's opinions and feelings are consulted when family decisions are made, and explanations and reasons are given for any punitive measures if these are imposed.

Research shows the children of such parents tend to be independent, self-assertive, friendly with peers, and co-operative with parents. They seem to enjoy life and have a strong motivation to succeed.

Authoritarian parents also attempt to control and assert their power over their children, but without warmth and nurturance. They attempt to set an absolute set of standards, and they value obedience, respect for authority, work, tradition and the presentation of order.

The children of such parents tend to be moderately competent and responsible but they also tend to be socially withdrawn and to lack spontaneity. The girls seem to be particularly dependent on their parents and to lack achievement motivation. The boys

	accepting responsive child-centred	rejecting unresponsive parent-centred
demanding controlling	authoritative	authoritarian
undemanding not controlling	indulgent	neglecting

Figure 4.1   Child-rearing practices
Source: after Maccoby and Martin 1983, in *Introduction to Psychology*, Atkinson R. (Harcourt Brace, 1993).

tend to be more aggressive than other boys. Some studies have found a link between authoritarian parenting and low self-esteem in boys (Coopersmith 1967).

Indulgent parents are accepting, responsive, child-centred parents who place few demands on their children and exercise little control.

The children of such parents tend to show more happiness and vitality than children of authoritarian parents, but their behaviour tends to be immature in that they lack self-reliance, social responsibility and impulse control over, for example, aggression.

Even though authoritarian and indulgent parents have completely opposed childrearing styles, both have children who tend to show little self-reliance, and may have problems with aggression.

Most *neglecting* parents do not neglect in the extreme sense that would be termed child abuse. But they are very parent-centred, concerned with their own interests and activities and uninvolved with those of their children. Typically, if their children are not at home they do not know where they are, who they are with, and what they are doing. They are uninterested in events at their children's schools, have few conversations with their children and do not consider their opinions.

The children of such parents tend to be moody, impulsive and aggressive. They tend to truant from school and may start drinking, smoking and dating at earlier ages than their peers.

Extreme neglect by parents consitututes emotional abuse. These parents are emotionally unavailable to their children. They are detached, emotionally uninvolved, often depressed and uninterested in their children.

Emotionally abused children show clear disturbance in their relationship and increasing deficits in all aspects of psychological functioning by age 2. Their deficits are actually greater than those of children whose parents physically abuse them (Egeland and Sroufe 1981).

Apart from cases of extreme behaviour in parents, as in severe neglect and child abuse,

it should be noted that links between parenting style and children's personality, though evident, are not as strong as researchers might expect:

- the two parents in a family might have different styles of parenting;
- the high divorce rate might mean that a woman has to change 'styles' when she has to work full-time;
- parents use different approaches at different times, so different children in the family have different experiences;
- following an unexpected family crisis, such as unemployment, accident or illness, child-centred parents might become more parent-centred;
- grandparents or other relatives who see the child regularly might provide aspects of parenting not provided by the mother or father.

STEREOTYPING PREJUDICE AND THE SELF-FULFILLING PROPHECY

What is stereotyping?

Originally a term from printing, a 'stereotype' is now used to mean a simplified image of a whole group of people, for example a racial, national, religious, sexual or occupational group. Stereotyping is the attribution of characteristics that are presumed to belong to a whole group of people to just one individual.

It seems that we need stereotypes in order to categorize somehow all the different people we meet, watch and read about. Stereotypes make useful pigeon-holes. Unfortunately they usually have value judgements, often negative, attached to them.

Educated people are nowadays more aware of stereotyping and its dangers. Try asking friends what is the stereotype of, for example, Scots, the elderly, an immigrant group, nurses. They will probably be reluctant or embarrassed to say what they think the stereotypes are, especially if they are negative or derogatory, and will say that they do not agree with them. This is encouraging, but nevertheless, the people you ask will probably be in accord about what the stereotype for each group is held to be. That is because stereotypes are very common in our society and are reinforced by sections of the media.

Stereotypes are learnt by children from their parents and the majority culture – newspapers, TV, comics, books and films. Out-of-date stereotypes are often perpetrated in children's books, written years ago, which are still popular.

Sex-role stereotyping

In the 'Thomas the Tank Engine' stories the engines are all male, while the silly clattering carriages are all female.

In 1982 J. Penrose complained to the *Guardian* that the Ladybird Key Words Reading scheme was guilty of traditional sex stereotyping. Peter made all the important decisions, took charge more often and spoke more frequently than Jane. He was active and adventurous, Jane was totally passive.

It is not surprising, therefore, to find rigid sex-role stereotyping among adults.

Racial stereotyping

Similarly, old children's books still hold out-of-date racial stereotypes. The Captain John Biggles stories show a corrupt world being kept in order by clean-living white English men; the villains are usually big negroes, harsh Prussian officers or fat, suave Eurasians.

The fact that racism is still, despite the anti-discrimination laws, more prevalent in England than in many other mixed-race societies must be in part due to the stereotypes that have been absorbed into our culture. D. Milner wrote: 'When racism has taken root in the majority culture, has pervaded its institutions, language, its social intercourse and its cultural productions, has entered the very interstices of the culture, then the simple process by which a culture is transmitted from generation to generation in the socialization process becomes the most important "determinant" of prejudice.'

Prejudice

Prejudice starts with a stereotype. Allport suggested five increasingly violent stages of behaviour which may take place against any minority group:

- Anti-locution – hostile talk, racial jokes, verbal denigration and insult.
- Avoidance – keeping a distance but without inflicting any harm.
- Discrimination – exclusion from housing, employment, schools, clubs. The Race Relations Act covers three kinds of discrimination: direct discrimination, indirect discrimination and victimization. Indirect discrimination is the most difficult to prove.
- Physical attack – violence against the person or property.
- Extermination – indiscriminate violence against a whole group.

Social identity theory

Tajfel and Turner put forward social identity theory to explain the development of prejudice. The basis of this theory is that people, particularly those with low self-esteem and an intense need for acceptance by others, will identify with a group that has a positive social image. The more positive the image of the group, the more positive will be their social identity, and therefore their self-image. By emphasizing how desirable the 'in group' is and how undesirable the 'out group', and by concentrating on those characteristics of the 'in group' which make it 'superior', people can make for themselves a satisfactory social identity, and it is this that lies at the heart of prejudice.

Scapegoating

This is put forward as another reason for prejudice. When there are problems in society like a shortage of housing and high unemployment, people find targets for their frustration and aggression. Minority racial groups are easy targets. The defence mechanisms of displacement and projection are involved in scapegoating.

The reduction of prejudice

To reduce everyday prejudice it is important:

- to meet people from discriminated groups on a personal level, and to see them performing in high-status occupations;
- to receive information from the media which breaks down the traditional stereotypes;
- to live in a society in which prejudice is actively discouraged.

Self-fulfilling prophecy and labelling

Stereotypes are not easily discarded. They influence our perceptions and our social interactions, and can lead us to interact with those we stereotype in ways that cause them to fulfil our expectations. Children are particularly vulnerable to this, but so too are adults who hold a low status in our society.

Many psychological studies have demonstrated this. The following are two examples.

1 In 1966 Rosenthal showed that expectations affect how much a child achieves. In one study, teachers in an American school were told that certain children (of average ability and randomly picked) would show dramatic improvements over the next year. After a year these children had shown dramatic improvements, presumably because the teachers, without realizing it, had started to treat these children differently, unconsciously giving them extra help and encouragement.

This self-fulfilling prophecy can work negatively as well, and most unconscious racism in British schools works in this way. If children are perceived to be less able, for example because of their accents, they may gradually come to believe, because of the way that they are treated, that they are less able, and will underachieve dramatically.

2 Aronson and Osherow (1980) reported an experiment with third graders (nine-

year-olds) in the USA, conducted by their teacher, Elliott.

She told her class one day that brown-eyed people are more intelligent and 'better' people than those with blue eyes. Brown-eyed students, though in the minority, would be the 'ruling class' over the inferior blue-eyed children, given extra privileges, and the blue-eyed students were 'kept in their place' by such restrictions as being last in line, seated at the back of the class and given less break time.

Within a short time, the blue-eyed children began to do more poorly in their schoolwork and became depressed and angry and described themselves more negatively. The brown-eyed group grew mean, oppressing the others and making derogatory statements about them.

The next day, Elliott announced that she had lied and that it was really blue-eyed people who are superior. The pattern of discrimination, derogation and prejudice quickly reversed itself; she then de-briefed the children.

Several similar studies have replicated this scenario with other populations.

Labelling a person can be self-fulfilling in this way, especially if the person is a child, and the people doing the labelling are 'significant others' such as parents or regular teachers. Up to adolescence, children believe what they are told by their carers. Therefore, if they are often described as, for example, lazy, difficult, clumsy, they may well absorb these labels into their developing self-concept and become these things. Fortunately, positive labels such as good, helpful, enthusiastic can also be self-fulfilling by the same means. At adolescence, children might reassess what they have been told they are, in the light of what they feel they are, but this process might involve considerable acting out and argument.

Labels and the caring professions

Labels have often been used by pepole who work in the caring professions. Before patients and clients were allowed by right to see their own medical or social work records, words such as 'nice' or 'difficult' tended to be put into reports. Such words would influence the perception of those reading the reports and the patient or client would be treated accordingly. Open access to records has put an end to this overt practice, but care workers must constantly be on their guard against the easy tendency to label and stereotype. It is important that people in the caring professions are aware of any stereotypes they hold in their own minds, so that they can overcome them. Such self-awareness is necessary, in order that all patients/clients are approached equally and with an open mind.

ACTIVITY

1 Look through children's books, old and new, tabloid newspapers, comics, and current TV programmes.

   List examples you have found where gender, racial, class or age stereotypes are being reinforced or deliberately reversed.

2 Another kind of individual stereotype involves inferring what somebody is like psychologically from certain aspects of their physical appearance. Attractive looking people are attributed with all kinds of positive characteristics (the 'halo effect').

   Using pictures cut from magazines, carry out an experiment to test the following hypothesis: 'that on first impression attractive looking people are attributed with positive characteristics and high status jobs, and unattractive people with negative characteristics and low status jobs'.

   What is the danger of this kind of stereotype to workers in the caring professions?

ACTIVITY W

1 Make notes on different attitudes patients/clients have to themselves and their health, focusing on one case study.

2 Make notes on cases you observe where professionals influence the way in which patients/clients view their own health, again focusing on one case study (NB respect confidentiality – do not use actual names).

STAGE 5: IDENTITY v. ROLE CONFUSION (12–18 yrs)

The growth spurt that proceeds ADOLESCENCE is rapid. Erikson has said that the previous trust in the body's mastery of its functions, enjoyed in childhood, is thereby disturbed. The adolescent has to learn to 'grow into' the new body. For a long time it will not feel comfortable or 'fit' properly.

At the social level, western culture, with its emphasis on extended education, has invented adolescence as a slow transition from childhood to adulthood.

The stereotype of storm and stress, conflict and rebellion which the western world has of adolescence is reinforced to a considerable degree by the media. Many magazines and sections of the clothing and music industry both serve it and profit from it. But research has shown that for many teenagers the adjustments and the negotiations of various freedoms are achieved relatively peacefully.

At the psychological level, adolescents re-experience the conflicts of early childhood as they seek to establish their own identity separate from that of their parents. The adolescent needs support and security at home. Unfortunately, many marriages break up as children reach adolescence, perhaps partly because of the shifts in family relationships at this stage.

An adolescent experiencing discord at home may turn to substance abuse or delinquent behaviour. An adolescent with a different personality type, from a different background, might develop an eating disorder.

A child who has been brought up in a minority culture, might at adolescence reject the customs he or she was brought up with in favour of the mainstream culture. Adolescents can be extreme in testing out various identities, so they might reject everything about their upbringing, only remembering the good things about it at a later stage.

The major developmental task of adolescence is for the individual to develop a sense of identity, by integrating all the images they have of themselves as son/daughter, pupil, friend, brother/sister, and reflecting on past experiences, thoughts and feelings. If adolescents are successful in this task, they will emerge from this stage with a clear sense of where they have been, who they are, and where they are going.

Those who came positively through the earlier stages of development are more likely to achieve an INTEGRATED PSYCHOSOCIAL IDENTITY at adolescence.

Whatever the final outcome of this stage, Erikson believes that some form of turmoil or upset of identity is inevitable: 'at no other phase of the life-cycle are the pressures of finding oneself and the threat of losing one-self so closely allied'. To have a sense of self-identity is to have a 'feeling of being at home in one's body, a sense of knowing where one is going and an inner assurance of anticipated recognition from those who count'.

ACTIVITY

1 Look at the styles of parenting described under Stage 4 above.

2 How might a child brought up in each of these styles act at adolescence?

STAGE 6: INTIMACY v. ISOLATION (20s)

For Erikson, the attainment of identity by the end of adolescence is a prerequisite of the ability to become intimate with another person. By this he means much more than just making love, and includes the ability to share with and care about another person. The essential need is to relate our deepest hopes and fears to another person and to accept another's need for intimacy in turn. The intimate relationship may indeed not involve sexuality at all and describes the relationship between friends as much as that between husband and wife.

Our personal identity only becomes fully realized and consolidated through sharing ourselves with another and, if a sense of intimacy is not established with friends or a marriage partner, the result in Erikson's view is a sense of isolation, of being alone without anyone to share with or care for.

Intimacy is normally achieved, according to Erikson, in the twenties (in young adulthood).

STAGE 7: GENERATIVITY v. STAGNATION (late 20s–50s)

According to Erikson, middle age – the thirties, forties and fifties – brings with it either generativity or stagnation (self-absorption).

GENERATIVITY means that the person begins to be concerned with others beyond the immediate family, with future generations and the nature of the society and world in which those generations will live.

Generativity is not confined to parents but is displayed by anyone who is actively concerned with the welfare of young people and with making the world a better place for them to live and work.

Failure to establish a sense of generativity results in a sense of STAGNATION in which the individual becomes preoccupied with his or her personal needs and comforts. Such people indulge themselves as if they were their own or another's only child.

Many writers believe that most adults never attain generativity: that men get 'stuck' in the industry stage and women in the adolescent stage.

Gould (1978) suggested that the major task of women in their mid-forties is to realize that they do not need a 'protector' to survive; it is time for women to reach full independence for the first time.

Sanguiliano (1978) interviewed women in depth and concluded that they achieve identity and intimacy in reverse order; agreeing with Gould, she found that women do not achieve a full occupational identity until much later than is typical for men. 'Indeed the typical life course for women is to pass directly into a stage of intimacy without achieving personal identity; most women submerge their identity into that of their partner and only at mid-life do they emerge from this to search for their own separate identity' (Gross). However, her sample was small, so the conclusion may not be generalizable.

There are also important social class differences. Working-class men and women tend to marry earlier and their careers may 'peak' sooner. Working-class men see an early marriage as part of the normal life pattern; their young adulthood (twenties) is a time for settling down, having a family and working to provide for them. But middle-class men and women see their twenties as a time to explore, and to try out different occupations; marriage comes later. 'Settling down' tends to be postponed until the thirties.

Many people in this stage of life have dependent children and increasingly dependent parents. A woman's psychological need to find her own identity may be prevented by the needs of DEPENDANTS. Many of this age are involved in full-time caring, perhaps of an infirm parent or a handicapped child.

In 1976 Gail Sheehy described a shift in our forties when men begin to explore and develop their more 'feminine' selves (e.g. they become more nurturant, affiliative and intimate), while women are discovering their more 'masculine' selves (e.g. they become more action-orientated, assertive and ambitious). This passing-by, in opposite directions, produces the distress and pain which characterize the 'MID-LIFE CRISIS', corresponding to an increase of testosterone in the female and a decline in the male.

However, too much can be made of this crisis – 'crises' can occur at every age. Later in middle age there is the 'empty nest syndrome' when all dependants go.

Thus the adult has to cope with a series of changing roles: starting work, marriage, parenthood, coping with dependants, the empty nest.

STAGE 8: EGO INTEGRITY v. DESPAIR (50s and beyond)

Anderson (1978) claims that old people face a painful wall of discrimination that they are often too polite or too timid to attack:

- they are not hired for new jobs despite long experience (age discrimination);
- they are edged out of family life.

The elderly have a very low status compared with both children and adults.

However, many 60-year-olds would not see themselves as elderly. Seventy-year-olds regard those over 80 as old, not themselves.

Some old people do withdraw from society, but Havighurst (1964) believes that the best way to age is to stay active and resist as far as possible the shrinkage of the social world that can happen after middle age. It is important for old people to maintain their 'role count' (the number of roles they play in society) in addition to friendships and family relationships. Mental abilities can be maintained if they are kept in practice.

In Erikson's view, the major task of ageing is to reflect on one's life, and to assess how worthwhile and fulfilling it has been. If on the whole the positive has outweighed the negative then the individual will end his or her life with greater ego integrity than despair. Individuals will achieve ego integrity:

- if they are convinced that life does have a meaning and does make sense;
- if they conclude that what happened in

their life was inevitable and could not have happened in any other way;

- if they believe that all of life's experiences had their value and that good and bad experiences were times of learning and psychological growth;
- if they come to see and understand their own parents better because they have now experienced adulthood and maybe raised children of their own;
- if they see that the cycle of birth and death is something they have in common with all other human beings, whatever the difference in culture, status, lifestyle. Understanding this makes it easier to face the prospect of death.

ACTIVITY

Take two children from different backgrounds and imagine their experiences through the life cycle. For example:

1 A Bangladeshi boy whose parents speak very little English and who live in a high-rise flat in a large, run-down council estate in an inner city. The father is unemployed, the boy has several siblings and other relatives living nearby. There is considerable unemployment in the area, and much racial abuse, especially against the Bangladeshi community. The boy is close to his parents, and intelligent.

2 Read again the case study of Tracy Congdon in Chapter 2. Try to predict her experience through the life cycle.

THREATS TO MAINTAINING INDIVIDUAL IDENTITY

At the various stages of life, people may undergo experiences that threaten their individual identity. This part of the chapter examines some of these:

- disruption and abuse suffered by children;
- eating disorders in (usually) young women;

- loss, grief and stress in adulthood.

Defence mechanisms

Coping with threats to one's identity may involve retreating from the problem in some way or confronting it. Freud used the term DEFENCE MECHANISMS to refer to the unconscious processes that defend a person against anxiety by distorting reality in some way. These strategies are emotion-focused. They do not alter a stressful situation, only the way a person sees it. Therefore all defence mechanisms involve some self-deception. Table 4.3 sets out the defence mechanisms that may be used in reacting to threats at the various life stages.

A more positive and constructive way of adapting to life event threats is PROBLEM-FOCUSED COPING, described later in this part of the chapter in the section on stress.

Disruption of children's attachment bonds

This can cause major distress to small children (0–3 years). They may be separated from their mother or mother substitute by death, divorce, moving house or hospitalization (of mother or child). Their distress will be greatly reduced if they can be with someone else to whom they are attached (e.g. grandmother, father, aunt).

Child abuse

The experience of the abused child has been compared to that of hostage victims and concentration camp inmates (Fillmore 1981). A few days as a hostage can change the whole psyche of an adult; this should indicate how much damage intermittent violence, emotional battery (criticism, shouting) and then occasional kindness, will inflict on an unknowing, inadequately verbal child. The abused child is asked to love and obey his or her warders, and protectors, but at the same time is psychologically and physically degraded, and often receives violence for no

Table 4.3 Coping with life event threats using ego defence mechanisms

Age group	Life event threat	Possible defence mechanism which might be used
Baby	Disruption of attachment bonds	Regression Denial
Child	Child abuse	Repression Denial Displacement Reaction formation
Adolescent	Delinquent behaviour Substance abuse Eating disorders	Displacement Regression Displacement Regression
Adult	Separation and divorce	Rationalization Projection
	Unemployment	Regression Displacement
Elders	Bereavement	Denial

consistent reason. As a result, the child internalizes feelings of self-blame, guilt, low-esteem and a need to fail.

EMOTIONAL ABUSE AND NEGLECT

Parents who neglect their children, who are cold, are too busy with their own lives, and who continuously fail to show their children love or affection, are abusing them emotionally. They may simply be uninterested, or they may continuously threaten, taunt, criticize or shout at a child.

The child feels unloved and unlovable, loses confidence and self-esteem, and becomes nervous and withdrawn. Children who are emotionally neglected usually show signs of being unhappy in some way. They may appear withdrawn or unusually aggressive, or they may have lingering health problems or difficulties at school. Emotional abuse hurts children very deeply. The effects on the child's personality can be very serious and make it hard for him or her to form successful relationships as he or she grows up.

The following extract is a description by a 9-year-old boy, Jamie, of his experience:

I used to get into bad tempers all the time because I wanted my mum and dad to love me and be interested in me, but they kept telling me I was a bad boy.

One day I made my mum so angry, she hit me. Later she told me she was sorry and that she had telephoned some people called the NSPCC who could help make us happy. I thought they would take me away. But they didn't. They said that I wasn't bad and that what had happened to me wasn't my fault.

We went to the NSPCC every week. My mum and dad talked about how they felt and I told them how angry I was. I know now that my mum loves me, and she shows it.

My mum and dad pay me lots more attention, and I'm so much happier now.

PHYSICAL ABUSE

Physical abuse occurs when parents or adults deliberately inflict injuries on a child, or knowingly do not prevent them. Abusing actions include hitting, shaking, squeezing, burning or biting. They also include using excessive force when feeding, changing or handling a child. Giving a child poisonous substances, inappropriate drugs or alcohol, and attempting to suffocate or drown a child, are also examples of physical abuse.

Physical abuse is on a scale which has a smack on one end and violent battering at the other. Punishments on the child, once started, tend to escalate. Sometimes just one child in a family is physically abused. Often a step-parent, who has not bonded down the years with a child, is involved. Sometimes highly aggressive and psychotic personalities are involved, who have little hope of becoming reasonable parents, and these cases are the ones reported in the press. In the majority of cases the children who have been battered can eventually be returned successfully to their homes. Frequently their parents desperately want to make a happy home for their family. Their motivation is high, but most are emotionally immature people who expect too much from their children and punish them too severely for 'faults' that are really just part of normal development. They may also fuss over them, sometimes with over-protective fanaticism.

In cases of child abuse, a detailed longitudinal family history should be obtained. When decisions have to be made about whether abuse has occurred, and what should be the future of the child and family, the parents' own family background will be taken very seriously into account. Worrying events in the parents' background would include:

- violent childhood (observed or experienced);
- inadequate or inconsistent parenting;
- significant periods in hospital/care;
- persistent truancy/under-achievement in school;
- lack of close adolescent friendships;
- left home when very young;
- poor employment record;
- no close friendships;
- brief cohabitations/marital relationships;
- record of criminal violence;
- obsessional personality traits;
- alcohol or drug abuse.

The opposite of these factors, or the absence of them, would be seen as hopeful signs.

Physical abuse can cause injuries including bruising, burns, fractures, internal injuries

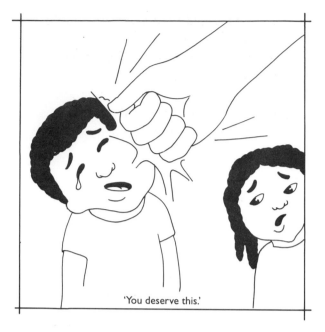

'You deserve this.'

and brain damage, and, in extreme cases, death. Shaking is more dangerous than people are aware and may cause brain damage or blindness. Beaten children often feel they are to blame and have low self-esteem. When they are older they tend to be aggressive and bully younger children, then aggressive towards their own children. Some forms of physical punishment are inbuilt in our culture, though this is not the case in other cultures. There is a link with criminality: John and Elizabeth Newson wrote in 1989: 'The measures which stand out as most predictive of criminal record before the age of 20 are having been smacked or beaten once a week or more at 11, and having a mother with a high commitment to corporal punishment at that age'.

Medical presentation

Some injuries presented at the surgery or casualty department could only have been caused by assault, but the majority of injuries are more difficult to assess – they could have been caused by abuse or by accident. The following characteristics would tend to imply abuse rather than accident:

- A long unexplained delay between the incident and presentation for treatment (in serious injuries).

- The injuries could not have happened in the way described.
- There may be injuries of different ages.
- There were no witnesses.
- The parents are touchy and hostile and have unrealistic expectations of the child.
- The parents might hint at other problems.

SEXUAL ABUSE

This takes place when an adult forces a child to take part in a sexual activity, using the child to satisfy his or her own sexual desires. This can involve actual sexual contact or exposing children to pornographic videos or magazines. Sexual abusers may be single men who are sexually attracted to children and the theory is that they feel inadequate in relationships with adults of their own age. They are capable of abusing very many children over the course of their adult life.

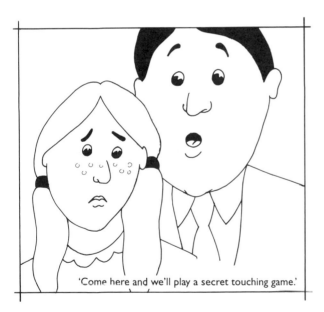

'Come here and we'll play a secret touching game.'

Imprisonment removes such offenders from society, but does not act as a deterrent to their behaviour. Some wish to stop offending but need professional help to do so.

Sexual abuse also occurs within the home. Theories about the origin of the problem relate in some way to the abuse of power, especially by men over their daughters. The pattern of family relationships varies significantly: isolated families in rural areas;

promiscuous families with a wide variety of sexual relationships between the different family members; or apparently highly moralistic and protective families, where the father turns to his daughter for sexual gratification because of marital problems no one wishes to acknowledge.

Sexual abuse can have very damaging and long-lasting effects. Children are confused because of their normal desire for physical affection and they feel that they are to blame for what has happened. They have to be told that they are never to blame. They may grow up feeling worthless and may, as young adults, become abusers themselves.

Finkelhor (1980) identified factors that might place a child at greater risk of sexual abuse. Many abusers are skilful in assessing and exploiting the emotional needs of vulnerable children. Finkelhor's factors include:

- living in a family with a stepfather;
- having lived at some time without the mother;
- not being close to the mother;
- having a mother who had a poor education;
- having no affection from the father;
- having two friends or fewer.

Note the importance of a close relationship with the mother as a protective factor.

THE WAYS IN WHICH ABUSE CAN THREATEN IDENTITY

The following are the ways in which abuse can threaten the identity of children, but adults suffering abuse (e.g. wife battering) will suffer in similar ways.

- Lack of trust in other people.
- Feelings of worthlessness.
- Loss of self-esteem and self-confidence.
- The child may feel he or she is to blame for what happened but is too ashamed to tell anyone for years. But the child's behaviour will still be affected.
- The child becoming an adult will have difficulty forming relationships and may

always expect or even seek out relationships which have an abusing content.

- If there has been no intervention, counselling help or personal reflection on the child's experience he or she may also become an abuser.
- The child is more likely to turn to alcohol or drugs than others.
- The child is more likely than others to turn to crime.

COPING WITH CHILD ABUSE

To cope with the stress of abuse, a child may adopt the following defence mechanisms (see Table 4.3 on page 141):

- *Repression*: A child may push the memory of the abuse out of consciousness, and forget what happened. But the repressed memory will still affect the child's behaviour; the child may, for example suffer recurrent nightmares.
- *Denial*: If a parent or older sibling was involved, a child may deny that anything happened, out of confused loyalty, and a need for security.
- *Displacement*: A child might act out what has happened to him or her with toys or smaller children.
- *Reaction formation*: A child might grow up fearing (in the case of physical or sexual abuse) any kind of physical contact from others at all.

METHODS OF PROTECTION FROM AND PREVENTION OF CHILD ABUSE

B. Gillham (1991) suggests three levels of prevention, particularly relating to child sexual abuse.

Primary prevention
- Increasing awareness of parents, teachers and other carers that child abusers are to be found at all levels of society, are often young or youngish men (and sometimes women), and may be in positions of responsibility towards children or may seek other involvement with children.
- Recognizing that boys are almost as much at risk as girls, *particularly after the age of 10*.
- Teaching children simple rules about dealing with approaches from strangers.
- Teaching children *specific* information about access to private/sexual parts of their body – rules can be made relatively simple.
- Establishing a more conspicuous social vigilance about child sexual abuse so that potential abusers might be deterred.
- Establishing a penal policy which removes from circulation serious and persistent child abusers because they represent a disproportionate and long-term risk to the child population.
- Providing children with education in personal and social relationships so as to sensitize them to interpersonal abuse in all forms.

Secondary prevention
- Creating an atmosphere in schools and families (by formal and informal means) whereby children feel able to report abuse; and providing them with a vocabulary – at least for body parts – which will enable and permit them to disclose abuse they are experiencing.
- Parents, teachers and others *acting* on their suspicions (which may result in *primary* prevention, if a persistent abuser is stopped).
- Teachers, in particular, being alert to signs of sexual abuse in children (principally oblique forms of disclosure) but *not* relying on supposed behavioural or psychological indicators, most of which are non-specific to any etiology, let alone sexual abuse.
- A clear recognition of the fact that children rarely lie about sexual abuse.
- Vigilance in the case of 'at risk' children, especially girls who are not with their natural fathers (an increasingly large category because of current rates of divorce and separation).
- When the offender is in the child's home, *removing him or her*, or, if that is impossible, removing the child.

Tertiary prevention

- Providing a sympathetic, undramatic, supportive response to the disclosure.
- Keeping formal interviewing and 'treatment' to a minimally intrusive level.
- Communicating to children that blame and responsibility are not theirs even if they 'co-operated' or 'consented'.
- Providing counselling services for adults who have current adjustment problems attributable to sexual abuse in childhood.

In a typical Social Services Department today there will be several specially selected and trained social workers working in conjunction with the police. The following outline of the course an investigation into child abuse might follow is taken from Surrey Social Services:

- police and social work team share their information and agree a course of action;
- team interview the informant;
- visit the family;
- seek parental consent to interview the child;
- joint social work/police interview;
- if consent is refused, consider whether a place-of-safety order should be sought and take legal advice about a medical examination;
- interview and take statements from witnesses;
- arrange a medical examination, if necessary;
- interview the suspect, usually at a police station.

For resources in the community for helping with child abuse and other life event threats – refugees, family units, etc. – see the book listed in the References and Resources section at the end of this chapter.

ACTIVITY

Choose one of the life stages described earlier in this chapter, then:

1 Collect as much information as you can about this life stage from newspapers, magazines and textbooks.

2 Prepare a poster illustrating individuals coping successfully/unsuccessfully with this life stage.

3 Find out the names of charities and helping agencies for this age group.

4 Answer the following questions as they apply to your chosen age group:

- What are the problems they most commonly have to deal with?
- Why do these problems arise?
- What help are the agencies able to offer?
- What social changes would the agencies like to see?

Eating disorders

ANOREXIA NERVOSA

Anorexia nervosa is a recognized eating disorder among women today. Between one in 100 and one in 250 women are likely to be affected; sufferers are most frequently found among the higher social classes in the developed world. The disorder is occasionally, but rarely, seen in men (only 10% of sufferers are men).

Anorexia nervosa is characterized by severe weight loss, wilful avoidance of food, and intense fear of being fat. It is popularly, but wrongly, called the 'slimmer's disease'. Features of the disorder are:

- weight loss;
- overactivity and obsessive exercising;
- tiredness and weakness;
- lanugo (baby-like hair on body; thinning of hair on head);
- extreme choosiness over food.

The criteria for diagnosis established by the American Psychiatric Association can be described as follows:

- intense fear of becoming obese which does not diminish as weight loss progresses;

- disturbance of body image, e.g. claiming to feel fat when emaciated;
- weight loss: at least 25% of original pre-illness body weight; or, if under 18 years of age, weight loss from the original pre-illness body weight plus projected weight gain expected from growth charts, which may be combined to make at least 25%;
- refusal to maintain body weight over a minimal normal weight for age and height;
- no physical illness that would account for the weight loss.

The causes of anorexia nervosa are much debated. The following are some theories:

- Dieting is seen by sufferers as a way of controlling their lives.
- Sufferers do not wish to grow up and are trying to keep their childhood shapes. In part, this may be influenced by the media obsession with achieving the 'perfect' (i.e. slim) body and also by the desire to defer the turbulence of adolescence.
- Some specialists see it as a true phobia about putting on weight.
- Feminist writers have suggested that the condition may be related to a new role for women within society.
- The development of eating disorders may be seen as the avoidance of adult sexual feelings and behaviours.
- The individual is over-involved in her or his own family so that when she or he enters adolescence there is a confrontation between the peer group and the family.
- Some specialists believe that the real cause is depression, personality disorder or, rarely, schizophrenia.
- Some doctors point to the hormonal changes related to weight loss and absence of menstruation and regard anorexia nervosa as a physical illness that is caused by a disorder of the hypothalamus (part of the brain concerned with hunger, thirst, and sexual development).

Hospital treatment is often necessary to help the sufferer return to a normal weight. Treatment is usually a combination of:

- a controlled re-feeding programme, sometimes via a naso-gastric tube in severe cases;
- individual psychotherapy;
- family therapy.

Occasionally drug abuse and alcohol abuse also occur and these require specific treatment. Drug treatment may be needed if there is a depressive or other illness.

Psychotherapy may be needed for months or even years after the sufferer has achieved a more normal weight. Relapses are common whenever there is the slightest stress.

About 50% of all patients treated for anorexia nervosa in a hospital continue to have symptoms for many years; 5–10% later die from starvation or suicide.

BULIMIA NERVOSA

Bulimia is often, but not always, a variant of anorexia nervosa. There has been a rise in the number of males suffering from this disorder, although most sufferers are girls or women between the ages of 15 and 30. Bulimia nervosa is characterized by episodes of compulsive overeating usually followed by self-induced vomiting.

As with anorexia, there is no single cause to account for the condition. Many of the theories advanced are linked closely to those put forward to explain anorexia nervosa, and include:

- a morbid fear of fatness;
- a constant craving for food developed after months or years of fasting.

Features of the illness include the following:

- The sufferer may be of normal weight or only slightly underweight.
- Bingeing and vomiting may occur once or several times a day.
- The sufferer may often become clinically depressed and even suicidal.
- In severe cases, repeated vomiting leads to dehydration and loss of the body's vital salts, especially potassium; this may result in weakness and cramps.

- The acid present in gastric juices may damage tooth enamel.

Often the bulimic carries out the bingeing and vomiting in secret, so the main difficulty in treating the illness lies in persuading the sufferer to accept treatment.

- Psychotherapy and/or anti-depressant drugs may be used.
- As with anorexia sufferers, supervision and regulation of eating habits is essential and there is often the need for hospital admission.
- Relapses are common and closely linked to stress.

ACTIVITY

1 Collect as many magazines aimed at women between the ages of 16 and 60, particularly issues for the months January to August, and list and analyse the different 'reducing' diets offered to their readers.

2 Find out how many magazines cater *specifically* for the person trying to slim?

3 Discuss the prevalence of slim role models on film and in television. Would it be 'healthier' if such media reflected society more honestly? NB 40% of adult women in the UK wear size 16 clothes.

Loss and bereavement

He who pretends to look on death without fear lies. All men are afraid of dying, this is the great law of sentient beings, without which the entire human species would soon be destroyed.

(Jean-Jacques Rousseau)

Loss is experienced in many ways, not necessarily involving the death of a loved one:

- growing up involves loss of infancy support networks;
- going to school involves temporary separation from parents;
- changing school involves loss of familiar surroundings.

Obviously, there are corresponding 'gains' here as well, e.g. the child gains new friends and experiences with each change in circumstance. Other life events that involve loss are:

- new siblings (loss of parental attention);
- death of a sibling;
- bereavement, as grandparents grow older and die;
- loss of parent through separation, divorce or death;
- ending or changing relationships;
- unemployment (either parent's, sibling's or one's own);
- miscarriage or stillbirth;
- disability (loss of a sense of the future and of security);
- birth of a handicapped baby (parents may grieve for the 'normal' child they have lost);
- caring for people with dementia or Alzheimer's disease.

Each loss may be seen as a preparation for greater losses. How the individual reacts to the death of a loved one will depend on how they have experienced other losses, their personal characteristics, their religious and cultural background and the support available.

GRIEF

Grief is a normal and necessary response to the death of a loved one. It can be short-lived or last a long time. Grief at the death of a husband, wife or child is likely to be the most difficult to get over. Grief can take the form of several clearly defined stages:

1 *Shock and disbelief.* Numbness and withdrawal from others enables the bereaved person to get through the funeral arrangements and family gatherings. This stage may last from three days to three months.
2 *Denial.* This generally occurs within the first 14 days and can last minutes, hours or

weeks. No loss is acknowledged; the bereaved person behaves as if the dead person were still there. Hallucinations are a common experience; they may consist of a sense of having seen or heard the dead person or of having been aware of his or her presence.

3 *Growing awareness.* Some or all of the following emotions may be felt and each conspires to make many people feel that they are abnormal to experience such harsh emotions:

- Longing: the urge to search, to try to find a reason for the death.
- Anger, directed against any or all of the following: the medical services; the person who caused the death, in case of accident; God for allowing it to happen; the deceased for abandoning them.
- Depression: the pain of the loss is felt, often with feelings of lack of self-worth. Crying, or letting go, usually helps to relieve the stress.
- Guilt: this may be guilt for the real or imagined negligence inflicted on the person who has just died; or the bereaved can feel guilty about his or her own feelings and inability to enjoy life.
- Anxiety, often bordering on panic, as the full impact of the loss is realized. There is worry about the changes and new responsibilities and future loneliness. There may even be thoughts of suicide.

4 *Acceptance.* This usually occurs in the second year, after the death has been re-lived at the first anniversary. The bereaved person is then able to re-learn the world and new situations with its changes without the deceased person.

The most meaningful help that we can give any relative – child or adult – is to share his feelings before the event of death and allow him to work through his feelings, whether they are rational or irrational.

(Elizabeth Kubler-Ross)

Research has shown that counselling can help to reduce the damage to physical and mental health which sometimes follows the loss of a loved one. Most people come through the healing process of grief with the help of relatives and friends. Those who may be in particular need of help are often those:

- with little or no family support;
- with young children;
- who have shown particular distress or suicidal tendencies.

Bereavement counsellors try to establish a warm, trusting relationship with the bereaved person. This is done initially by listening with patience and sympathy; accepting tears as natural and even desirable. Bereavement counselling should not be undertaken by individuals working alone. The support of a group under professional guidance is crucial as close contact with intense grief can be very stressful and emotionally demanding.

HOW TO HELP SOMEONE WHO IS SUFFERING FROM LOSS

- DO be available
- DO let your concern show
- DO allow them to cry if they want
- DO allow them to talk about their loss as much as they want
- DO reassure them that they did everything that they could

- DON'T avoid them because you feel awkward
- DON'T say you know how they feel
- DON'T change the subject when they mention their loss

The following poem was written by 'Kate', who was unable to speak, but was occasionally seen to write. After her death, her locker was emptied and this poem was found. It was first printed in the *Sunday Post* in 1973 and has since appeared in newspapers and magazines all over the world.

KATE

What do you see nurses
What do you see?
Are you thinking
When you are looking at me,
A crabbit old woman
not very wise,
Uncertain of habit
with far-away eyes,
Who dribbles her food
and makes no reply,
When you say in a loud voice
'I do wish you'd try'
Who seems not to notice
the things that you do,
And forever is losing
a stocking or shoe,
Who unresisting or not
lets you do as you will
with bathing and feeding
the long day to fill,
Is that what you're thinking,
is that what you see?
Then open your eyes nurse,
You're not looking at me.
I'll tell you who I am
as I sit here so still,
I'm a small child of ten
with a father and mother,
Brothers and sisters who
love one another,
A young girl of sixteen
with wings on her feet,
Dreaming that soon now
a lover she'll meet;
A bride soon at twenty,
my heart gives a leap,
Remembering the vows
that I promised to keep;
At twenty-five now
I have young of my own
Who need me to build
a secure and happy home.
A young woman of thirty
my young now grow fast,
Bound to each other
with ties that should last;
At forty my young ones

now grown will soon be gone,
But my man stays beside me
to see I don't mourn;
At fifty once more
babies play round my knee,
Again we know children
my loved one and me.
Dark days are upon me,
my husband is dead,
I look at the future
I shudder with dread,
For my young are all busy
rearing young of their own,
And I think of the years
and the love I have known.
I'm an old woman now
and nature is cruel,
'Tis her jest to make
old age look like a fool.
The body it crumbles,
Grave and vigour depart,
There now is a stone
where once I had a heart:
But inside this old carcase
a young girl still dwells,
And now and again
my battered heart swells,
I remember the joys
I remember the pain,
And I'm loving and living
life over again,
I think of the years
all too few – gone too fast,
And accept the stark fact
that nothing can last.
So open your eyes nurses
Open and see,
Not a crabbit old woman
look closer – see ME.

ACTIVITY

1 Explain the idea of loss in its widest sense, giving examples of loss experienced at all life stages.

2 How would you explain the death of a loved grandparent to a child of 6 years?

3 Outline the stages of grief that are normally experienced following a bereavement.

4 Find out about support services for the bereaved in your area.

5 Interview anyone who has suffered a bereavement and make brief notes.

Stress

Many of the stressors mentioned in this section, e.g. bereavement, migration or the birth of a child, involve prolonged, major changes in the patterns of people's lives. The possible negative effects of these changes on both physical and mental health are explored. Stress represents an inadequate adaptation to change, or an unsuccessful attempt on the part of individuals to cope with, and adapt to, the changed circumstances of their lives. The stress response is affected by a number of factors which include:

- the characteristics of the individuals;
- their physical environment;
- the social support available to them;
- their economic status;
- their cultural background.

Not all these factors present as negative factors in relation to the stress response. The importance of each factor lies in each individual's ability to adapt and respond to the stressor.

STRESS AND PERSONALITY

Different people can tolerate different levels of arousal.

At one end of the scale are those who actively seek out maximum stress, who take life-threatening risks, for example stunt performers, racing drivers, mountaineers. Such people are characterized by, among other things, a very low level of anxiety and a high degree of emotional control.

At the other extreme are those who find too much arousal in everyday life and seek to minimize it. Some people who find ordinary life too stressful may develop panic attacks or phobias and need psychological treatment.

Phobias are treated in three ways:

- Systematic desensitization: the client and the therapist draw up a list of frightening situations and put them in order. For example: most frightening – a spider crawling up your skin; least frightening – a spider seen on a TV programme. The client is then trained in relaxation, and if he or she can remain relaxed through the least frightening situation, he or she will move up to a slightly more frightening situation. The process is repeated up the scale.
- Implosion therapy or 'flooding': here the client faces the thing he or she is most frightened of, perhaps is put in a room with some spiders. This provokes a strong emergency reaction but the client cannot flee. Arousal cannot last indefinitely at its maximum level. After a while it will die down and the client will feel calmer and more able to face the thing that frightens him or her.
- Modelling: here the client watches someone dealing confidently with the frightening object – for instance, lifting a spider out of the bath, showing it to children, putting it gently outside. This works best if the model is like the client (similar stage of life, same sex).

Too high arousal – excessive stress – leads to poor performance. Too much stress affects a complex task more than a simple task but very high arousal will affect performance of the simplest task. This relationship between performance and arousal is known as the Yerkes Dodson Law (see Figure 4.2).

ACTIVITY

Too high arousal may be controlled by advance planning and rehearsal of the stressful situation. Levels of arousal are cumulative, so a lot of minor 'hassles' will add to the overall level of arousal.

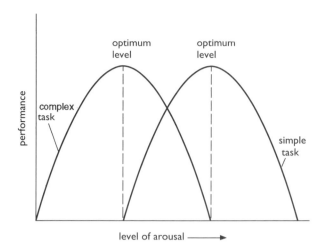

Figure 4.2   The Yerkes–Dobson law of arousal

1 Think of a stressful situation coming up, e.g. important interview, examination, driving test.

2 Think of all the stressful things that have happened in previous interviews and list them.

3 Then make a list of stressful things that might happen, e.g. for an interview:

- *stressful things that happened in previous interviews*: couldn't answer the questions; clothes felt wrong;
- *stressful things that could happen in this interview*: might get up late and miss the bus; might not be able to find the interview room.

4 Go through your lists and work out a way of being absolutely sure that none of these things would actually happen at your important interview.

ACTIVITY

Answer the following questions to clarify the physiological basis of stress.

1 Provide a short definition of biological stress.

2 What is homeostasis? How may the stress reaction be considered as a homeostatic response?

3 List the role of the following in the response of the human body to stress:

- sympathetic nervous system
- hypothalmus of the brain
- pituitary body
- adrenal gland

Draw an annotated diagram to show how the roles of these parts of the body are linked in the reactions to stress.

4 Find ten physiological responses to stress (changes in functions of the body which occur when it is stressed). For each one note how it is brought about. Also show how it is an adaptive response to stress. How does it help the body in stressful situations?

5 These physiological responses of the body to stress may no longer be appropriate to our modern life style. What does this mean?

6 The physiological and biochemical changes that occur in stressful situations may be doing us harm. Note six long term effects of stress; these may be considered as stress-related symptoms and diseases. Show how the symptoms are related to the original response to stress.

THE EFFECT OF LONG-TERM STRESS

H. Seyle (1976) described the changes brought about by stress as the General Adaptation Syndrome. This has three stages:

- *Alarm*: The alarm reaction.
- *Resistance*: If the stressor is not removed the body begins to recover and to cope but there is still a large output of adrenalin.
- *Exhaustion*: The stressor is still not removed

and the body's resources are now becoming depleted (the adrenal gland can no longer function properly; blood glucose levels drop). It is at this stage that psychosomatic disorders develop, for example high blood pressure, ulcers.

HOW WE COPE WITH STRESS

Lazarus and Folkman (1984) found two major forms of coping strategies:

- emotion-focused coping, using ego defence mechanisms;
- problem-focused coping.

Defence mechanisms were introduced earlier in this chapter (see Table 4.3 on page 141). A more detailed description is given in Table 4.4. They are means of emotion-focused coping; while useful in the short term, they are unhealthy and undesirable in the long term.

CASE STUDY 4: A FAMILY UNDER STRESS

A woman describes her situation to a member of the Social Services Department:

I've come with my little one who's having terrible nightmares and wetting the bed. We've got no money, my husband's been made redundant, it's completely changed him, he just sits around watching old films on TV. His temper is terrible too, he keeps shouting and slamming doors. My eldest boy is all right, but they keep ringing up to say he's not attending school, well why should he if there's no jobs to go to afterwards, they're even concerned he might be trying drugs – well, not my boy, I don't believe that – the school just pick on him, his teacher is always criticizing, she's useless. Why don't they think of me? I can't take much more.

Table 4.4 Examples of ego defence mechanisms

Defence mechanism	Description	Example
Repression	Repression of painful or frightening memory out of consciousness (But repressed memories can still affect behaviour)	A child who has been abused may push the memory out of consciousness but then be disturbed for years by bad dreams
Rationalization	Making an excuse and believing it. Not giving the real reason	'I can't speak in public because I've got a cough'
Reaction formation	Concealing a motive from oneself by giving strong expression to the opposite motive	People who crusade with fanatical zeal against loose morals, alcohol etc. may have themselves at one time had difficulty with these problems
Projection	Protects us from recognizing our own undesirable traits by assigning them in exaggerated amounts to other people	'I hate that group of people' becomes 'they hate me'. An element of paranoia and prejudice
Intellectualization	Used to distance oneself suffering	Used by e.g. doctors
Denial	When a reality is too unpleasant to face, an individual may deny it exists	Someone refusing to accept they have a serious illness, or that a relationship is over
Displacement	Choosing a substitute object for expression of feelings	When angry with parents/partner, slam the door or kick the cat
Regression	Returning to an old childhood habit	Eating or curling up in bed when upset
Sublimation	Finding a substitute activity to express an unacceptable impulse. This is a constructive defence mechanism and could be called problem-focused	Rechannelling aggression by playing sport

ACTIVITY

1 Read case study 4 of a family trying to deal with its problems using emotion-focused coping.

2 Identify the defence mechanisms being used by the family members.

3 What are the possible strengths in this family?

4 What might a counsellor suggest as more conscious and constructive ways of dealing with their problems?

Role-play is a possibility here (for example, one person could take the role of the mother and one person could take the role of the counsellor).

Table 4.5

Coping mechanism	Description
Objectivity	Separating feelings from thoughts
Logical analysis	Analysing problems; making plans
Concentration	Putting aside upsetting thoughts to concentrate on the matter in hand
Empathy	Seeing how others feel in a situation and taking account of this
Suppression	*Not* repression: this is holding feelings back consciously until the time is right to express them
Substitution of thoughts and emotions	*Consciously* to substitute thoughts for how we really think in order to deal with a difficult situation

PROBLEM-FOCUSED COPING

These are *conscious* ways of trying to adapt to stress in a positive and constructive way. They include:

- searching for information;
- problem solving;
- seeking help from others;
- recognizing true feelings;
- establishing goals and objectives.

Grasha (1983) described the problem-focused mechanisms as in Table 4.5.

PATIENTS UNDER STRESS

Carers both in hospital and at home should be aware of the factors causing stress in a patient's life. Admission to hospital (even a planned admission may be stressful) may entail any or all of the following stressors:

- unexpected events, if admission is as a result of an accident or sudden illness;
- unpleasant symptoms, e.g. pain or vomiting;
- loss of function, e.g. loss of mobility or sensation;
- loneliness;
- unfamiliar surroundings and relationships;
- altered status and role.

ACTIVITY

See how many stressors you can identify in a patient or client. Record your observations, remembering to preserve confidentiality.

There are many ways in which a carer can reduce the harmful effects of these stressors:

- Give patients information about their environment and what will happen to them. However busy a ward is, time must be allowed to welcome patients; to show them where their 'home' will be and where they can find facilities, e.g. toilet, telephone, assistance.
- Promote understanding of the patient's physical and psychological symptoms. Medical jargon should be translated into simple-to-understand language.
- Offer treatment to alleviate symptoms. Many carers now appreciate the benefit

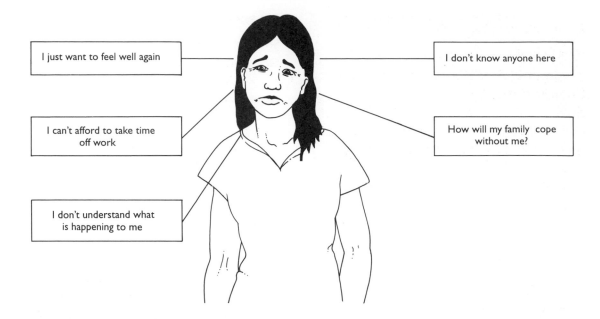

I just want to feel well again

I don't know anyone here

I can't afford to take time off work

How will my family cope without me?

I don't understand what is happening to me

of a more holistic approach and can offer massage, aromatherapy, and other relaxation techniques.

- Offer support and companionship with others. Most patients gain valuable support from those with similar problems. 'A problem shared is a problem halved.'
- Suggest different and more positive ways of perceiving what is happening to the patient.
- Provide aids to increase physical strength and functioning. Physiotherapists and occupational therapists are trained in methods of enabling patients to regain function following a stroke or visiting the patient's home prior to discharge to install physical aids such as grip rails in the bathroom.

It is essential that *all* advice given to patients is closely monitored by trained personnel.

RELATIVES UNDER STRESS

Most of the stressors described above are felt equally by relatives, who may be unable to visit their loved one as often as they would wish and who perceive hospital as a strange and threatening environment.

Carers can minimize their stress:

- simply by showing relatives that the patient

is being cared for as well as possible;
- by explaining everything that is being done for the patient;
- by asking the relative how he or she is feeling.

Relatives undertaking individual care at home may be under more stress. There are many reasons for this:

- feeling inadequate, i.e. lacking the expertise to interpret symptoms or to relieve pain when oral medication fails;
- fatigue – sleep may be interrupted by the patient's poor sleep patterns or hallucinations;
- guilt – if the carer can no longer cope, then the relative may have to be admitted into hospital.

The community nursing staff can help by regular visits to give both practical help and advice and by being on call to sort out problems, e.g. with medication.

ACTIVITY

In each of the following case studies:

1 Identify the stresses each person mentioned would be under.

2 Indicate how carers can help.

CASE STUDY A

A woman aged 38 is living in a high-rise flat in an inner-city area. She has three children aged 5, 6 and 10. She works part-time. She lives close to her mother who is now restricted to a wheelchair due to a recent accident. She calls on her mother regularly. Her mother used to help her with baby-sitting. Her husband's firm is under threat of closure and he may face redundancy as a consequence. She is going into hospital shortly for a hysterectomy.

CASE STUDY B

A young couple aged 32 and 35 have two children, a son of 3 and a daughter of 1½. Both of them are engaged in demanding professions – the husband is a solicitor and the wife is an advertising executive. They live near a country town and are very independent, as they have no relatives living nearby. They have had a live-in nanny to look after the children.

CASE STUDY C

A father aged 48 has two boys of 9 and 11. They go to a local primary school. The mother died two months ago after having been in hospital for two years. They live on a housing estate.

CASE STUDY D

A woman of 52 and her husband, aged 54, are both from a West Indian background. The husband works locally in a government office. She works part-time in a department store. They have four children, three daughters and one son. The father is very authoritarian. The eldest daughter has become very independent. She works in a bank and has married an English boy. The parents are not happy about this situation and as a consequence have become very strict with the other two daughters. Their son, aged 13, has developed a kidney problem and is likely to require regular hospital visits.

STRESS-RELATED ILLNESS

Stress and how we manage our own stress levels has a direct link to our general well-being. Various illnesses may be said to be either caused or triggered by stress, including:

- Stomach ulcers, which may sometimes be caused by too much acid being produced in the stomach at a time of anxiety or worry.
- Heart attacks: it is thought that the fat released into the bloodstream when the body responds to demands gets trapped in the walls of the heart's own vessels. This gradually narrows these tubes, and when increased demand is placed on the heart, the narrowed tubes prevent the flow of oxygen, causing the heart muscle to die.
- Skin disorders such as eczema and psoriasis.
- Myalgic encephalomyelitis (ME): the role of stress has been well documented in this very distressing condition.

Myalgic encephalomyelitis is sometimes called post-viral fatigue syndrome. In April 1990, it was estimated that 150,000 people in the UK were affected by ME, and studies affirmed that people in the caring professions made up the largest group affected, with three times as many women as men suffering from ME. Thus the label 'yuppie flu' was given to ME by the press, although it was rejected by ME victims as insulting. The media have given relatively little attention to ME compared with other illnesses affecting a similar proportion of the population.

No one definite cause is known, but theories have suggested the following:

- persistent viral infection;
- damage to the immune system following a viral infection;
- a neurotic disorder, e.g. hyperventilation.

The main symptoms are:

- muscle fatigue
- exhaustion
- headaches

- dizziness

Other symptoms common to many people with ME are:

- muscular pains
- fever
- depression
- bowel and digestive problems

There is no diagnostic test, although enteroviruses can be traced in the colon of more than half of ME sufferers. Diagnosis is by process of elimination of other illnesses and diseases.

The medical profession has little to offer in terms of scientific explanation or treatment of ME. The following treatments are among the more common:

- Anti-depressants: these are often prescribed, but the long-term use of these drugs is not recommended.
- A sugar- and yeast-free diet: many sufferers follow this, in common with sufferers from *Candida Albicans*, a yeast infection of the gut. It is thought that stress can lead to a weakening of the immune system, thus allowing this infection to flourish.
- Relaxation techniques such as meditation, the Alexander technique and yoga are often practised.
- Homoeopathy.
- Acupuncture.
- Herbal treatments, with e.g. evening primrose oil.
- Counselling: this can enable a person to lead a less stressful lifestyle, thereby reducing his or her propensity to further bouts of ME.

CASE STUDY 5: HOLLY

Before becoming ill with ME, Holly, aged 32, had led an active life both at work as a social worker and outside her job, having many interests which occupied most of her spare hours. She made little time for relaxation and her diet was high in sugar and carbohydrates. Her emotional history had been stressful. When she became ill, she suffered from most of the common symptoms of ME and was bedridden for three months. After numerous setbacks and relapses, she is now in the fifth year of her illness and has used diet, homoeopathy, herbal treatments and counselling as her path to recovery. The most difficult experiences for Holly were the financial implications of being ill. She lost her job and has been living on state benefits; she has found her practical circumstances difficult to reconcile with her need for relaxation and a reduction in stress. After five years out of work it will be difficult for her to find a job, particularly with this history of ill-health. She says that counselling has empowered her to face the stresses and difficulties which the future might hold, without becoming ill again.

ACTIVITY

Study Holly's story, then answer the following questions:

1 What advice and recommendations should be made to a person with ME pre-disposal factors, to avoid contracting ME?

2 What support should be made available to people with ME by (a) the NHS; (b) the DSS; (c) the workplace; (d) friends and family?

3 Many ME sufferers feel isolated as there is still a lot of ignorance about the illness. How could this be combated?

THE RELATIONSHIP OF SOCIAL AND ECONOMIC FACTORS TO HEALTH

The political context

With politicians arguing that the amount of money which can be spent on health and social care services for people is limited, pressing questions on the relationship between health and social and economic circumstances become a prominent element in public and political debates. For example:

- What are the choices, or lack of them, which arise for individuals and families in relation to their health as a result of the income and other ECONOMIC RESOURCES (savings, winnings, inheritance, etc.) available to them?
- Can people be said to be contributing to their own ill-health by choosing to spend their money on an unhealthy lifestyle, by making the wrong choices in their diet and by showing a defeatist and passive response to difficult life situations?
- Alternatively, how might people's health be affected by social and economic factors outside their control?
- Even if there were total agreement upon what a healthy lifestyle was, would everyone be equally able to choose to follow it?
- What impact could differing levels of income and economic resources have on people's lifestyles, their resulting health and their ability to cope with life-event threats?

Government health education campaigns have generally targeted the individual and his or her lifestyle, exhorting us to exercise more frequently, eat less fat, avoid dangerous drugs and so on: in other words, implying that good health is to a very great extent within the grasp of anyone.

In Britain the right of everyone to health care is increasingly being questioned, raising ethical dilemmas for medical and social workers about who should be treated or helped. Two articles reproduced here illustrate some of the current debates:

BEING ECONOMICAL WITH HEALTH

I am a first year undergraduate at the London School of Economics. I receive a London weighted grant of £2,845. In January I was diagnosed as having a kidney disease and a leaking heart valve and I have to take prescribed medication indefinitely. Also, my heart complaint means that I have to take prescribed antibiotics prior to dental treatment.

In the summer I have to make two visits to London to see consultants which will cost over £30 in rail fares. I did apply for help with NHS costs but as one who is not the 'most vulnerable' I have to pay £4.25 per prescription, dental charges up to £60 per course of treatment and travel costs up to £21 per week. Your leader writer is obviously not in my shoes. When s/he writes (May 21) that they have 'no quarrel' with prescription charges of £4.25.

(letter to the Guardian, 25 May 1993)

HEART SURGERY COULD BE LIMITED TO NON-SMOKERS

More hospitals are likely to adopt a formal policy of limiting vital heart surgery to non-smokers because of financial pressures and increasing waiting lists, a leading specialist on medical ethics said yesterday.

Commenting on reports that heart surgeons in Manchester and Leicester are turning away smokers who refuse to give up, Dr Richard Nicholson said: 'This is not surprising. In the long term it is the kind of decision that will be made much more frequently as the pressure on society not to waste health-care resources increases'. Similar policies are already in operation informally in hospitals around the country.

Dr Nicholson, editor of the *Bulletin of Medical Ethics*, said such policies were similar to those adopted in the early days of liver transplants, when alcoholics were excluded. 'It is an interesting ethical question for much wider debate', he said.

In a letter to the *British Medical Journal*, the Manchester surgeons said treating smokers was 'pointless'. They spend longer in hospital, were less likely than smokers to make a full recovery and more likely to need another operation.

(The Independent, 24 May 1993)

ACTIVITY

1 The letter to the *Guardian* reproduced in the text was written in response to government proposals in May 1993 to increase prescription charges to £4.25 per item. In what way does this writer believe that his or her ability to maintain his/her health is affected by his/her income?

2 What other groups (besides students) in the population of this country may face difficulties in paying for health and welfare services if they are not provided free of charge?

3 Investigate and make a list of charges which are now made for health services and treatments within the NHS – for example, many dentists now refuse to take on new NHS patients and most dental treatments other than routine check-ups for adults now involve charges for most patients.

4 The article about heart surgery from the *Independent* quotes some Manchester surgeons as saying that 'treating smokers was "pointless" '. Do you agree that treatment should be withheld from those who could be argued to have contributed to their own ill-health?

5 Arrange a debate along the lines of question 4, both immediately before and after embarking upon a study of this unit of work. In discussing the issues raised above, sociological evidence relating to income, class, poverty and unemployment will be discussed.

Differences in income, economic resources and wealth

A wide range of official reports covering the distribution of income, of personal wealth,

of work and earnings and of the regional distribution of income all confirm that the gap between the rich and the poor in Britain is growing wider.

In their book, *Income, Poverty and Wealth*, Thomas Stark and Giles Wright use official statistics and the results of government surveys to show how, throughout the 1980s, the share of disposable income taken by the top 10% of the population has steadily risen while the poorest fifth of all households suffered a fall in their average income between 1987 and 1989. This trend was confirmed by a Labour Commission on Social Justice report in July 1993 which suggests that nearly two-thirds of the population has an income below the family average of £250 a week and that extremes of income are wider than at any time since 1886.

There are also marked and widening regional differences in average household income. Greater London in the late 1980s was

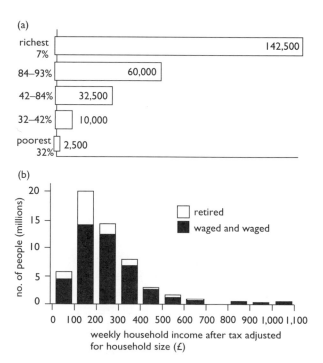

Figure 4.3   Wealth and income distribution
Source: *Guardian*, 20 July 1993; wealth statistics from Inland Revenue, income distribution statistics from Institute for Public Policy Research.

the most prosperous region, with average incomes 26% above the national average. At the other end of the scale, the least well-off regions – namely Northern Ireland and Wales – had average incomes only 73% and 82% respectively of the national average.

Personal wealth remains concentrated among the richest 10% of the population.

Poverty

There is no official definition of poverty. Two poverty lines drawn from official and quasi-official data are commonly used:

- Income Support level;
- 50% of average income after housing costs.

In her book, *Poverty: The Facts*, Carey Oppenheim suggests that:

- Using either poverty line, between 11 million and 12 million people in the UK were living in poverty in 1988/9.
- In 1988/9, 4.4 million people were living below the level of the government's 'safety net' of Income Support. A principal reason for this is the low take-up of benefits. According to government figures, one in four of those eligible for Income Support do not claim it and around one in two do not claim Family Credit to which they are entitled.
- Certain groups face especially high risks of poverty: 50% of lone-parent families, 42% of single pensioners, 69% of families where the breadwinner(s) are unemployed and 26% of families with an adult in part-time work lived in poverty (defined as below 50% of average income after housing costs) in 1988/9. There are no poverty figures broken down by ethnic origin, but Afro-Caribbeans and Asians have much higher rates of unemployment and are more likely to have low wages or to rely on inadequate benefits.
- Between 1979 and 1988/9 the composition of the poorest 10% of the population changed: pensioners fell from 31% to 14% of the poorest 10%; families with children grew from 50% to 54%; and single people without children more than doubled from 10% to 22%.

ACTIVITY

Examine the points made about those in poverty.

1 Work out what proportion of the total population of the UK are below the 'poverty line'.

2 Suggest reasons why the take-up of benefits is low.

3 Why do certain groups face a higher risk of poverty than others?

4 What factors could account for the changing composition of the poorest 10%?

Children are more at risk of poverty than the rest of society. Children growing up in lone-parent families have a much higher risk of poverty. In 1989, over three-quarters (76%) of children in lone-parent families – 1.4 million – were living in poverty (defined as on or below Income Support level), compared to 13% of children in two-parent families – 1.35 million.

Women are more at risk of poverty than men. The Child Poverty Action Group estimates that in 1989 around 5.1 million women were living in poverty (defined as on or below Income Support level), compared to 3.4 million men. Low wages, lone parenthood and inadequate social security benefits and childcare provision all contribute to women's poverty.

ACTIVITY

The statistics quoted here give only the briefest introduction to the debate about

---

levels of income, wealth and inequality in Britain. Use secondary sources to investigate these issues in more depth.

How have these factors been studied in relation to health?

The broad conclusion of most studies investigating the relationship between levels of income, economic resources and health is that deprivation and inequality in income, housing and employment status contribute to inequalities in health. Key pieces of research include the Black Report on *Inequalities in Health* (1980), *The Health Divide* by the Health Education Council (1987) and *The Nation's Health* (1988). (For details see the References list at the end of the chapter; see also Chapter 5.)

Drawing mainly on data published in the 1970s, the Black Report concluded that despite the existence for more than thirty years of a health service expressly committed to offering equal care for all, there remained a marked class gradient in standards of health, with substantial increases in the rates of both mortality and morbidity (illness) as one moves down the social class scale from class I (professional workers) to class V (unskilled manual workers). Moreover, not only did the report draw attention to the large inequalities in health between the social classes, it also argued that these differences were not declining. Indeed, the report pointed out that social class differentials in mortality, as measured by standardised mortality ratios (SMRs), had *increased* since the 1930s.

The extent of the class inequalities in health was perhaps most dramatically illustrated by the calculation of what the Black Report called 'excess deaths'. Using data for England and Wales, it calculated that if classes IV and V had had the same mortality rate as class I, then during the three-year period from 1970–72, the lives of 74,000 people under the age of seventy-five would not have been lost. This estimate included the 'excess' deaths of almost 10,000 children.

(Waddington 1989)

SOCIAL CLASS is the most widely used indicator of the social and economic circumstances of individuals. In the study of health inequalities, social class is used to show how social and economic circumstances are related to the health experiences and expectations of individuals.

There are different ways of defining social class, but for the purposes of research, social scientists carrying out large-scale research have tended to measure social class in terms of one single factor: OCCUPATION.

The Black Report and many other pieces of research have used occupational class scales such as the Registrar-General's Scale.

Table 4.6 Registrar-General's classification of social class

Social class		Examples of occupations
I	Professional	Lawyer, doctor
II	Intermediate	Teacher, nurse, manager
III(NM)	Skilled non-manual	Typist, shop assistant
III(M)	Skilled manual	Miner, cook, electrician
IV	Semi-skilled manual	Farm worker, packer
V	Unskilled manual	Cleaner, labourer

According to this classification:

- Men are allocated a social class according to their own occupation.
- Married women are ascribed the social class of their husband.
- Children in two-parent families are ascribed the social class of their father.
- Single women living alone, or with their children, are allocated a social class according to their own occupation.

As Clare Blackburn writes, many criticisms have been directed at the use of this measurement of class:

Some groups are poorly described by measures of social class based on occupations, for example, those who have never had a job, those who do not have a job now and married women who are classified according to their husband's social class.

The Registrar-General's classification is based on a hierarchy that reflects the traditional status of male occupations. It does not always accurately reflect the status or experiences associated with women's occupations.

It ascribes to all members of the same family the same social class. Thus it fails to recognize that some members of a family may experience poorer social and economic circumstances than others.

Social-class measures do not reflect that social class experiences are different for Black people and white people, just as they are for men and women.

(Blackburn 1991)

Other researchers have also suggested that there is a need to find better measures of inequality in populations. Illsley has suggested that the top 20% of the population should be compared with the bottom 20%. Others have argued that large-scale research should at least be supplemented with smaller-scale studies which look in more depth at how inequalities are generated and sustained in everyday life.

ACTIVITY

1 Do you consider yourself as belonging to a particular social class? If so, which one? Use this question to start a discussion about people's definitions of class. How could or should it be defined?

2 There is no official definition of poverty. Would you agree with the definitions of poverty adopted in Oppenheim's study (those relying on Income Support or those who receive only 50% of the average national income after housing costs)?

3 The following is one attempt by social scientists to draw up a list of conditions which could be held to represent

'underprivilege' (the Jarman 8 underprivileged area index). The more factors which apply to a household from the list, the more likely they are to be underprivileged. Do you agree that this list could be a useful way to measure underprivilege? Could you write a better one?

- elderly living alone
- under five years old
- one-parent household
- unskilled head of household
- unemployed
- lacking exclusive use of a basic amenity
- a household with more than one person per room
- has moved house within twelve months
- was born in the New Commonwealth or Pakistan

Trends in income, class and health

- At almost every age, people in the poorer social classes (IV and V) have higher rates of illness and death than people in wealthier social classes (I and II).
- A study by Smith *et al.* 1990, reported in the *British Medical Journal*, argued that the disparity in death rates between the social classes is widening and that as changes in income distribution continue to occur, such disparities can be expected to increase. Good health and longevity are most directly related to levels of affluence.
- Blaxter (1990), analysing data from the Health and Lifestyles Survey, has found that the apparent strong association between social class and health was primarily one of income and health. Other studies have shown how changes in income levels can correlate with changes in health. This may explain how social class differences in health can widen, despite rises in absolute income and living standards. Around the

year 1950, the proportion of the population living in relative poverty was at its lowest level since 1921, with only 8% of the population living in relative poverty. By 1987 the number of people living in poverty had risen to 28% of the population. With overall rises in living standards over the century, death rates for the poor have not fallen as fast as death rates for the rich. Being healthy seems, then, to require a level of income which allows families to enjoy similar living standards and participate in a similar way as families with higher incomes (adapted from Blackburn 1991).

The following trends are taken from Blackburn (1991):

- In 1986, babies born to social class IV and V families were 148% more likely to die in the perinatal period than babies born to social class I and II families.
- In 1986, babies born to parents in social classes IV and V had a 178% greater chance of dying in the post-neonatal period than babies of social class I and II parents.
- Two-thirds of all low-birth-weight babies are born to working-class mothers.
- The mortality rate for all causes of death tells us that children aged 1–5, from social classes IV and V, are twice as likely to die as their counterparts from social classes I and II.
- Large-scale longitudinal studies show that children from manual classes suffer more respiratory infections and diseases, ear infections and squints, and are likely to be of shorter stature than their counterparts in non-manual classes.
- Children from manual social classes are also more likely to have less healthy teeth. In 1983, children from manual social classes had twice as many decayed teeth as their counterparts in non-manual classes.
- Surveys indicate that class inequalities in health experiences between classes are greatest for limiting long-standing illnesses, with unskilled manual classes

reporting rates that are double those of professional classes, less steep for long-standing illness and only evident for acute illness reporting at age 45 and over.

ACTIVITY

1 Carry out research, using secondary sources, into the differences in levels of MORBIDITY and MORTALITY by social class for illnesses not mentioned here, such as cancers, heart disease, high blood pressure, obesity, arthritis, haemorrhoids, alcohol-related disease and mental illness.

2 What possible explanations can there be for the trends illustrated above?

Unemployment and health

Most research shows beyond doubt that there is an association between unemployment and ill-health. Mortality rates, rates of long-standing illness, rates of disability and rates of psychological disturbance have all been shown to be higher among the unemployed than among those with jobs. A higher risk of suicide and diseases such as stomach ulcers have also been traced in part to the effect of unemployment.

Ill-health may occur as a result of:

- the threat of job loss;
- the actual event;
- the state of being out of work.

ACTIVITY

An important question, of course, is whether poor health leads to or results in unemployment or whether the reverse effect occurs. Read the extract below and discuss the issue in relation to this case.

When news filtered through last May of possible mine closures – Westoe among them, Mr Frelford, whose job was looking after the skip-loading plant, started to worry.

Work was hard to come by in a borough where unemployment is 26.7 per cent. There was a time when he might have got a job in the shipyards as an electrician, but Swan Hunter's failure to win a £170 million contract for a Royal Navy helicopter carrier ruled that out. Younger men might retrain, but he was 39. Colleagues took jobs as security guards, or cleaners for £1.60 an hour – but they worked 80-hour weeks, and he had a family.

Black October came and went. The 800 miners at Westoe were told that the colliery might shut in six weeks or six months. Some were ecstatic: they were the older ones, looking forward to a handsome redundancy payoff and an early retirement. Mr Frelford did not take the news well. For the next six months of uncertainty he suffered from not being able to plan, of thinking 'this week is the last week'.

There were reports that he had taken time off work for 'anxiety', that he had had a breakdown and been taken into hospital.

He came back to work looking normal. He worked as conscientiously as ever. 'But it played on his mind,' said Michael Meughen, 44, a colleague. 'It must have done. But I didn't know anything about it.'

He was the kind of man who drank three pints at most, exchanged a few words about football and then went off home to the wife.

Last Wednesday, David Frelford took his children to school, as he did every day, and went in to see John Pattinson, Mowbray Junior School's headteacher. 'He was showing genuine concern about Jack', said Mr Pattinson. 'There were no problems mentioned. I knew he had been made redundant . . . but he seemed perfectly happy.'

On Thursday morning, David Frelford dropped his children off, went home, put the chain on the front door and bolted the back door at the top and bottom. Then he wrote a note, climbed the stairs, went into the bathroom, poured petrol over his clothes and, with a match, set himself alight.

Independent, 24 May 1993

Housing and health

People who live in unhealthy homes usually suffer from other forms of social and economic disadvantage, so it becomes difficult to disentangle the effect of housing conditions on health from other factors. Moreover, there may be links between housing conditions and health not necessarily linked to poverty. For example, it has been suggested that the trend towards centrally heated homes with fitted carpets has increased the likelihood of allergies resulting from 'dust mites'.

Nevertheless, the strong relationship between health and housing can be related to four aspects of that housing:

- geographical location – where people live;
- patterns of tenure;
- the poor layout and design of homes;
- costs of fuel and other essential services.

GEOGRAPHICAL LOCATION

Low-income families, especially one-parent families and black families, are much more likely to be housed in neighbourhoods that are unattractive, densely populated, with poorly maintained houses and few communal areas and amenities.

The concept of ENVIRONMENTAL POVERTY can be used to refer to housing areas where there is a lack of, or lack of access to, gardens, parks, play space, shopping facilities, health centres, etc. Pollution from noise, litter, dirt and airborne pollutants such as metal particles (e.g. lead) can also be a factor in environmental pollution in inner cities and areas near industrial plants. Psychological and stress-related illnesses may be higher in environmentally poor areas along with respiratory illnesses, chesty coughs, etc. Infections caused by poor hygiene facilities may also be increased.

Child accident rates are higher among poorer social groups and can be linked to the difficulties of supervising children in environmentally poor areas. The Child Accident Prevention Trust estimates that

250,000 childhood accidents a year can be attributed to bad housing design.

Homelessness may be considered under this heading. Surveys of the living conditions of families in hotel accommodation and their health status (see Table 4.7) show that this accommodation is often overcrowded and insanitary with poor access to cooking facilities.

In 1990 there were 55,300 families officially classed as homeless by local authorities and placed in temporary accommodation.

Table 4.7

	1966	1990/91
Number sleeping rough	683	2,703
Households in temporary accommodation	2,558	55,300
Mortgages 6–12 months in arrears	N/A	162,210
Estimated number of homes considered unfit	2m	1m
'Hidden' households (estimate of households sharing with another host household)	N/A	760,000
Percentage of government expenditure on housing	5.3	2.6
House completions:		
Local authority	157,000	13,434
Private sector	157,000	130,132

Source: Shelter

PATTERNS OF TENURE

Research shows that owner-occupiers are likely to have the lowest death rates and council tenants the highest. A study by Kogevina (1990) showed that male council-house tenants were more likely to die from cancer of the face, oesophagus, stomach, larynx, bladder and lungs, and women tenants were especially more likely to die from cancer of the cervix, than owner-occupiers.

Damp is a major health hazard in certain types of rented accommodation, especially when families cannot afford to heat their homes. Spores from fungi in damp or dilapidated housing appear to lead to a greater frequency of respiratory symptoms, e.g. wheezing, runny noses, sore throats, headaches, fever and irritability. If children are adversely affected, their progress and development at school may also be impeded by frequent absence. Certain viruses also appear to thrive in damp conditions.

POOR LAYOUT AND DESIGN OF HOMES

Children who live in flats have higher incidences of respiratory infections than children who live in houses.

People who live in flats have higher incidences of emotional disturbances and mental health problems. Parents worry about the safety of their children. Vandalism, graffiti, racial and sexual attacks are increased where flat or block design is poor and there is no clear responsibility for communal areas or walkways.

People with disabilities often have great difficulty adapting small houses to their needs: for example, rooms are often too small to accommodate wheelchairs.

Lack of privacy and storage space in overcrowded homes can lead to considerable domestic tensions and physical and psychological problems.

COST OF FUEL AND OTHER ESSENTIAL SERVICES

Where low income affects housing choice, it also affects the 'choice' of fuel for many families. Owner-occupiers may more often be able to choose the form of heating they prefer. Tenants usually cannot. Fuel bills are often high because of damp conditions, condensation and poor insulation. They usually account for a greater proportion of the expenditure of low-income families than of higher-income families. They are often a major source of debt; gas disconnection rates have risen since 1981. A newer source of debt and disconnection for lower-income families is failure to pay water rates. With rising rates of water disconnections in the news, some people are asking whether this may soon become an additional and serious source of health risk to low-income families.

Physiological, psychological and behavioural effects of poverty

The following outlines a few of the main effects on health of low income, poverty and lack of economic resources. It should be used as a basis only for further discussion and research.

PHYSIOLOGICAL EFFECTS: POVERTY AND DIET

In June 1991 the National Children's Home charity commissioned a survey on the eating habits of low-income families in Britain. The results suggested that one in five parents regularly denied themselves food through lack of money, and one in ten children under the age of five went without enough to eat at least once a month. The report claimed to have found a direct relationship between those on the lowest income and those with the poorest diet.

Studies such as these have often provoked politicians into claiming that, with careful planning and shopping, one could eat a very healthy diet on Income Support levels.

PSYCHOLOGICAL EFFECTS

Poverty appears to increase the number of stressful life events for families and makes it more difficult to overcome the stresses.

Poverty can mean relative powerlessness and lack of control over events which can increase a sense of helplessness and depressive illness.

The coping mechanisms to which people may resort to overcome stress may lead to worse problems, e.g. drug abuse, heavy consumption of alcohol, smoking.

BEHAVIOURAL EFFECTS

Here we return to the questions posed at the beginning of this section. The poor are often chastised and urged to act more responsibly by choosing healthier lifestyles and behaviours.

Is this a realistic and fair criticism?

ACTIVITY

Politicians often claim that it is possible to eat healthily on Income Support level.

1 How far do you agree with this claim?

2 In a group in your school or college, design a diet to feed yourselves for three or four weeks on the amount of money you would have if you were on Income Support.

REFERENCES AND RESOURCES

Atkinson, R.L. (1993), *Introduction to Psychology*, 11th ed. US: Harcourt Brace Jovanovich College Publishers.

Black Report (1980), *Inequalities in Health*. London: Penguin.

Blackburn, C. (1991), *Poverty and Health: Working with Families*. Oxford: OUP.

Dobraszczyc, U. (1989), *Sickness, Health and Medicine*, Sociology in Focus series. London: Longman.

Eysenck, H. (1991), *Know Your Own Personality*. London: Penguin.

Gillham, B. (1991), *The Facts about Child Sexual Abuse*. London: Cassell Educational.

Gross, R. (1992), *Psychology: The Science of Mind and Behaviour*, 2nd ed. Sevenoaks: Hodder and Stoughton.

Hayes, N. (1984), *A First Course in Psychology*. Walton-on-Thames: Nelson.

Hayes, N. and Orrell, S. (1993), *Psychology: An Introduction*, 2nd ed. London: Longman.

Health Education Council (1987), *The Health Divide*. London: HEC.

Jones, D.N. and Pickett, J. (1993), *Understanding Child Abuse*, 2nd ed. London: Macmillan Educational.

Leach, Penelope, 'Should parents hit their children?' in *The Psychologist*, vol. 6, no. 5, May 1993.

Oppenheim, C. (1993), *Poverty: The Facts*. London: Child Poverty Action Group.

Robertson, J. and J. (1989), *Separation and the Very Young*. London: Free Association Books.

Rutter, M. (1988), *Maternal Deprivation Re-assessed*. London: Penguin.

Social Services Yearbook 1993. London: Longman Community Information and Reference.

Tucker, N. (1990), *Adolescence*. London: Wayland.

Waddington, I. (1989), 'Inequalities in Health', *Social Studies Review*, January.

HEALTH PROMOTION

HEALTH AWARENESS

What is health?

The World Health Organization defines health as 'a state of complete physical, mental and social well-being and not merely the absence of disease or infirmity'.

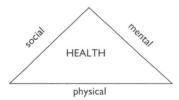

Figure 5.1   The three aspects of health

A person can be described as healthy provided the three sides of the triangle – social, mental, physical – remain intact; if the natural equilibrium is damaged then a state of ill-health, often only temporary, results.

The risks to health in society today differ greatly from those of the past. Diseases which were once major threats to life at all stages have been either eradicated or controlled:

- *Smallpox*: More than half the people of Europe would probably have had smallpox in their lifetime before Edward Jenner discovered the remedy, vaccination, in 1796.
- *Cholera*: the Public Health Acts in the 1870s halted the spread of cholera in the UK by improving water supplies and sewage disposal.
- *Tuberculosis*: in 1862 Robert Koch isolated the TB bacillus, leading to the development

of a vaccine. (However, this disease is once again increasing in the 1990s, both in the developed and in developing countries – see Chapter 3).

- *Diphtheria*: The anti-toxin was first used in 1890. Before then, death from diphtheria was common (see Figure 5.2).

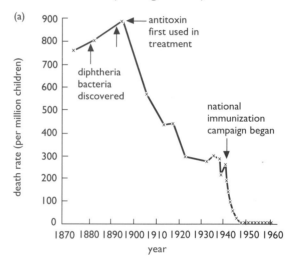

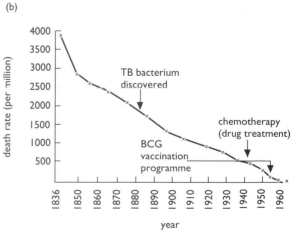

Figure 5.2   Decline in annual death rate from (a) diphtheria and (b) tuberculosis, England and Wales

Source: L. Hartley, *History of Medicine* (Blackwell).

Health problems today

Medical advances such as the development of new drugs, improved health services and high technology have not managed to deal with a new generation of diseases – the CHRONIC DEGENERATIVE DISEASES:

- heart disease
- cancers
- stroke
- arthritis

All these represent the effect of wear and tear on the human body. In addition, new bacteria and viruses have emerged within the last 20 years:

- legionnaire's disease
- campylobacter enteritis
- helicobacter pylori gastritis (duodenal ulcer)
- human immuno-deficiency virus (HIV-AIDS)
- bacterial spongiform encephalitis (BSE)

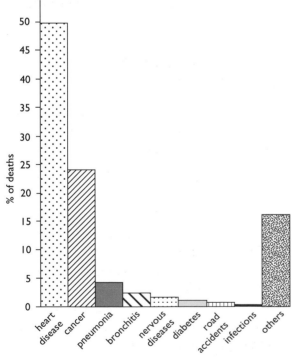

Figure 5.3 Causes of death in Britain in the 1980s
Source: L. Hartley, *History of Medicine* (Blackwell).

Health education

Health education is a method of self-empowerment, i.e. it enables people to take more control over their own health, and over the factors which affect their health. HEALTH PROMOTION is a term used to include all aspects of health education, but placing greater emphasis on changes in health policy and POSITIVE HEALTH as opposed to the rather negative prevention of ill-health.

The nursing profession has evolved over the last two decades into a research-based profession; care plans and nursing procedures are continually modified to take account of the latest research findings. Health promoters need access to all kinds of health information before they can identify the needs, goals and methods appropriate to their task.

ACTIVITY

1 Who are the health promoters in society?

2 How much should society interfere with the freedom of the individual, e.g. smoking at work, the sale of alcohol at concerts etc.?

3 How effective do you think the shock-horror tactics were of the campaigns popular in the 1970s and 1980s, e.g. pictures of cancerous lungs and photos of emaciated drug addicts? Discuss the campaigns memorable to you and the reasons for their success.

During the latter part of the twentieth century, the shift of emphasis has moved from cure to prevention.

Effects of lifestyle on health

It is now recognized that people's lifestyles and behaviour are causative factors in most of the diseases mentioned above.

Important factors are:

- diet
- exercise and maintaining mobility
- stress
- recreation/leisure activities
- smoking
- alcohol and substance abuse
- sexual behaviour
- housing and sanitation

SELF-EMPOWERMENT

Throughout life we are faced with decisions regarding our lifestyle and behaviour. Self-empowerment, or genuine informed decision-making, starts with parental and family influences and ideally should be developed through formal education.

ACTIVITY

1 List some reasons why people may not adopt a healthier lifestyle. Consider: foods which constitute a healthy diet; smoking; alcohol; exercise.

2 Collect some advertisements for alcohol, cigarettes and 'fast' or 'junk' food and discuss their effectiveness. What are the advertisers promoting? Which social groups are they targeting?

TOBACCO AND SMOKING

An estimated 110,000 people die in Great Britain each year directly from smoking-related illnesses. Meanwhile, tobacco companies spend an estimated £12 million each year sponsoring sports, such as motor racing, which would be hardest hit by a ban forbidding the display of brand logos.

The Nation's Health: A Strategy for the 1990s was an independent UK-wide report produced in 1988 by the King Edward's Hospital Fund for London. It examined current patterns of disease and of health-related behaviour and asked how they could be changed for the better. It concluded by proposing a health

strategy for the 1990s and identified 17 priorities for public health action. One of these concerned the use of tobacco. The report sets out the general objectives:

- to create a physical and social environment where non-smoking is the norm;
- to support the creation of a generation of non-smokers;
- to maximize public awareness of the risks of smoking across all sectors of the community;
- to support the efforts of those who wish to stop smoking.

One of the targets set by the report – to be achieved by the year 2000 (or earlier) – is:

- to increase the proportion of children under 16 who are non-smokers to at least 95% and
- to reverse the trend towards increased smoking in girls.

According to the Law of Primacy, primary socialization is both more powerful and more enduring than later socializing influences; research shows that a child is more likely to smoke if one or both parents smoke.

Why do people start smoking?

Smoking usually begins in adolescence. There are various factors which might tempt a young person to smoke:

- If cigarettes are readily available at home, there is a greater temptation to start smoking.
- Smoking is thought to be a social habit which gives confidence.
- A young person may start smoking as a gesture of defiance against authority.
- If role models, e.g. parents, teachers and friends smoke, there is a desire to conform and copy their behaviour.

Studies have shown that a teenager who smokes just two or three cigarettes has a 70% chance of becoming addicted.

ACTIVITY

1 Set up a role-play scene in which one of you refuses to join friends in smoking, then is persuaded to give in. Notice what arguments are put forward and whether they appeal to the intelligence or to the emotions.

2 Set up the same scene. This time the non-smoker succeeds in persuading one other person to quit. Again, notice the language used.

3 Write to or visit your local Health Promotion Office. Ask for details on (a) helping addicted people to stop smoking and (b) teaching materials for use in junior schools.

4 Calculate the cost of smoking 20 cigarettes a day for one year.

How smoking affects your body

Figures 5.4 and 5.5 show the physical effects of smoking. In addition to the diseases noted in Figure 5.3, many other diseases and health problems are caused or complicated by smoking, including:

- cancer of the mouth, lip, larynx, oesophagus, lung, pancreas, cervix, stomach, bladder and kidney (the direct evidence that cigarette smoking causes cancer of the lung is clear: fewer than 10% of lung cancers occur in non-smokers);
- emphysema;
- stroke (CVA or cerebro-vascular accident);
- leukaemia;
- chronic lung disease – bronchitis and COLD (chronic obstructive lung disease);
- fertility problems;
- early menopause;
- cataracts;
- male impotence;
- sickle-cell anaemia;
- stomach ulcers.

There are also diseases and health problems associated with PASSIVE SMOKING, i.e. inhaling the smoke from other people's cigarettes. MAINSTREAM SMOKE is that delivered directly to the smoker by inhalation. It tends to be filtered whereas the SIDESTREAM SMOKE emitted into the atmosphere from the burning end of

Nicotine $C_{10}H_{14}N_2$

Nicotine is the drug in tobacco that causes addiction. It is a 'mood-altering' drug which can give so-called pleasurable effects. It is an organic compound (i.e. it contains carbon), occurring naturally in the tobacco plant, especially in the leaves.

Key
○ nitrogen
● hydrogen
CH₃ (methyl group)

Entering the body

cigarette

inhaled fumes

smoke particles

nicotine

As the tobacco burns, the nicotine from the tobacco leaf passes into the smoke and is inhaled into the lungs along with the tar (smoke particles). The nicotine then passes through the wall of the tiny air sacs, or alveoli (singular alveollus), in the lungs, into tiny blood vessels (capillaries). It enters the bloodstream and is carried around the body.

semi-permeable wall between alveolus and capillary

inhaled fumes

alveolus

capillary

1 Oxygen, nicotine and other smoke components (under high pressure in alveolus move across semi-permeable walls into the capillary.

2 Carbon dioxide (under high pressure in the capillary) moves the other way.

Figure 5.4 How smoking affects the body (1)

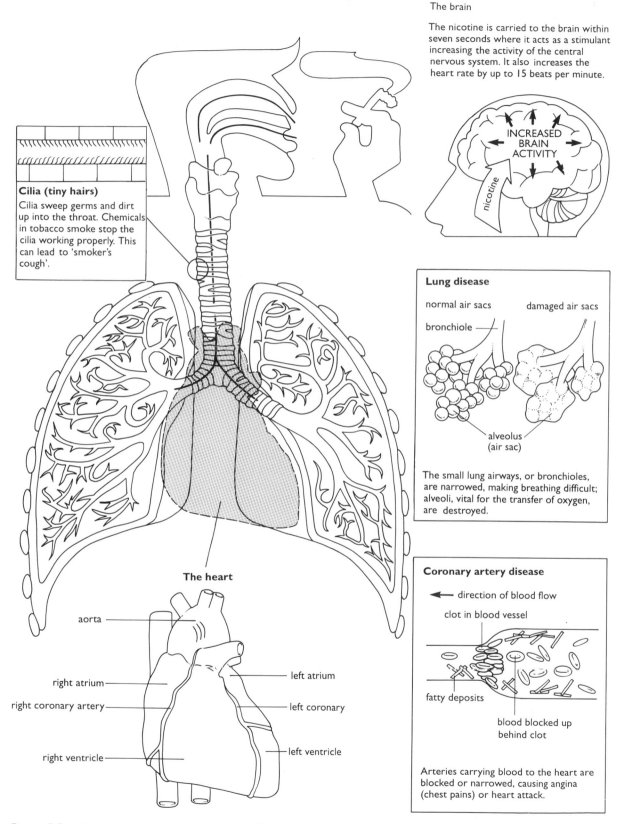

The brain

The nicotine is carried to the brain within seven seconds where it acts as a stimulant increasing the activity of the central nervous system. It also increases the heart rate by up to 15 beats per minute.

INCREASED BRAIN ACTIVITY

nicotine

Cilia (tiny hairs)

Cilia sweep germs and dirt up into the throat. Chemicals in tobacco smoke stop the cilia working properly. This can lead to 'smoker's cough'.

Lung disease

normal air sacs   damaged air sacs

bronchiole

alveolus (air sac)

The small lung airways, or bronchioles, are narrowed, making breathing difficult; alveoli, vital for the transfer of oxygen, are destroyed.

The heart

aorta

right atrium

right coronary artery

right ventricle

left atrium

left coronary

left ventricle

Coronary artery disease

← direction of blood flow

clot in blood vessel

fatty deposits

blood blocked up behind clot

Arteries carrying blood to the heart are blocked or narrowed, causing angina (chest pains) or heart attack.

Figure 5.5   How smoking affects the body (2)
Source: Imperial Cancer Research Fund.

a cigarette is unfiltered and contains a higher proportion of CARCINOGENS than mainstream smoke. Diseases caused are:

- lung cancer
- bronchitis
- heart disease
- low birth weight
- respiratory disease in children

Quick facts

- 33% of the adult population of the UK are smokers.
- Almost one in three of all school-leavers are regular smokers.
- Out of 1,000 smokers who die each year, one will be murdered, six will die on the roads and 250 will die from smoking-related disease.
- On average, babies whose mothers are smokers weigh 200 g less at birth than the babies of non-smokers.
- Out of every 10 smokers, six say they would like to give up; they also say they need the support of a health professional.
- Giving up smoking reduces the risk of premature death; the risks return to those of a non-smoker within 5–10 years.

ACTIVITY

Set up a 'No Smoking' campaign in college.

- Obtain posters from the local Health Promotion Unit or make some using the 'Quick Facts' section.
- Choose a prominent site to display posters and fact sheets.
- Obtain several PEAK FLOW METERS. Learn how to use them and to instruct others in their use. (NB follow the rules of hygiene.)
- Ask each volunteer if he/she smokes and offer them a chance to test their own peak flow.

- Record results from smokers and non-smokers on separate charts.
- At the end of the session, analyse the results and present them on a poster.

Giving up smoking

The Health Education Council gives the following advice to those who wish to give up smoking:

- Cut out the first cigarette of the day to start with, then the second, and so on.
- Start by cutting out the most 'enjoyable' cigarette of the day, like the one after a big meal.
- Give up with a friend.
- Tell everyone you are giving up smoking.

Think about the reasoning behind each piece of advice.

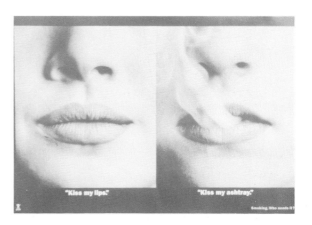

"Kiss my lips."   "Kiss my ashtray."

DRUGS

A drug is any chemical substance which changes the function of one or more body organs or alters the process of a disease. Drugs may be:

- prescribed medicines
- over-the-counter remedies
- alcohol, tobacco and caffeine
- illegal drugs

DRUG ABUSE is the use of a drug for a purpose other than that for which it is usually prescribed.

DRUG DEPENDENCE is the compulsion to continue taking a drug, either to produce the desired effects that result from taking it, or to prevent the ill-effects that occur when it is withdrawn. There are two types of drug dependence:

- psychological
- physical

A person is psychologically dependent if he or she experiences craving or emotional distress when the drug is withdrawn. A person is physically dependent when the body has adapted to the presence of the drug and symptoms of withdrawal syndrome are caused when the drug is withdrawn.

DRUG TOLERANCE develops when the body becomes almost immune to the drug and requires larger doses in order to achieve the original effect.

There are four main groups of drugs which are commonly abused:

- stimulants ('uppers')
- depressants ('downers')
- psychedelics or hallucinogens
- narcotics

Stimulants

These drugs increase arousal and make the user feel temporarily more euphoric, alert and wide-awake. They are rarely prescribed for any 'medical' problem. Examples are:

- *Caffeine*, found in coffee, tea, chocolate and cola drinks. High daily dosages (such as six cups of coffee, i.e. 600 mg of caffeine) can induce agitation, tremor, insomnia and irregularities of the heart rhythm.
- *Cocaine*, derived from the leaves of *erythroxylum coca* trees. Cocaine was widely used in the nineteenth century (Sigmund Freud was an enthusiastic user and an advocate of its powers). In its purified

form, it is usually taken intranasally ('snorted').
- *Crack*, a highly purified form of cocaine which is usually smoked or mixed with heroin and injected.
- *Nicotine*, a mild stimulant derived from the tobacco plant and usually smoked in cigars and cigarettes.

Depressants

Drugs which depress the central nervous system produce a calming or relaxing effect. As the dose is increased, this feeling gives way to drowsiness and sleep. Tolerance develops to all the depressant drugs and they also cause physical and psychological dependence to a varying degree. Examples are:

- alcohol
- sleeping tablets or hypnotics
- tranquilizers
- solvents (abused in glue-sniffing)

ALCOHOL

Alcohol (ethanol or ethyl alcohol) has been used and abused since prehistoric times and is probably the most commonly abused drug in the developed world. It is absorbed into the body through the stomach and intestines and distributed throughout the body by the bloodstream. In pregnant women, alcohol crosses the placental barrier to reach the developing baby.

Doctors recommend that sensible weekly limits on intake are up to 21 units of alcohol for men and up to 14 units for women. (See Figure 5.6 for what constitutes a unit.)

Alcohol problems occur at all educational and social levels and in every age group. There are several signals that a person is having difficulty controlling his or her alcohol intake:

- drinking for relief from pain and stress;
- pattern drinking (drinking every day or every week at a certain time, particularly in the morning);
- making alcohol the centre of life or of all pleasurable, relaxing activities.

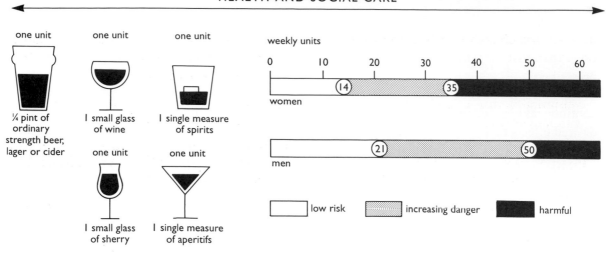

Figure 5.6   How much is too much?

Some quick facts on alcohol:

- After heart disease and cancer, alcohol is the third biggest health hazard today.
- Up to 30% of men admitted to hospitals are either 'problem drinkers' or physically dependent on alcohol.
- Drink is commonly believed to be an aphrodisiac, but, as Shakespeare wrote, it 'provokes the desire but takes away the performance'.
- There are many proven links between alcohol and violence. Alcohol is associated with 60–70% of homicides, 75% of stabbings and 70% of beatings.
- Recent research in the UK and America shows a connection between child abuse and problem drinking.
- Only 13% of single homeless people are heavy drinkers. Half of all single homeless people are light drinkers or abstain completely.
- A third of all deaths on the road are caused by drunken drivers.

In *The Nation's Health*, the authors have set out

Table 5.1   How does alcohol affect physical and mental behaviour?

No. of drinks	Quantity of alcohol	Effects
1 pint of beer	30 mg	Likelihood of having an accident starts to increase
1½ pints of beer or 3 whiskies	50 mg	A feeling of warmth and cheer; impairment of judgement and inhibition
2½ pints of beer or 5 whiskies	80 mg	Loss of driving licence if discovered driving a vehicle
5 pints of beer or 10 whiskies	150 mg	Loss of self-control; exuberance; slurred speech; quarrelsomeness
6 pints of beer or 13 whiskies	200 mg	Stagger; double vision; memory loss
¼ bottle of spirits	400 mg	Oblivion; sleeplessness; coma
1 bottle of spirits	500 mg 600 mg	Death possible Death certain

the following objectives in relation to alcohol use:

- to promote patterns of alcohol consumption that minimize its harm without jeopardizing its benefits;
- to create an environment which minimizes pressures to drink excessively and maximizes choice of non-alcoholic alternatives;
- to improve understanding of the adverse medical, psychological and social effects of excessive drinking and to promote a better understanding of what constitutes 'safe' drinking patterns;

- to support the efforts of those with alcohol problems who wish to cut down on their drinking or remain abstinent.

The long-term effects of alcohol on the body are shown in Figure 5.7.

ACTIVITY

1 Find out why women are more sensitive to comparable doses of alcohol than are men.

2 Find out what treatment or therapy is available for people with drinking

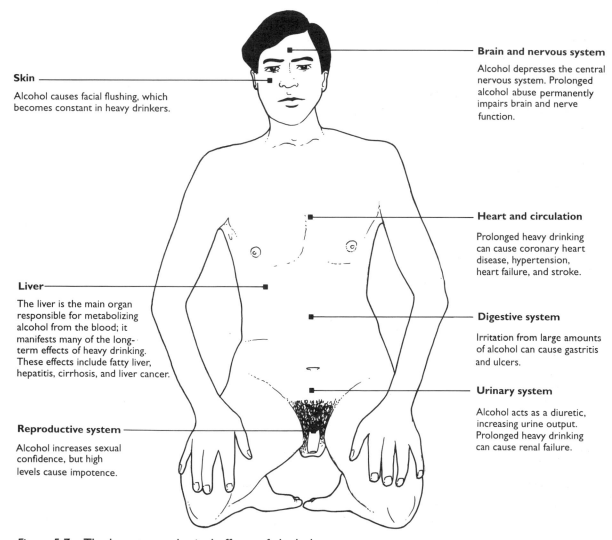

Skin

Alcohol causes facial flushing, which becomes constant in heavy drinkers.

Brain and nervous system

Alcohol depresses the central nervous system. Prolonged alcohol abuse permanently impairs brain and nerve function.

Heart and circulation

Prolonged heavy drinking can cause coronary heart disease, hypertension, heart failure, and stroke.

Liver

The liver is the main organ responsible for metabolizing alcohol from the blood; it manifests many of the long-term effects of heavy drinking. These effects include fatty liver, hepatitis, cirrhosis, and liver cancer.

Digestive system

Irritation from large amounts of alcohol can cause gastritis and ulcers.

Urinary system

Alcohol acts as a diuretic, increasing urine output. Prolonged heavy drinking can cause renal failure.

Reproductive system

Alcohol increases sexual confidence, but high levels cause impotence.

Figure 5.7 The long-term physical effects of alcohol

problems (alcoholism) in your area? What does the self-help group Alcoholics Anonymous offer?

ACTIVITY

1 Describe some of the ways in which people who drink excessive amounts of alcohol endanger (a) themselves and (b) other people.

2 Collect advertisements for drink from magazines, and also the posters and advertisements put out by bodies such as the Health Education Council which warn of the dangers of heavy drinking. Which posters are more effective? Design your own posters.

3 Research the condition known as foetal alcohol syndrome. How many babies are affected each year in the UK and what problems does it present?

SOLVENT ABUSE

Solvent abuse is the practice of inhaling the intoxicating fumes given off by certain volatile liquids. Glue sniffing is the most common form of solvent abuse, but lighter fluid and paint thinner may also be used.

- The usual method of inhalation is from a plastic bag containing the solvent.
- It is usually a group activity and is common among boys from poor urban areas.
- Effects are similar to becoming drunk or getting 'high'.

Solvent abuse can cause:

- hallucinations
- headache
- vomiting
- stupor
- confusion and coma

Occasionally, death occurs due to a direct

toxic effect on the heart or by inhalation of vomit. Signs and symptoms are:

- a flushed face;
- intoxicated behaviour;
- ulcers around the mouth;
- a smell of solvent;
- personality changes, e.g. edginess or moodiness.

Acute symptoms such as vomiting or coma must be treated following the basic principles of first aid:

- Maintain airway, breathing and circulation.
- Arrange urgent removal to hospital.
- DO NOT attempt to induce vomiting. It is often ineffective and may harm the casualty further.

Psychedelics or hallucinogens

Drugs in this category produce disturbances of perception and a changed state of consciousness and awareness. The feelings experienced range from terror to ecstasy. Some, like LSD, are manufactured; others occur naturally as plants and fungi. As many as 25% of users of hallucinogens will experience a 'flashback' or return of the hallucinatory and delusional experience even months after the drug has been taken. The episode is usually brief, lasting only minutes, but it is often frightening and disturbing. Aldous Huxley wrote *The Doors of Perception* in 1954 whilst under the influence of the hallucinogen mescaline. Other examples of hallucinogens are:

- LSD (lysergic acid diethylamide). This is usually taken as tiny tablets. Its effects are unpredictable and depend very much on the individual. LSD is used socially in groups, with one person not 'using' to keep an eye on others.
- *Cannabis* (or marijuana or hashish). This is produced from the plant Indian hemp. Visible effects of the drug includes

reddening of the eyes caused by dilation of the blood vessels. Effects on the mind and emotions vary. In general perception is altered and ideas flow more quickly. This drug is not addictive and there is no evidence that it harms the body. Usually cannabis is smoked but it can also be made into cakes and eaten. There have been frequent calls for legalizing the sale and use of cannabis, as has been done in the Netherlands.

- *Ecstasy* (MDMA). This substance was originally marketed as an appetite suppressant in 1914 and has been used in the 1970s by US psychotherapists to improve talking. It appeared in the UK in the 1980s and is mostly used in clubs. It is very expensive and comes in a variety of coloured tablets with exotic names such as Tangerine Dreams, California Sunshine, etc. Ecstasy is not addictive but has been known to cause death. Dancing for six hours at a stretch under its influence is not unusual. Excessive sweating leads to loss of fluid, hyperthermia and eventual collapse. The immediate effect is a rush – a feeling of warmth towards everyone. This may lead to unsafe sex with a stranger. There may also be a 'come down' the next day with feelings of depression and panic attacks.

Narcotics

Narcotics are ANALGESIC drugs (painkillers) used to treat moderate and severe pain. Abuse of narcotic drugs for their euphoric effects often causes tolerance and physical and psychological dependence. Examples are:

- heroin
- morphine
- pethidine
- methadone
- codeine
- opium

HEROIN

Heroin is more potent than morphine and is

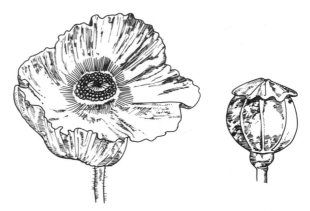

Figure 5.8   The poppy (*Papaver somniferum*) from which heroin is derived

derived from opium, which is harvested from the flower of the poppy, *Papaver somniferum* (see Figure 5.8). It is most active and effective when given by injection. Tolerance and physical dependence develop rapidly. Withdrawal symptoms are particularly unpleasant, and include:

- agitation;
- restless disturbed sleep;
- abdominal cramps;
- watering eyes and a running nose;
- dilated pupils;
- tremor.

These withdrawal symptoms last for a week or more.

Heroin addicts have a mortality rate 15 times higher than normal and, although death is not usually due to the direct effects of heroin use, it may result from:

- an overdose;
- mixing heroin with other substances;
- physical debility due to neglect;
- illness associated with unclean injection techniques, including venous thrombosis, septicaemia, hepatitis, HIV/AIDS.

Most users recognize the dangers of injection (mainlining) and yet prefer this method because of the 'rush' or intensity of the experience. Many users now choose to smoke heroin. The drug is placed in a strip of tinfoil

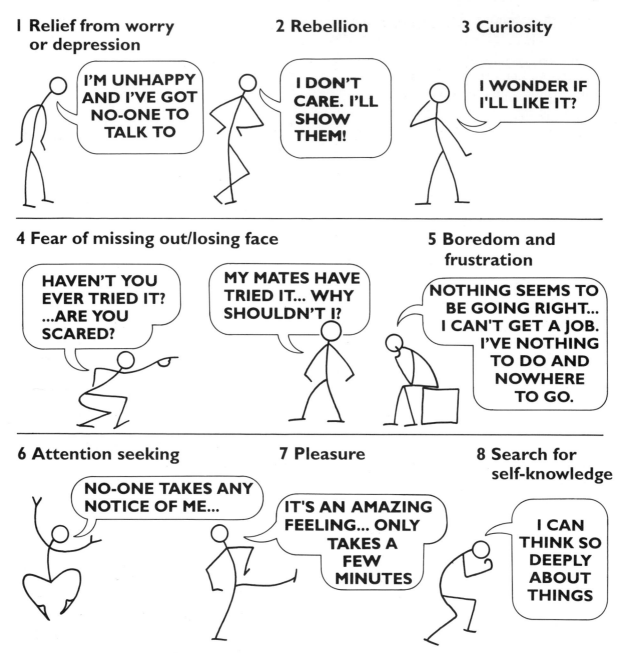

Figure 5.9 Why do people take drugs?
Source: BPI, Biology resource book.

and heated until it gives off smoke which is inhaled. The substance writhes above the foil while it is being heated, giving rise to the colourful phrase 'chasing the dragon'.

Methadone is a synthetic opiate which is much longer-acting than heroin, but still addictive. It is usually taken orally as a syrup and is often prescribed by clinics in maintenance therapy.

Why do people take drugs?

Obviously no one knows for certain why people abuse drugs, but Figure 5.9 shows some of the reasons which might be involved.

ACTIVITY

1 Draw up a chart showing the 'pleasant' and 'unpleasant' effects of Ecstasy, heroin, amphetamines and cocaine.

2 Choose one of the following drugs and research it:

- alcohol
- tobacco
- cocaine
- heroin

Include as much up-to-date information as you can; use your library's resources centre. The project should cover:

- What is the drug and what are its effects?
- Who uses the drug and why?
- How can health promoters change the patterns of drug abuse?

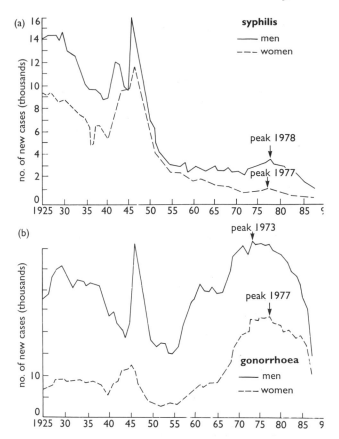

Figure 5.10   Incidence of (a) syphilis and (b) gonorrhea, 1925–90
Source: D. Taylor, Human Physical Health (CUP, 1989).

SEXUALLY TRANSMITTED DISEASES

These are infections transmitted primarily, although not exclusively, by sexual intercourse. Until about 30 years ago, STDs were commonly called venereal diseases (VD) and were thought to be limited to three specific infections:

- syphilis
- gonorrhoea
- chancroid

However, gonorrhoea and syphilis account for only about 10% of the cases of STD treated in clinics today (see Figure 5.10). Changing attitudes towards sex may be correlated with the changes in incidence of STDs.

ACTIVITY

Examine Figure 5.10. Discuss in groups why there are two rises in the figures and why the trend is now downward for both diseases

(NB: Syphilis is 10 times more prevalent among homosexual men than heterosexual men. Gonorrhoea is three times more prevalent.)

Since the 1970s in Britain, there has been an increase in the viral diseases:

- herpes;
- hepatitis;
- genital warts;
- AIDS (acquired immune deficiency syndrome), a 'new' viral disease.

Other diseases on the increase are:

- non-specific genital infections (NSGI), often called non-specific urethritis (NSU).

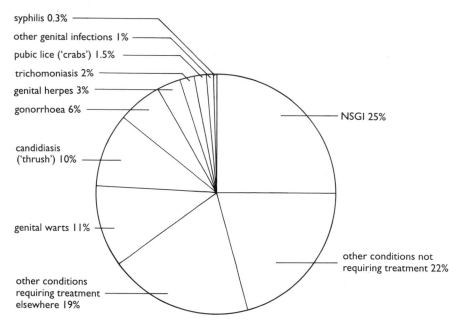

syphilis 0.3%
other genital infections 1%
pubic lice ('crabs') 1.5%
trichomoniasis 2%
genital herpes 3%
gonorrhoea 6%

candidiasis ('thrush') 10%

genital warts 11%

other conditions requiring treatment elsewhere 19%

NSGI 25%

other conditions not requiring treatment 22%

Figure 5.11   New cases seen at NHS genito-urinary medicine clinics in England and Wales, 1986
Source: D. Taylor, *Human Physical Health* (CUP, 1989).

In about 50% of cases of NSGI, the causative agent is a bacterium called *chlamydia trachomatis*. The most common STD in Britain today is chlamydia;

- candidiasis (thrush);
- trichomoniasis (caused by a protozoan called *trichomonas vaginalis*);
- pubic lice (pediculosis).

Gonorrhoea

Although there is a decreasing trend of reported cases of this disease (commonly known as 'the clap'), the worldwide trend is increasing. Statistics are very unreliable for this disease as 50% of cases in women present no symptoms and are therefore not reported. However, in the 1970s 60 million new cases were being reported each year worldwide.

CAUSE

The bacterium *neisseria gonorrhoeae*, or gonococcus, infects the lower part of the urethra in men and the cervix (or neck of the womb) and urethra in women. Infection of the rectum is possible in homosexual or

bisexual men and in some cases the rectum of women may be affected even if anal sex has not occurred. Gonorrhoea can affect the throat where oral sex is practised.

SIGNS AND SYMPTOMS

- The incubation period is 2–10 days, usually about 5 days.
- In men: pain on passing urine and slight urethral discharge.
- In women: 50% have no symptoms, but when they are present symptoms include vaginal discharge and discomfort on urinating. There may also be slight headaches and fever.
- A baby exposed to infection in the mother's reproductive tract during childbirth may acquire gonococcal ophthalmia, a severe inflammation affecting one or both eyes.

COMPLICATIONS

Untreated gonorrhoea may spread to other parts of the body.

- In women, the infection may travel up through the uterus and into the Fallopian tubes, causing pelvic inflammatory disease

(PID). There is an increased risk of ectopic pregnancy and of infertility.

- In men, infection may spread to the prostate and testes, causing inflammation and sometimes sterility.
- Occasionally infection spreads through the bloodstream to cause gonococcal arthritis, with pain and swelling of joints around the body.
- Multiplication of bacteria in the bloodstream causes septicaemia which, if it affects the brain or heart, can prove fatal.

DIAGNOSIS

Laboratory tests are carried out on a sample of the discharge or on swabs taken from the urethra, cervix and sometimes the rectum. Diagnosis is only confirmed by isolation of gonococci from infected tissue.

TREATMENT

One oral dose of penicillin is usually sufficient to cure the disease. If the patient is allergic to penicillin, other antibiotics may be used. Unfortunately, strains of the bacterium are developing partial and sometimes total resistance to penicillin.

ACTIVITY

Discuss which groups of people are most at risk of contracting gonorrhoea.

What do you consider is the best way to combat the spread of gonorrhoea?

Syphilis

Syphilis was first recorded as a major epidemic in Europe in the 1490s following the return of Columbus from America. It is most common in certain South American and African countries, where infection rates are several hundred times higher than in Britain. The history of reported cases in Britain from 1925 to 1987 is shown in Figure 5.10. Today all expectant mothers in the UK are tested for syphilis, although it is rare.

CAUSE

Syphilis is caused by the bacterium *treponema pallidum*. It belongs to an unusual group of bacteria called spirochaetes, which have a long, slender spiral shape. The organism dies quickly in dry conditions and has proved impossible to culture in the laboratory.

There are two forms of syphilis:

- Congenital, transmitted from an infected mother across the placenta to the foetus while it is still in the uterus. Often this results in spontaneous abortion or stillbirth.
- Acquired, by sexual contact. The bacterium penetrates broken skin or mucous membranes in the genitalia, rectum or mouth during sexual intercourse. The risk of infection during a single contact with an infected person is about 30%.

SIGNS AND SYMPTOMS

In congenital syphilis, if the baby is born alive, it may suffer the following problems:

- syphilitic rash, particularly in the genital area;
- bone abnormalities;
- inflammation of the nose – persistent snuffles;
- mental retardation.

Untreated syphilis usually passes through several stages, summarized in Table 5.2.

DIAGNOSIS

Primary syphilis is easily diagnosed by finding active spirochaetes during microscopic examination of a smear taken from the chancre serum. Blood tests confirm the diagnosis.

TREATMENT

Treatment should ideally be given in the primary stage. All forms of the disease are treated by penicillin injections. However, organ damage already caused by the disease cannot be reversed.

For congenital syphilis, treatment before the sixth month of pregnancy will always

Table 5.2   The stages of syphilis (untreated)

| | 'Early stage' (infectious stage) | | | | | |
	Primary syphilis	Secondary syphilis	Latent stage	Tertiary syphilis	Cardiovascular syphilis	Neuro-syphilis
Time from original infection	2 to 4 weeks	8 to 12 weeks	2 years	3 to 10 years	10 to 20 years	30+ years
Duration	up to 4 weeks	2 years	approx. 1 to 10 years	approx. 10 years	until death	until death
Typical signs and symptoms	1 chancre (a highly infectious sore) at site of infection, painless	Non-itchy pink rash on trunk, face, limbs (palms and soles) lasting several weeks. Swollen lymph nodes. Lesions in warm, moist areas, e.g. groin	No signs or symptoms	Many parts of body affected. Gummas (large lesions/ulcers) in skin, mouth, nose, throat. Bones and joints painful and crippled	Occurs in approx. 10% of untreated patients. Degeneration of base of aorta, coronary thrombosis, other complications	Insanity, blindness

prevent infection of the unborn child. A syphilitic mother who is not treated within this period has only one chance in six of having a healthy child.

ACTIVITY

1   Construct a brief questionnaire to find out how much people know about syphilis.

2   Find out where one would go for help in your area if symptoms of syphilis were apparent.

Non-specific genital infection

Non-specific genital infection (NSGI) is the commonest sexually transmitted disease in Britain. It is otherwise known as NSU or non-specific urethritis.

CAUSE

In about 50% of cases of NSGI, the causative agent is a small bacterium called *chlamydia trachomatis*. An estimated 5% of cases of NSGI are caused by the *ureaplasma* bacterium and the remaining 45% of cases have no known cause.

SIGNS AND SYMPTOMS

- Incubation usually takes two to three weeks.
- In men, there is slight pain on passing urine and there may be a slight discharge from the penis.
- In women, there are usually no signs or symptoms but there may be a slight increase in vaginal discharge and discomfort when urinating.

COMPLICATIONS

- If untreated, men may develop swelling of the testes which in turn may cause infertility.
- In women, infection may spread to the fallopian tubes (salpingitis) and, rarely, lead to the development of pelvic inflammatory disease (PID), which may cause infertility. (NB: PID can be caused by other factors, e.g. pregnancy, the insertion of intra-uterine contraceptive devices (IUCDs) and with abortion.)
- A child born to a woman with a chlamydial infection may acquire an acute eye infection called neonatal ophthalmia.

TREATMENT

- A technique known as immuno-fluorescence is used to diagnose chlamydial infections, but the lack of symptoms in women means that many are unaware that they have an infection.
- Treatment is with antibiotic drugs, usually tetracycline or erythromycin, and is very effective.

Genital warts

If you refer to Figure 5.11 on page 180 you will see that genital warts account for 11% of new cases seen in genito-urinary medicine (GUM) clinics. Latest figures show them to be a rapidly increasing disease.

Genital warts are soft warts found on the vulva or penis and around the anus.

CAUSE

- The papillomavirus is responsible for infection.
- They are transmitted by sexual contact.

SIGNS AND SYMPTOMS

- The warts are similar in appearance to warts found on other parts of the body.
- There may be an interval of up to 18 months between infection and the appearance of the warts.

TREATMENT

- A special anti-wart paint may be applied.
- Removal by surgery may be necessary.
- There is a tendency for the warts to recur.

NB: Genital warts have been linked with cases of cervical cancer. A woman who has had genital warts – or whose partner has – should have annual cervical smear tests.

Genital herpes

CAUSE

- Caused by a virus, herpes simplex: type 1 causes cold sores on the lips, type 2 causes genital herpes.

- Transmitted by sexual intercourse with an infected person.

SIGNS AND SYMPTOMS

- Incubation period is about one week.
- Itching, burning, soreness and small blisters in the genital area. These blisters burst to leave painful, red ulcers which heal within 10 to 21 days.
- In the case of homosexuals the anus is affected.
- Fever, malaise and swollen lymph nodes may also occur.
- Once the virus enters the body, it stays there for the rest of the person's life. Symptoms disappear after two weeks but return at irregular intervals in about 50% of patients.

TREATMENT

- Genital herpes cannot be cured.
- Anti-viral drugs help to reduce pain and promote faster healing of the ulcers.
- During attacks, sexual intercourse should be avoided to prevent transmission of the disease.
- If a pregnant woman has an attack of genital herpes when the baby is due, a caesarian section is performed to prevent the baby being infected during delivery.

Candidiasis (vaginal thrush)

CAUSE

- Caused by the yeast Candida Albicans, a unicellular fungus.
- It can be contracted by sexual intercourse with an infected partner. It is much more common in women than in men.

SIGNS AND SYMPTOMS

- Vaginal candidiasis may cause a thick, white 'cottage cheese' discharge from the vagina and/or vaginal soreness and irritation.
- There may be pain when urinating.

- Men rarely show signs or symptoms, but may suffer mild irritation of the foreskin.
- A woman is more susceptible if she is diabetic, pregnant, taking oral contraceptives or anaemic.

The fungus is normally present in the vagina and mouth. Its growth is kept under control by the bacteria usually present in these organs. If a course of antibiotic therapy kills too many of the bacteria, the fungus may multiply excessively.

TREATMENT

- Antifungal suppositories or cream may be inserted into the vagina via a special applicator.
- Antifungal tablets may be taken by mouth.
- Hygiene is important as the fungus thrives in damp conditions. Cotton underwear is advisable and sexual intercourse should be avoided until cured.
- A non-hormonal contraception method may be prescribed.

Trichomoniasis

Trichomonal infections are common and may occur in conjunction with other sexually transmitted diseases.

CAUSE

- Trichomoniasis is caused by the protozoan (single-celled micro-organism) *trichomonas vaginalis*.

SIGNS AND SYMPTOMS

- In women, painful inflammation of the vagina; a profuse frothy, yellow, unpleasant-smelling discharge from the vagina.
- In men, signs and symptoms are usually absent.

TREATMENT

- Drug treatment (metronidazole) is usually effective.
- Both sexual partners should be treated.

ACTIVITY

Make a chart to present the information on the sexually transmitted diseases described on the preceding pages. Use the following headings:

- incidence (refer to Figure 5.11 on page 180)
- cause
- signs and symptoms
- treatment
- complications

The principles of prevention of sexually transmitted diseases

SEXUAL ABSTINENCE

The greater number of sexual partners a person has, the greater the risk of contracting disease. Promiscuity, a changing moral climate and the advent of the contraceptive pill are just some of the reasons for the periodic rise in sexually transmitted diseases. Celibacy is probably not a feasible option but reduction in the number of sexual partners is a realistic objective.

THE PROMOTION OF 'SAFER SEX'

Some measure of protection is afforded by the use of the condom (sheath) as a contraceptive. This physical barrier around the penis reduces the chance of a pathogen passing to and from the female.

TRACING OF CONTACTS

The patient must try to identify the person from whom the disease was caught as well as anyone he or she may have infected. At genito-urinary medicine clinics (formerly called special clinics), trained health workers interview patients after their diagnosis to explain the disease in detail, how it is transmitted and the complications that might occur if the disease is left untreated. Patients are also given printed leaflets which they are recommended to give to their sexual contacts and which advise the contacts of the need for treatment.

EDUCATION

In Britain, sex education is a compulsory part of the secondary school curriculum. Such education should encompass the moral and social sphere as well as the biological one. Further information is available from Health Promotion Units, from GP practices and from the media.

ACTIVITY

1 Visit your local Health Promotion Unit and collect posters and leaflets on sexually transmitted diseases.

2 Prepare a display board with the aim of raising awareness in college. Include information on where to go for advice.

HIV INFECTION AND AIDS

- AIDS stands for acquired immune deficiency syndrome.
- HIV stands for human immunodeficiency virus.
- The HIV virus has now been identified as the cause of AIDS.

What is HIV?

The AIDS virus was identified in 1983 as an RNA virus of the type known as retroviruses. The disease known as AIDS was first noticed among homosexual men in New York and California in 1981. It has received enormous publicity worldwide because it is a disease affecting relatively young people and is, at present, usually fatal.

Read through the sections of Chapter 3 dealing with transmission of disease and particularly the section describing viruses.

The genetic blueprint of most viruses is stored

in the form of the chemical DNA. RETROVIRUSES differ from this pattern, however, since their genetic material is stored in the form of a related but different chemical called RNA. One sub-family of the retroviruses is known to cause leukaemia in humans, but the sub-family to which HIV belongs was previously only known to cause fatal diseases in sheep, horses and goats. HIV affects the IMMUNE SYSTEM, replicating in a particular type of lymphocyte called the T4 cell. T4 cells or 'helper cells' induce other T-cells to fight invading organisms. Without them the body's immune system breaks down, leaving the patient exposed to a variety of diseases.

It is important to realize that infection with HIV does not necessarily result in AIDS. Some people are carriers of the disease while remaining symptom-free. The disease has been discovered too recently to know whether all people with HIV will eventually have AIDS.

Student quiz: what do you already know about HIV and AIDS?

Put a ring round the correct statement for each question.

1 *By the end of 1991 there were:*
   (a) 823
   (b) 2,536
   (c) 5,065
   cases of AIDS recorded in the United Kingdom.
2 *How many people are thought to be infected with HIV in the United Kingdom?*
   (a) 2,000–6,000
   (b) 20,000–50,000
   (c) 50,000–80,000
3 *How can the HIV virus be transmitted?*
   (a) by vaginal intercourse
   (b) by blood transfusion
   (c) by kissing or touching another person
   (d) by sharing utensils, e.g. cups, glasses, with other people
   (e) by anal intercourse
   (f) by use of shared injecting equipment
   (g) in swimming pools
   (h) across the placenta

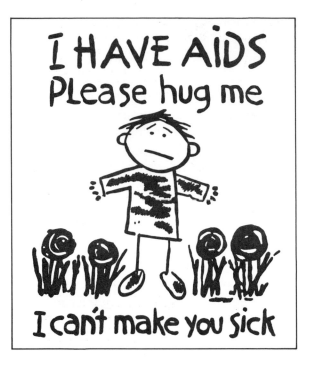

• By transfer of blood, blood products or organs.

The virus cannot survive outside the body (unlike the flu virus, for example) and is destroyed by acid in the stomach.

Signs and symptoms

• Incubation period is normally six weeks to several months but may extend for years.
• First symptoms are a short flu-like illness, followed by no signs or symptoms for months or years.
• Because of a defect in the IMMUNE RESPONSE, other OPPORTUNISTIC INFECTIONS follow (see Figure 5.12).

Treatment

There is no known cure for AIDS.

Antibiotics may be prescribed to treat symptoms such as pneumonia and radiotherapy used to treat the various cancers, but these treatments do not constitute a cure.

Research is aimed at developing a drug to inactivate the virus and/or a vaccine to provide immunity to HIV. A successful vaccine has been developed against feline leukaemia virus, which bears similarities to HIV. Until such measures are found, prevention is the most effective method of controlling the spread of AIDS.

Prevention

In 1991 the Order for Science in the National Curriculum was revised in the UK and the requirement to teach 11–14-year-olds about the HIV virus was introduced. One of the key ideas is that children should appreciate that they need to take more responsible attitudes towards their own well-being and that of others.

SAFER SEX TECHNIQUES

• Reduce the number of sexual partners.
• Ideally, sex should be restricted to partners whose sexual history is known.

   (i) by intercourse with an infected person
   (j) by mouth-to-mouth resuscitation

4 *Who can be affected by HIV?*
   (a) drug users
   (b) homosexual men
   (c) haemophiliacs
   (d) anyone

5 *The method of contraception that offers some protection against HIV is:*
   (a) The coil
   (b) The pill
   (c) The condom/sheath
   (d) The cap/diaphragm

6 *HIV is found in the following body fluids:*
   (a) semen
   (b) vaginal secretions
   (c) blood
   (d) saliva
   (e) tears

Answers on page 187

How is HIV transmitted?

• During unprotected penetrative sex.
• By sharing needles and syringes used for injecting drugs.
• From mother to baby across the placenta during birth and via breast milk.

Symptoms of AIDS

AIDS is a 'syndrome' and causes a number of different diseases. It can make people lose weight very quickly and feel as though they have very little energy.

It can give them headaches and fevers, often at night, and make them weak and ill, especially in the later stages.

HIV can cause skin diseases. People sometimes find purple patches on their skin. This is a symptom of Kaposi's sarcoma, a cancer that affects many AIDS patients. It is not usually painful.

More painful are cold sores, which are caused by a virus and are found on the face, neck, mouth and glands.

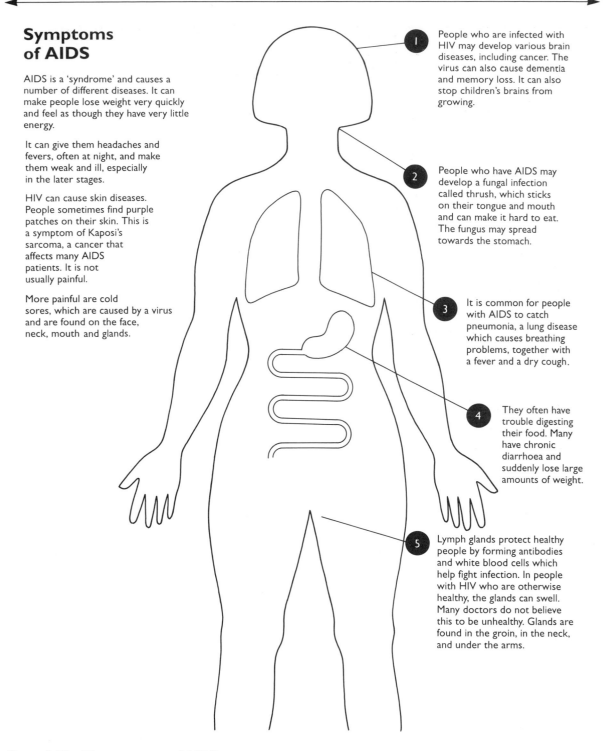

1. People who are infected with HIV may develop various brain diseases, including cancer. The virus can also cause dementia and memory loss. It can also stop children's brains from growing.

2. People who have AIDS may develop a fungal infection called thrush, which sticks on their tongue and mouth and can make it hard to eat. The fungus may spread towards the stomach.

3. It is common for people with AIDS to catch pneumonia, a lung disease which causes breathing problems, together with a fever and a dry cough.

4. They often have trouble digesting their food. Many have chronic diarrhoea and suddenly lose large amounts of weight.

5. Lymph glands protect healthy people by forming antibodies and white blood cells which help fight infection. In people with HIV who are otherwise healthy, the glands can swell. Many doctors do not believe this to be unhealthy. Glands are found in the groin, in the neck, and under the arms.

Figure 5.12 The symptoms of AIDS

- Use of a condom is recommended for both anal and vaginal intercourse.
- Intravenous drug users should not share needles or syringes.

See also the section on prevention of sexually transmitted diseases.

Answers to Quiz

1 (c). **2** (b). **3** (a), (b), (e), (f), (h) and (i). **4** (a), (b), (c), (d). **5** (c). **6** (a), (b), (c), (d) and (e). However, there is no good evidence that anyone has contracted HIV from saliva or tears.

ACTIVITY

- Study Figure 5.13. Draw a bar graph or pie chart to show the distribution of HIV infections.
- Women are more vulnerable to HIV than men, because of their subordinate social status in most of the world. Look at the posters (Figure 5.14a–c) and try to design a poster to highlight the fact that HIV/AIDS is now a family problem.

ACTIVITY

Investigate your own feelings about the spread of AIDS and prepare to debate the following issues in a group session:

- Should it be legal to sample and test blood for HIV antibodies without a patient's knowledge or consent?
- Should life insurance companies discriminate against homosexuals, or those who have had HIV tests, even if the tests proved negative?
- Should there be compensation for those who have been infected by blood transfusions, notably haemophiliacs?

Quick facts

- At least 80% of cases of HIV/AIDS are in the developing world; the people most at risk are the poorest.
- 40% of the 12 million HIV-infected adults today are women; three years ago, women accounted for only 25% of adult infections.
- In Africa, TB has already become the leading cause of death in adults with HIV.
- Within the next three years, AIDS will cause more deaths in children in sub-Saharan Africa than either malaria or measles.
- A successful vaccine against HIV is not expected before the year 2000.

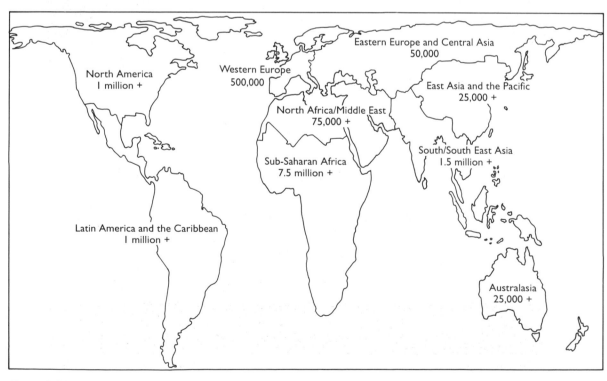

Figure 5.13   Estimated cumulative adult HIV infections, end 1992

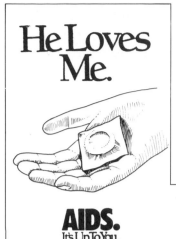

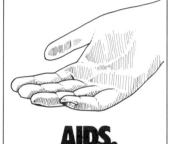

(a)

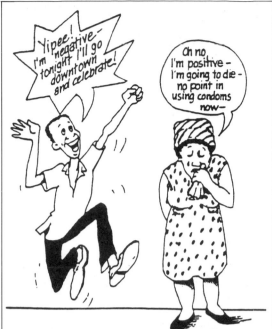

(b)

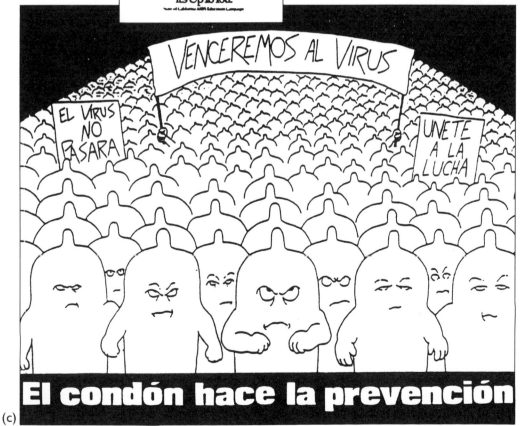

(c)

"We'll beat the virus"   Condoms are for prevention

Figure 5.14

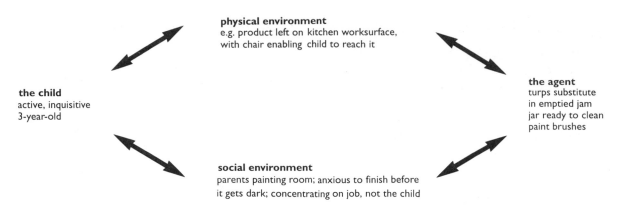

Figure 5.15 An accident waiting to happen

ACTIVITY

1 Find out what AIDS control policies are being adopted by your government. Are there plans for wide-ranging compulsory testing of selected groups? How would such plans affect a citizen's human rights?

2 Tuberculosis (TB) has become a major threat to public health, and is linked to HIV/AIDS. What is being done to counter this threat?

RISKS TO PERSONAL SAFETY

Many people believe that, as individuals, they have little control over risks to their health due to large-scale environmental problems such as acid rain or industrial pollution. While it is true that many environmental issues require global policies to be dealt with effectively, risks in one's immediate environment *can* be controlled.

Safety at home

Although the most dangerous place for accidents is the road, the home is the setting for many *preventable* accidents (see Table 5.3).

Of all accidents resulting in death in the 0–4 year age group, the majority take place in the home.

ACTIVITY

Arrange the following 'accidents waiting to happen' into the format outlined in Figure 5.15.

1 A six-year-old boy runs out into the road to retrieve his football which a friend kicked out of his hands.

Table 5.3 Causes of accidental death

Age (yrs)	Chief causes of accidental death (as % of total)	Commonest other causes (in order of frequency)
Under 1	Choking and suffocation (70%)	Falls; fire; road accidents
1–4	Road accidents (37%)	Fire; drowning; choking and suffocation
5–9	Road accidents (57%)	Drowning; fire; falls
10–14	Road accidents (53%)	Drowning; choking and suffocation; falls
15–24	Road accidents (76%)	Poisoning; falls; drowning
25–44	Road accidents (53%)	Poisoning; falls; choking and suffocation
45–64	Road accidents (44%)	Falls; poisoning; fire
Over 64	Falls (61%)	Road accidents; fire; poisoning

2 A ten-month baby, sitting in her high chair, has been given a peeled banana to eat. Her mother is speaking on the telephone; the baby is silently choking.

Assuming that the worst happens, i.e. the six-year-old sustains a head injury, and the baby stops breathing because her airway is obstructed,

- State first aid measures you would take.
- How could the accident have been prevented?

Accidents in the home have a number of causes, varying with each age group involved. A young child's curiosity, an adult's care-lessness or an old person's slower reactions may all be factors.

In addition to these mental and physical factors, accidents can be caused by:

- badly designed houses;
- faulty equipment;
- incorrect storage and use of dangerous substances.

Electrical injuries

Contact with high-voltage current, found in power lines and overhead high-tension (HT) cables is usually immediately fatal.

The passage of electrical current through the body may cause breathing and even the heart to stop.

HIGH-VOLTAGE CURRENT

- The power must be cut off and isolated before the casualty is approached.
- Call the emergency services immediately (dial 999).
- The casualty will be unconscious; check breathing and pulse; resuscitate if necessary.
- Treat burns and take steps to minimize shock.

LOW-VOLTAGE CURRENT

Many injuries result from faulty switches, frayed flexes and defective domestic appliances. Water is a very good conductor of electricity. The risk of electrical injury is far greater if one has wet hands or is standing on a wet floor.

- Do not attempt first aid until contact with the electrical current has been broken. Pull the electric plug out. If this is impossible, stand on a dry, insulating object, e.g. rubber mat or thick pile of newspapers. Push the victim away using a broom or wooden chair.
- Check breathing and pulse; resuscitate if necessary.
- Cool any burns with plenty of cold water.
- Place in recovery position and wait for arrival of ambulance.

ACTIVITY

1 Suggest two methods of ensuring that an electrical accident does not occur in the home.

2 Find out the correct first aid treatment for burns and scalds.

Drowning

Every year, about 350 people die in the UK from drowning. The victim is usually swimming or playing in water, although some deaths result from falling into water.

NB: Infants can drown in a few centimetres of water.

PREVENTION

- Wear a lifejacket or buoyancy aid for all water sports, e.g. sailing and windsurfing.
- Never jump into deep water without ensuring there is a safe way out.
- Always obey the safety rules operated by lifeguards at pools and beaches.
- Do not drink alcohol before swimming or taking part in water sports.

- Never leave a child alone in the bath and always supervise water play.
- Children should never walk on an iced-over pond unless the ice has first been tested by an adult.

SYMPTOMS AND SIGNS

General signs of asphyxia:

- difficulty in breathing;
- frothing around the mouth, lips and nostrils;
- confusion;
- possible unconsciousness;
- cyanosis (blueness of face, lips and fingernails).

TREATMENT

- Remove obstructions (e.g. seaweed) from casualty's mouth and check for breathing and pulse.
- Do not waste time trying to expel water from the casualty's lungs.
- Resuscitate if necessary.
- As soon as casualty begins breathing, place in recovery position.
- Keep casualty warm; if necessary, treat for hypothermia.

Poisoning

A poison is a substance that, in relatively small amounts, disrupts the structure and/or function of cells, causing temporary or permanent damage.

Poisons enter the body by various routes. They may be:

- swallowed, e.g. contaminated foods, drugs or corrosives;
- inhaled, e.g. gases, solvents, vapours or fumes;
- absorbed through the skin, e.g. pesticides;
- injected under the skin, e.g. insect stings or snake bites.

Poisons may also originate within the body itself; for example, disorders such as liver failure may cause toxins to be produced.

INDUSTRIAL POISONS

Most cases of industrial poisoning involve poisonous fumes. Factories using potentially dangerous gases or chemicals may keep oxygen equipment, and must display notices indicating action to be taken in an emergency.

POISONOUS PLANTS

There are numerous different poisonous plants, including some common garden or house plants (see Table 5.4). Most cases of poisoning occur in young children who are attracted to brightly coloured berries and seeds and are liable to eat them.

Table 5.4   Plants that are poisonous if swallowed

Mushrooms	Seeds, bulbs and rhizomes	Berries
Death cap	Laburnum	Deadly nightshade
Spotted fly agaric	Lupin	Holly
Cortinarius speciosissimus	Daffodil	Laurel
	Iris	Mistletoe
	Foxglove	Yew
		Wild arum

ACTIVITY

1 A four-year-old child complains of 'tummy-ache' and you notice some red berries in her mouth. What action would you take? Use the first aid manual to help you.

2 Statistics show that there is a higher accident rate among boys than among girls. The discrepancy starts at the age of eight months and continues until the age of 14 years, when accident levels are again the same for the sexes. Suggest three reasons for this discrepancy.

3 Prepare a poster or leaflet warning parents of the dangers of poisons commonly available (remember tablets, medicines, bleaches, etc.).

4

Where would you expect to see the labels above, and what do they tell us?

Occupational disorders

DUST DISEASES

- *Pneumoconiosis*, or fibrosis of the lungs, is caused by the inhalation of organic and inorganic dusts. Those affected work in mining industries – coal and quartz mining and china clay factories – and in metal grinding and foundry work.
- *Asbestosis* is a similar hazard in the asbestos industry and is also a problem in the demolition industry (where buildings have involved the use of asbestos).

The most dangerous dusts are usually the ones so small that they cannot be seen with the naked eye. In general, the smaller a dust particle, the further it goes into the lungs and the more damage it causes. Less well-known sources of dust include wool, cotton, hay (fungal spores may cause farmer's lung), fibreglass, talcum powder and detergents.

CHEMICAL POISONING

- *Cadmium fumes* (used in the welding and electroplating industries) may cause kidney damage.
- *Carbon tetrachloride* and *vinyl chloride* (used in the manufacture of chemicals and plastics) may cause liver disease.
- *Lead compounds* and *benzene* can damage the bone marrow, leading to anaemia.

NOISE

Regular exposure to loud noise over a long time leads to increased deafness. Any noise above 90 decibels may cause damage (see Figure 5.16). Prolonged tinnitus (ringing or buzzing in the ears) occurring after a noise has ceased indicates that some damage has already occurred.

Regulations governing maximum noise levels apply to all places of work. Where exposure cannot be avoided (e.g. workers using pneumatic drills) ear protection should be worn.

RADIATION HAZARDS

- *Radiation from the sun*: people with outdoor occupations in sunny climates are at increased risk of skin disease, e.g. skin cancer.

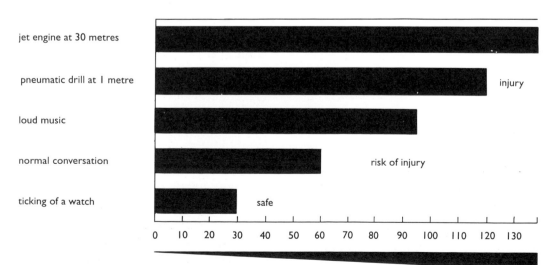

Figure 5.16 Comparative noise levels

- Ionizing *radiation*: X-rays and radiation from nuclear waste may cause cancer (particularly leukaemia) if levels of exposure are not controlled. Controlled radiation, or radiotherapy, is however useful in the treatment of some cancers.

REPETITIVE STRAIN INJURY (RSI)

This is a newly discovered hazard caused by repetitive movement of part of the body. The strain is felt in the joints and muscles, e.g. tennis elbow. Typists, assembly line workers and musicians may all experience pain and stiffness in the affected joints and muscles.

Symptoms usually disappear with rest.

ACTIVITY W

1 Find out about the Safety at Work Act.

2 When you are working in a health or social care setting, ask to see how accidents are reported and dealt with by staff.

REFERENCES AND RESOURCES

British Medical Association (1992), *Complete Family Health Encyclopedia*. London: Dorling Kindersley.

Ewles, Linda and Simnett, Ina (1993), *Promoting Health: A Practical Guide to Health Education*. Chichester: John Wiley and Sons Ltd.

First Aid Manual (1992). London: Dorling Kindersley.

Open University (1989), *Drug Use and Misuse: A Reader*. Chichester: John Wiley and Sons Ltd.

Smith, Alwyn and Jackson, Bobbie (eds) (1988), *The Nation's Health: A Strategy for the 1990s* (A report from an Independent Multidisciplinary Committee). London: King Edward's Hospital Fund for London.

Taylor, Dennis (1989), *Human Physical Health*. Cambridge: Cambridge University Press.

USEFUL ADDRESSES

Health Education Authority
Hamilton House
Mabledon Place
London WC1H 9JP
Tel.: 071 631 0930

Help for Health Trust
Highcroft Cottage
Romsey Road
Winchester
Hants SO22 5DH
Tel.: 0962 849100

Royal Society for the Promotion of Health
RSH House
38A St George's Drive
London SW1V 4BH
Tel.: 071 630 0121

British Heart Foundation
14 Fitzhardinge Street
London W1H 4DH
Tel.: 071 935 0185

British Red Cross Society
9 Grosvenor Crescent
London SW1X 7EJ
Tel.: 071 245 6315

St John Ambulance
1 Grosvenor Crescent
London SW1X 7EF
Tel.: 071 235 5231

MIND (National Association for Mental Health)
22 Harley Street
London W1N 2ED
Tel.: 071 637 0741

Mencap
123 Golden Lane
London EC1Y 0RT
Tel.: 071 454 0454

Disability Alliance
1st Floor East
Universal House
88–94 Wentworth Street
London E1 7SA
Tel.: 071 247 8763

Comprehensive directories of groups and organizations are included in the following publications, available at your local reference library:

Directory for Disabled People, 6th ed. (1991). Woodhead-Faulkner.

Directory of Black and Ethnic Community Health Services in London (1990). London: MIND.

Disability Alliance (1993).

Disabled Rights Handbook (1993–94).

People Who Help, 3rd ed. (1992). Profile Publications.

The Voluntary Agencies Directory, 13th ed. (1993). NCVO Publications.

For free literature about HIV and AIDS, telephone 0800 555 777.

STRUCTURE AND PRACTICES IN HEALTH AND SOCIAL CARE

THE STRUCTURE OF HEALTH AND SOCIAL CARE PROVISION

Provision of health and social care is through a combination of STATUTORY, VOLUNTARY and PRIVATE organizations.

ACTIVITY

What do you understand by the terms

- statutory,
- voluntary,
- private?

Give examples of each.

Health care

STATUTORY PROVISION

The central government department responsible for health and personal social (welfare) services is the DEPARTMENT OF HEALTH (DoH). Each government department is headed by a Minister, who may be designated Secretary of State.

The Secretary of State for Health is responsible for the broad policy and central administration of health and welfare services.

ACTIVITY

1 Who is the current Secretary of State for Health?

2 What do you know of their actions in this role?

On a local level the provision of health services is the responsibility of the regional and district health authorities of the National Health Service (NHS), and the welfare services are provided through Personal Social Services (or social work) departments of local authorities.

The NATIONAL HEALTH SERVICE was created in 1948. The structure of the NHS is constantly changing. Eight English regional health authorities were set up in April 1994, replacing the previously existing 14 (see Figure 6.1a). More changes are to follow and it is currently proposed that district health authorities will be merged with family health service authorities from April 1996. This book explains the structure of the NHS as it exists at the time of publication (see Figure 6.1b), but the reader should always be aware of any actual or proposed changes.

ACTIVITY

1 Find out what health provision was available before the foundation of the NHS in 1948.

2 Find out what changes to health provision are now being made.

The Welsh Office, Scottish Office and Northern Ireland Office, each of which is headed by its own Secretary of State, are responsible for health services in their respective areas. There are no Regional Health Authorities.

- Wales has nine District Health Authorities

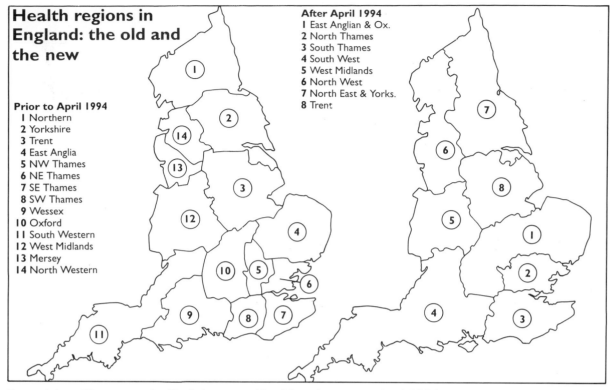

Health regions in England: the old and the new

After April 1994
1 East Anglian & Ox.
2 North Thames
3 South Thames
4 South West
5 West Midlands
6 North West
7 North East & Yorks.
8 Trent

Prior to April 1994
1 Northern
2 Yorkshire
3 Trent
4 East Anglia
5 NW Thames
6 NE Thames
7 SE Thames
8 SW Thames
9 Wessex
10 Oxford
11 South Western
12 West Midlands
13 Mersey
14 North Western

Figure 6.1a Changes to the English regional health authorities in April 1994
Source: Guardian, 22 October 1993.

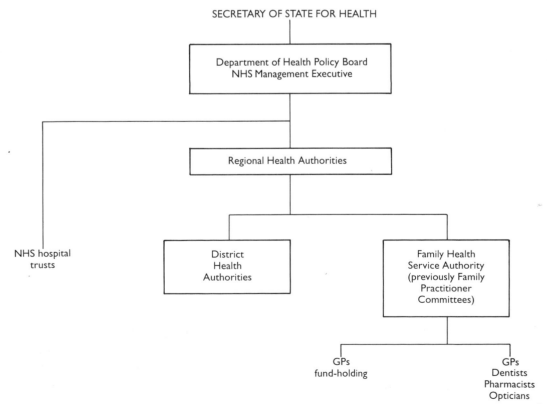

Figure 6.1b The current structure of the NHS in England

and eight Family Health Services Authorities (FHSAs).

- Scotland has 15 Health Boards. (These combine the role of District Health Authorities and FHSAs.)
- Northern Ireland has four Health and Social Services Boards, which look after personal social services as well as health.

Regional Health Authorities

England is divided into eight Regional Health Authorities. The functions of the Regional Health Authority are:

- Determination of regional priorities (e.g. how much kidney transplant surgery should be done).
- Regional planning (e.g. location of specialities such as neurosurgery).
- Allocation of resources to District Health Authorities, Family Health Services Authorities and fund-holding general practitioners.
- Monitoring District Health Authorities' activities and relative costs.
- Provision of major building projects.
- Securing co-ordination among District Health Authorities.
- Employment of medical and dental consultants and senior registrars (except in health teaching areas where there is a university medical school).

District Health Authorities

Each region contains a number of District Health Authorities, 210 in all. The functions of the District Health Authorities are:

- Assessing local health needs.
- Employment of medical and other staff.
- Planning and administering the appropriate health services (under guidance from the Regional Health Authority): for example, they have to make annual contracts with hospitals agreeing in advance the services the hospitals will provide and the price to be paid for them.

Each District Health Authority is responsible for the hospitals and Community Health Services in the district.

ACTIVITY ⬛ **W**

Use your local activity and workplace visits to answer the following questions.

1 What is the name of your Regional Health Authority?

- Draw a map to show the area it covers.

2 What is the name of your District Health Authority?

- Draw a map to show the area it covers.
- Can you find any information on the age structure of this population?

Hospitals

In England and Wales there are approximately 2,500 hospitals, in Scotland 355 and in Northern Ireland 59.

In April 1991, major changes were made to the organization of the NHS. The emphasis was put on health authorities becoming purchasers of the health services their residents need, and local hospitals and other units becoming providers of those services. Hospitals could choose to remain directly managed by health authorities, or to become NHS trusts. These trust hospitals became responsible for managing their own affairs without intervention from district or regional management. In the NHS and Community Care Act 1990, trusts were given freedom to exercise the following powers:

- to employ staff on terms they consider appropriate;
- to buy and sell property;
- to enter into NHS and other contracts;
- to undertake, commission or make facilities available for research;
- to provide, or make facilities and staff available for, staff training;
- to carry out functions jointly with other bodies;
- to treat private patients and generate income subject to this not interfering with other obligations;

- to accept money, land and other property on trust.

For further information on NHS Trusts, contact the NHS Trusts Unit at the Department of Health (for address see list at end of chapter).

ACTIVITY

1 How many NHS hospitals are there in the area covered by your District Health Authority?

- Are any of these trust hospitals?

2 If you have access to a trust hospital:

- Interview a member of staff to find out what they consider to be the advantages and disadvantages of trust status (a) to staff and (b) to clients.
- Design and use a questionnaire to find out whether members of the public are aware of the trust status of their local hospital, and, if they are, their perceptions of the advantages and disadvantages of this.

3 Are any of the hospitals in your area (NHS or trust) specialized, for example, for maternity, mentally disordered or long-stay patients?

4 If possible, visit one of the hospitals in your area (see appendix) and prepare a report on its organization. To help you with this, first prepare a description of its physical layout and structure and then find out about the following (use formal interviews, informal chats, printed leaflets and notice boards as sources of information):

- catchment area
- size – number of patients
- staffing levels
- management structure
- departments (make a chart): pathology, accident/emergency, outpatients, pharmacy, speech and language therapy, etc.

Write down what you think each department does, and then find out what they really do.

Include in your report a brief description of the hospital's history and development, and its plans for the future.

Community Health Services

The purpose of the Community Health Service is to deliver local health care. Its aims are to provide the following:

- a personalized service;
- a client-centred approach to care;
- accessible services available to all;
- a quality service to agreed standards;
- a highly trained workforce to deliver such a service;
- a widely available written statement of service provision;
- an integrated service with other agencies.

ACTIVITY

Find out how your local Community Health Service is organized. (Your local library or Health Clinic will probably have the relevant information):

- Is it divided into neighbourhoods?
- How many clinics are there?
- What type of nurses make up the nursing team?
- What liaison is there between the Community Health Service and GPs?

• Which of the services below does your Community Health Service provide?

Alcohol counselling	Diabetic service	Opthalmic services
Dietician	Ante-natal	Orthoptic clinic
Enuresis (bedwetting)	Parentcraft	AIDS
Audiometry	Family planning	Physiotherapy
Baby clinics	Footcare	Psychosexual counselling
Bio-mechanics	General advice	Psychologist
Health visiting	Child health	Post-natal
Hearing aid batteries	Chiropody	Speech and language therapy
Child protection	Health promotion	School nursing
Dentistry	HIV/AIDS	Toddlers' clinic
Immunization	Terminal care	District nursing
Incontinence services	Welfare foods	Drug abuse
Older persons' clinic	Well woman clinic	

Family Health Services Authorities

The Family Health Service Authority is responsible for purchasing the front-line or PRIMARY CARE services.

These services have important preventative as well as diagnostic and curative roles to play in medical care.

The providers of these services are:

• general practitioners (there are about 32,000 GPs in Britain);

• dentists (there are about 17,000 dentists);

• opticians (there are about 9,000 opthalmic opticians);

• pharmacists (there are about 12,000 retail pharmacies under contract for prescriptions with the NHS).

ACTIVITY

In the area covered by your Family Health Services Authority, find out:

1 About GPs:

• How many of the residents are registered with a GP?

• How many GPs are there in the area? (How many males/females?)

• Calculate the average number of patients per GP.

• How many practices are there in the area?

• How many of the practices have wheelchair access?

• How many of the practices have practice nurses; health visitors; district nurses; a psychiatric nurse; chiropodist; speech and language therapist; other health professionals?

• How many of the GPs carry out minor surgery?

• What percentage of women are screened for cervical cancer?

• What other screening services do the GPs in the area provide?

• What percentage of children are immunized?

• How many of the GPs offer a family planning service?

2 About dentists:

• How many dentists are there in the area? (How many males/females?)

• How many of these dentists give NHS treatment?

• How many of these dentists will take on new NHS patients? (NB: Some will take new children on for NHS treatment, but not new adults.)

• Find out how much dentists are paid

for various treatments, (a) under the NHS, (b) privately.

3 About pharmacists:

- How many pharmacies are there?
- What is the role of the pharmacist?

4 About opticians:

- How many opticians are there? (NB: The FHSA has no control over the location of opticians.)
- Distinguish between opthalmic opticians; opthalmic medical practitioners; dispensing opticians.

GP fund-holders

Since 1990 GPs working in large practices of 7,000 or more patients have been offered the opportunity to become 'fund-holders'.

The fund is given to GPs by the regional health authority. It can be used to purchase services (e.g. hospital treatments, out-patient services and diagnostic tests) which would usually be paid for by the district health authority. It is also supposed to cover most of the drugs that GPs prescribe. The amount each GP receives depends on factors such as their past drugs budget and which providers of services they use.

This money is used to purchase most drugs prescribed, diagnostic tests, and hospital care for their patients. Like District Health Authorities, fund-holding GPs can make their own contracts with hospitals and decide themselves where to have their patients treated.

GP SURGERY FIRST TO BE STRIPPED OF FUNDHOLDING

A family doctor practice in Sheffield has been stripped of its fundholding status after running up a reported £100,000 deficit and placing a block on the referral of non-urgent patients.

The medical centre was among the surgeries that set the pace for the Government's NHS changes, opting for fundholding status and the power to control its own budget in April 1991. It is the first practice to have fallen foul of Department of Health rules and guidance governing fundholding.

The move is bound to embarrass Virginia Bottomley, Secretary of State for Health, who has consistently proclaimed fundholding as one of the success stories of the NHS changes and the split of service functions into purchasers and providers of health care.

Helen Jackson, Labour MP for Sheffield Hillsborough, is pressing the all-party Commons public accounts committee to investigate the finances of the practice. Last year, the centre, which serves 12,000 patients, set up a company which provided medical treatment to the practice. Critics argued that such companies made a nonsense of the purchaser-provider split. Ms Jackson said: 'I understand the practice ran out of money at the end of last year, but nobody wrote to inform the patients as far as I know.'

(The Independent, 10 March 1993)

ACTIVITY

1 Read the extract from *The Independent* on this page, which gives an example of problems which may be encountered with fund-holding.

2 If possible speak to a fund-holding GP to find out what advantages and disadvantages of the system he or she has identified.

3 What do you consider to be the possible advantages and disadvantages?

PRIVATE PROVISION

It is estimated that expenditure on private health treatment in Britain is the equivalent of about 5% of NHS expenditure. The private sector falls into three categories.

1 'Off-the-shelf' products

Commercial 'off-the-shelf' sales of medicines, drugs and appliances in chemists'

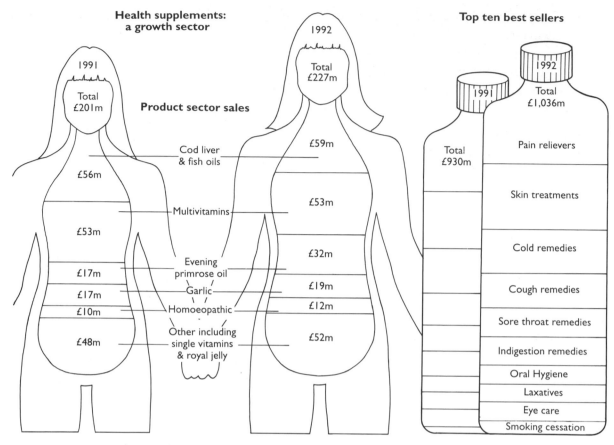

Figure 6.2 Over-the-counter pharmacy sales, 1991 and 1992
Source: Independent, 2 June 1993.

shops and supermarkets (informal or self-care) has an estimated annual value of £1,036 million. NHS prescription charges have risen to a level that makes many commonly prescribed medicines cheaper to buy directly over the counter from a pharmacist. (See Figure 6.2.)

2 Private treatment by doctors

Private treatment is provided by some family practitioners and specialists who are mainly hospital based.

Frequently, private treatment is financed by insurance (70% of private hospital admissions are covered by insurance).

There are about 200 private hospitals and nursing homes in Britain, and private treatment is also given in some NHS hospitals. 'Pay beds' may be reserved by hospital doctors for their private, fee-paying patients. Patients using 'pay beds' are generally in single rooms, and may be offered more attractive food than standard NHS food, but the treatment they receive will be the same as that given to an NHS patient.

ACTIVITY

1 Carry out a survey of the amount spent per month on 'off-the-shelf' health products. How does this vary with age? NB Think carefully about confidentiality before carrying out your research.

2 Find advertisements for private health insurance schemes and compare the services offered.

- How do the costs vary with the age of the insured?
- Can you find examples of large organizations that provide health insurance for their employees?

3 If possible, interview a person who has had hospital treatment privately. Compare his or her experiences with a patient having similar treatment in an NHS hospital.

- Why did the first person choose private treatment?
- Did it meet his or her expectations?

4 Organize a debate, or role play a debate, on the motion: 'The private sector should be phased out of health care in this country.' Each side should be given time to prepare a list of the main advantages/disadvantages of a private health sector.

3 Complementary medicine

Some areas of complementary medicine practised by well-trained professionals, such as osteopathy and chiropractic, which provide treatment where orthodox medicine has often been weak, are quite well established. Other areas of complementary medicine are less widely accepted and scientific.

There is no law controlling the qualifications of practising complementary therapists. This means it can be difficult to choose a reputable therapist, although some organizations can give some guidance (for example, the Institute for Complementary Medicine and the Council for Complementary and Alternative Medicine: for addresses see list at end of chapter). An increasing number of GPs are now practising alternative therapies, such as acupuncture and homoeopathy.

ACTIVITY

1 Have a 'brainstorming session' to list all the areas of complementary medicine you can think of.

2 Question people who have used complementary medicine to find out:

- why they chose complementary medicine
- how they chose their therapist
- if they were happy with their treatment.

VOLUNTARY PROVISION

A VOLUNTARY ORGANIZATION is an association or society which has come into existence of its own accord; it has been created by its members rather than being created by the state. Within voluntary organizations some workers are salaried (i.e. voluntary organizations are not staffed solely by volunteers). The volunteer organizations play a relatively minor role in health care provision compared with the NHS. However, with the introduction of the 1992 Community Care (Residential Accommodation) Act, they are increasingly important providers of certain services.

ACTIVITY

1 In a group 'brainstorming' session, generate a list of voluntary organizations concerned with health care provision (e.g. British Red Cross, Multiple Sclerosis Society, League of Friends of local hospitals . . .)

2 Complete your list by checking with your local library, hospital and health care centre.

3 What do you think are the characteristics of a good volunteer? What do you think a person gains from doing voluntary work?

ACTIVITY   **W**

Select one (or a few) organization/s each,
and find out about:

- the services provided
- the roles of salaried and volunteer staff
- staff training
- how the organization is financed
- the history of the organization

Social care

STATUTORY PROVISION

At the start of the chapter it was explained
that the Department of Health is responsible
for the broad policy and central administration of welfare services, which are
provided on a local level through the Personal
Social Services (social work) departments of
local authorities.

These local Social Services Departments
provide caring services to improve the quality
of life of:

- elderly people
- people with disabilities
- people with learning disabilities
- people with mental health problems
- children and young people

and their families and carers, so they can live
as independently and as safely as possible.

The services provided include:

- assessing needs
- providing personal help
- social work
- day care facilities
- residential and respite care facilities
- occupational therapy (OT)
- rehabilitation
- supplying specialist equipment
- an emergency service, 24 hours a day, 365
  days a year

ACTIVITY

Write a paragraph to demonstrate that you
understand what is meant by each of the
services listed in the text. For example,
what are respite care, occupational therapy
and rehabilitation?

ACTIVITY   **W**

1 Look at Figure 6.3, which outlines
  different client groups and the services
  generally available to them through the
  Social Services Department.

2 Choose one client group, and investigate
  the social services available to them in
  your locality. (Within the class of
  students it may be possible to cover each
  of the client groups, and for the
  information gathered to be shown on a
  series of posters.)

The Department of Health is not the only
government department concerned with
social care provision. The Department of
Social Security (DSS) also plays a major role.

This department is responsible for the
national administration of social security,
which includes:

- National Insurance
- war pensions
- Child Benefit
- Child Support Maintenance
- Attendance Allowance
- industrial injuries
- Mobility Allowance
- Care Allowance
- Family Credit
- Housing Benefit
- Income Support

The DSS has regional and local offices.

ACTIVITY

1 Use information from your local DSS
  office, Citizen's Advice Bureau or library
  to find out what financial help may be

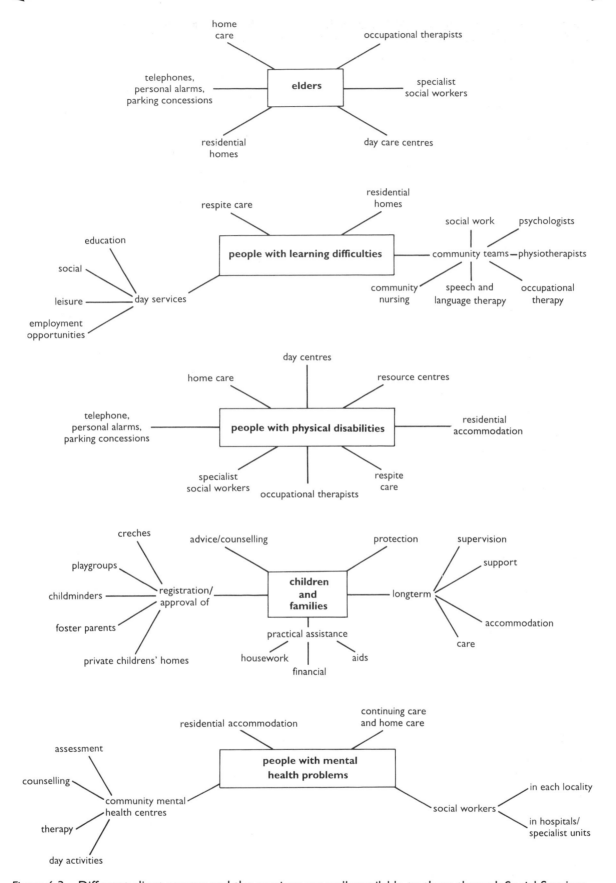

Figure 6.3   Different client groups and the services generally available to them through Social Services

available to the particular group of clients you chose to study above (see Figure 6.3). Present this in poster form.

2 Anyone getting Family Credit or Income Support is automatically entitled to receive help with NHS costs. Others on a low income may also be entitled to this help. Find out which NHS costs may be covered.

3 Mary Smith lives alone with her 4-year-old daughter. She works 20 hours a week as a cleaner at the local hospital, for which she earns £100. She has no savings and her rent is £50 per week.

- To what benefits are she and her daughter entitled?
- Under what conditions would a cold weather payment be made to them?
- Mary's cooker stops working and she urgently wants to buy a new one. What help may she obtain from Social Security?

PRIVATE PROVISION

Some social care is delivered through private provision. For example, of the elders living in old people's homes, only about half are in local authority homes. The remainder are in private and voluntary homes. The number of private homes has increased by over 200% since 1979 (see Figure 6.4).

Local authorities may pay for children to be cared for in private community homes, or, more widely, to be privately fostered. Private day nurseries and child-minding are further examples of private care for children.

Although privately run as profit-making schemes, these arrangements are regulated by Acts of Parliament and they have to be registered and inspected by the local authority. For example, private old people's homes are regulated by the Registered Homes Act 1984, which dictates that local authorities must carry out an annual inspection. The Foster Children Act 1980 dictates that all foster homes must register with the local authority and must be open to inspection.

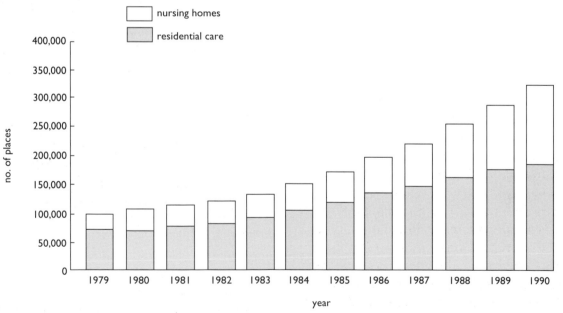

Figure 6.4   Private residential and nursing home places, 1979–90

Source: Audit Commission, *Community Care: Managing the Cascade of Change* (HMSO, 1992), after Laing's review of private health care 1990/1, reproduced by permission of the Controller of Her Majesty's Stationery Office.

ACTIVITY W

1 Find out what private provision for social care is available to your chosen client group:

- nationally
- locally

2 If possible find out the cost to the client of using services provided through local private provision. Where appropriate (e.g. day nurseries, old people's homes), compare this cost with that of using state provision.

3 What links with the local authority do these private establishments have?

4 What do you consider to be the advantages and disadvantages of the private provision of social care for your client group?

VOLUNTARY PROVISION

The provision of social care by voluntary bodies, charities and volunteers is considerable.

Much care is undertaken informally by CARERS: for example, the care of disabled elders by children, neighbours, etc. Some statutory support and support from voluntary bodies and charities may be available to these carers.

SELF-HELP GROUPS are common. These are organized, formally or informally, to protect and promote the interests of their members; they include, for example, tenants' groups, and mother-and-toddler groups. The National Self-Help Support Centre (for address see list at end of chapter) was set up in 1986 to support the work of local centres and increase awareness of self-help at a national level.

There are many formally organized voluntary bodies and CHARITIES involved in social care. Examples include The Samaritans, NSPCC, Relate, Shelter, MIND, Mencap, Dr Barnardo's, the WRVS and the Spastics Society.

Organizations may be pressure groups aiming to bring about changes in statutory care, or they may directly provide care to clients. Most organizations combine these two functions. With the introduction of the Community Care Act, Social Services Departments are now increasingly contracting out some of their services to local voluntary organizations, so that care can be provided on a domiciliary basis (in the home) instead of in a more expensive residential setting.

ACTIVITY W

1 What do you think are the advantages and disadvantages of voluntary organizations and volunteers providing social care, compared with statutory and private provision?

2 What voluntary provision is there for social care for your chosen client group:

- nationally?
- locally?

3 For the voluntary organizations involved, find out about:

- the services they provide
- the roles of salaries and volunteer staff
- how they are financed
- the history of the organization

4 Is there any contracting out of services for your client group to voluntary organizations by the local Social Services Department? Can you find any evidence for the success or failure of these schemes?

One important voluntary organization which you have probably already used in the course of your research is the CITIZEN'S ADVICE BUREAU (CAB). The CAB was set up in 1939 to provide the following:

- accurate information and skilled advice to

individuals on the personal problems that arise in life generally;

- explanation of legislation;
- help to allow the citizen to benefit from and to use widely the services provided by the state;
- counsel to men and women in the many difficulties which beset them in an increasingly complex world.

There are approximately 1,200 Citizen's Advice Bureaux throughout the UK, staffed mainly by trained volunteers. Many bureaux offer on their premises legal advice from solicitors and financial advice sessions. Many CABs are under pressure, with an increasing number of people seeking help and advice, and so have requested statutory, and not voluntary, local authority funding.

A volunteer may offer a client advice, or may refer them on to other statutory or voluntary agencies.

ACTIVITY

What would you do if you were working as a volunteer in your local CAB and people came in with the following problems?

1 A woman has been made redundant. Her partner is unemployed; they have three children and are now unable to afford their rent.

2 A woman tells you that her partner is violent towards her and her young child. She says she cannot afford to move out of the family home.

3 A teenager has just started a Saturday job because he needs the money to enable him to study at college. However, his colleagues at work constantly make racist remarks and he wants to hand in his notice, but is prevented from doing so because of his financial situation.

4 A man tells you that his teenage daughter

has given up college and spends most of the day in bed. He suspects she has a drugs problem.

Health and social care personnel

There is a wide variety of careers in the health and social care structures outlined above.

ACTIVITY

1 Have a 'brainstorming' session to produce a list of as many careers in health and social care as you can. Check your list against the following.

- care assistant
- chiropodist
- dietician
- health service manager
- homoeopath
- housing officer
- district nurse
- health visitor
- hospital nurse
- midwife
- occupational therapist
- osteopath
- physiotherapist
- probation officer
- psychologist
- social worker (field)
- social worker (residential)
- speech and language therapist
- teacher: special educational needs
- volunteer organizer
- warden: accommodation
- youth and community worker

2 For each of the careers, produce a profile including qualifications needed for entry, length of training, prospects and personal qualities. You may wish to divide the research between a group of you (e.g. choose a few careers each).
   Suggested sources of information: college

careers libraries, local careers offices and local libraries will have useful books, videos and computer programs. The list of addresses at the end of the chapter can be used to obtain further information.

3 Choose a career and devise a questionnaire about it. Use this to interview a professional about their work.

4 Use the information from this interview, and your careers profiles, to produce a 'careers resource pack'.

5 If facilities permit, make a short promotional video of 'caring careers'.

6 If you have the opportunity, set up a 'caring careers' stall at your college, using appropriate material.

7 Evaluate the effectiveness of the material you have produced.

ACTIVITY **W**

If you have the opportunity to observe and interview people at work (for example, during work experience) find out what you can about the following aspects of employment:

- the role of trade unions;
- levels of staff provision;
- hours worked per week;
- the gender balance in different occupations;
- the differences between working in statutory, voluntary or private provision.

ACTIVITY

Study Figure 6.5 overleaf, which shows the roles of key personnel in caring for an elderly patient. Consider the needs of the

other client groups shown in Figure 6.3 (page 205) and then draw diagrams to illustrate the roles of the key personnel involved in meeting these needs.

Users' access to health and social care provision

ACCESS TO HEALTH CARE

Referral through professionals

The first professional a person will generally visit if they have a health problem is a GENERAL PRACTITIONER (GP). A person should be registered with a GP to obtain regular health care. Every person has the right to be registered with a GP.

To register with a GP:

- Contact the FHSA, who will provide a list of GPs. (NB: Children under 16 must be registered by their parents.)
- Take your medical card which shows your NHS number to the practice you choose and tell the receptionist you wish to register.
- If you are accepted, the FHSA will send you a new medical card, and your medical records will be sent on to your new GP.
- If you are not accepted (e.g. if the GP's list is full), try at least two other GPs.
- If you are still not accepted, contact the FHSA who will allocate you a GP.

NB: If you are staying in an area for less than three months you can be treated as a temporary resident by a local GP.

ACTIVITY

1 What factors would you take into consideration when choosing a GP?

2 Use a questionnaire to find out how other people have chosen their GP.

At any time a GP can remove a person from their list without giving a reason. The patient also has the right to leave a GP and register

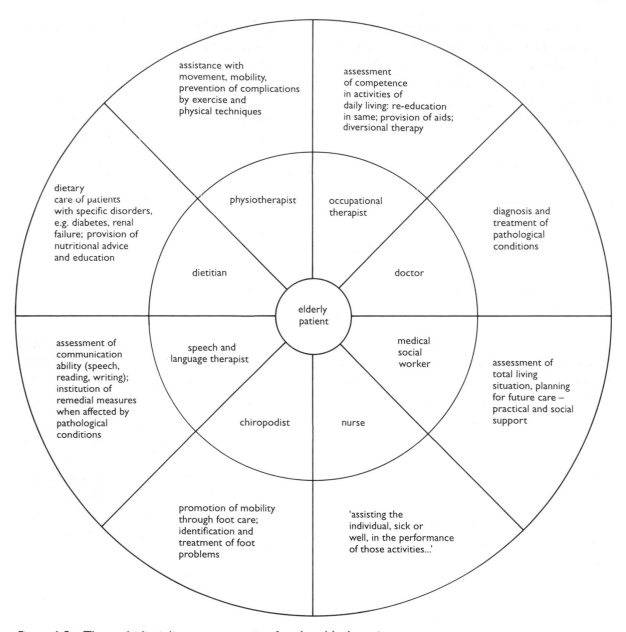

Figure 6.5 The multidisciplinary team caring for the elderly patient
Source: The Essentials of Nursing: Health Needs of the Elderly (Macmillan, 1987).

with another without asking permission or giving a reason. If the patient cannot find another, the FHSA is obliged to find one, who must accept the patient for a minimum of three months.

Most general practices operate on an appointments system. Some practices have an 'open surgery' when patients can turn up and be seen on a first come, first served basis.

Most practices operate a combination of these two systems.

A GP only has to carry out a home visit if 'the condition of the patient so requires'. Out-of-hours home visits may be carried out by the GP, or he or she may make arrangements to provide alternative medical cover, for example, for other local doctors to work on a rota system.

A GP may refer a patient to a SPECIALIST. Generally, the professional to whom a GP will refer a patient will be a CONSULTANT. Unlike GPs, consultants are salaried employees of the NHS, although they may also have private patients. Consultants are specialists in particular:

- *diseases*, e.g. oncologist (cancer care);
- *age groups*, e.g. geriatrician (care of elders);
- *parts of the body*, e.g. urologist (bladder, prostate and kidney surgery).

In a hospital the consultant normally heads a small team of doctors. In descending order of priority this team includes a senior registrar, a registrar, a senior house officer and a house officer.

It is the GP, and not the patient, who decides whether specialist attention is needed. If the patient disagrees with the GP about the need for an appointment with a consultant, he or she can request a second opinion (e.g. from another GP in the same practice).

If the GP thinks referral to a consultant is necessary, the following procedure is followed:

1 The GP writes a letter to a consultant to request an outpatient appointment. (Most GPs choose consultants in the hospitals with which their district health authority has a contract. GP fund-holders have their own contracts with hospitals and may also pay for consultants to hold outpatient clinics at their health centres.)
2 The hospital writes directly to the patient with notification of the date and time of the outpatient appointment. (The waiting time for this appointment is generally about six weeks, or less if urgent.)
3 The patient attends an outpatient clinic where he or she will be seen by a consultant or registrar.
4 If the specialist finds it necessary to admit the patient for treatment (for example, an operation) he or she will be put on a waiting list. The Patient's Charter states that patients have 'the right to be guaranteed

admission for treatment by a specific date not later than two years from the day when your consultant places you on a waiting list'. Even two years may be considered an unacceptably long wait. Hospitals and health authorities are given targets and incentives by the Department of Health to keep their waiting lists within limits.
5 The consultant will send a letter to the GP to notify him or her of the proposed course of action.
6 After hospital treatment, the patient will receive care from his or her GP, and may also be given further appointments at the consultant's outpatient clinic.

ACTIVITY W

1 Give as many examples as you can of specialists working in each of the three areas noted in the text (diseases, age groups, parts of the body).

2 In some countries, e.g. the United States and Germany, a patient can often go directly to a specialist without consulting the family doctor first. What do you think are the main advantages and disadvantages of the British system compared with the other?

3 Discuss the reasons for long waiting lists, and try to find out how hospitals are trying to cut them.

There are two hospital departments for which the patient does not require professional referral:

- Accident and Emergency departments
- Sexually Transmitted Diseases clinics

In an emergency which is not life-threatening, the patient's GP should be the first point of contact. However, in a real emergency the 999 service should be called and an ambulance requested. The Patient's Charter states that an ambulance should arrive within 14 minutes in urban areas, and within 19 minutes in rural areas. Emergency ambulance crews are trained in emergency medical techniques, although the importance of basic first aid training for all members of the public cannot be over-emphasized.

In a large general hospital the ACCIDENT AND EMERGENCY DEPARTMENT ('casualty department') is open 24 hours a day. Usually the condition of the patient will be assessed initially by a nurse, who will either recommend immediate treatment or indicate the length of the waiting time before a doctor will see the patient for treatment.

A patient does not have to arrive at Accident and Emergency in an ambulance but treatment may not be given if it is thought the problem is not urgent and can be dealt with by their GP.

SEXUALLY TRANSMITTED DISEASES (STD) CLINICS are usually, but not always, attached to main hospitals. They give free, confidential advice and treatment to people of all ages with genito-urinary infections (for example, gonorrhoea and syphilis). They will also give HIV antibody tests. Telephone numbers of STD clinics are listed in the phone book, and some clinics will see patients without them having to make appointments.

Before patients undergo invasive treatment (for example, surgery or radiotherapy), they are usually asked to sign a CONSENT FORM. An example is given in Figure 6.6.

The standard NHS form includes the following:

- name of proposed treatment/operation;
- a statement that the nature and purpose of the treatment have been explained to the patient;
- a clause which gives consent for any other procedures which may be necessary if there is an urgent or unexpected complication.

In an emergency (i.e. if the patient is unconscious) permission will be sought from the patient's next of kin, if possible.

ACTIVITY

List the questions you would wish to be answered before you signed a consent form.

Consent is required from parents if their child is too young to have a full under-standing of the treatment in question. If a doctor thinks consent is being withheld unreasonably, he or she can apply for a court order. However, a court order would be likely to go against parents' wishes only in life-and-death cases.

It is very rare for the wishes of an adult refusing to give consent for life-saving treatment to be overruled. For example, Jehovah's Witnesses, who believe that by accepting blood transfusions they will be denied eternal life, have had their wishes respected, even when this proves fatal. In the US courts an adult's refusal to accept a transfusion has been overridden only when the validity of the withholding consent was doubtful (for example, undue pressure had been put on the patient by relatives), or when the patient was a pregnant woman whose foetus was at risk, or whose child would be motherless. In the UK few cases have reached the courts, but instances of controversy from time to time make the news, as the following letter to the *Guardian* illustrates:

Doctor [name deleted] should not have the trauma of having to weigh the legal points about a Jehovah's Witness who does not wish for a blood transfusion, and may die as a result of not having it. Nor should there be expensive legal court cases on the point.

The medical establishment should ensure that all those who treat the sick and injured know that the patient's wish is paramount. There is no argument about it. If the Jehovah's Witness would prefer to die than accept someone else's blood, it is decided in the whole ethic of his or her life; there are countless thousands of people who would rather die than lose something they

CONSENT FORM
For medical or dental investigation, treatment or operation

Health Authority .... Patient's Surname ....
Hospital .... Other Names ....
Unit Number... Date of Birth..
Sex: (*please tick*)   Male ☐   Female ☐

DOCTORS OR DENTISTS (*This part to be completed by doctor or dentist. See notes*)

TYPE OF OPERATION INVESTIGATION OR TREATMENT

I confirm that I have explained the operation investigation or treatment, and such appropriate options as are available and the type of anaesthetic, if any (general/regional/sedation) proposed, to the patient in terms which in my judgement are suited to the understanding of the patient and/or to one of the parents or guardians of the patient

Signature .... Date .../.../.......
Name of doctor or dentist ....

PATIENT/PARENT/GUARDIAN

1. Please read this form and the notes very carefully.

2. If there is anything that you don't understand about the explanation, or if you want more information, you should ask the doctor or dentist.

3. Please check that all the information on the form is correct. If it is, and you understand the explanation, then sign the form.

I am the patient/parent/guardian (*delete as necessary*)

I agree	■ to what is proposed which has been explained to me by the doctor/dentist named on this form.
	■ to the use of the type of anaesthetic that I have been told about.
	■ to be examined, whilst under anaesthetic by no more than two students.
I understand	■ that the procedure may not be done by the doctor/dentist who has been treating me so far.
	■ that any procedure in addition to the investigation or treatment described on this form will only be carried out if it is necessary and in my best interests and can be justified for medical reasons.
I have told	■ the doctor or dentist about any additional procedures I would *not* wish to be carried out straightaway without my having the opportunity to consider them first.

Signature   ....
Name   ....
Address   ....
(*if not the patient*) ....
....

NOTES TO:

Doctors, Dentists

A patient has a legal right to grant or withold consent prior to examination or treatment. Patients should be given sufficient information, in a way they can understand, about the proposed treatment and the possible alternatives. Patients must be allowed to decide whether they will agree to the treatment and they may refuse or withdraw consent to treatment at any time. The patient's consent to treatment should be recorded on this form (further guidance is given in HC(90)22 (*A Guide to Consent for Examination or Treatment.*)

Patients

■ The doctor or dentist is here to help you. He or she will explain the proposed treatment and what the alternatives are. You can ask any questions and seek further information. You can refuse the treatment.

■ You may ask for a relative, or friend, or a nurse to be present.

■ Training health professionals is essential to the continuation of the health service and improving the quality of care. Your treatment may provide an important opportunity for such training, where necessary under the careful supervision of a senior doctor or dentist. You may refuse any involvement in a formal training programme without this adversely affecting your care and treatment.

Figure 6.6   An example of a consent form

hold precious, whether it is their freedom or anything else.

I had thought it was perfectly understood that anyone is at liberty to refuse any form of medical treatment, when they are conscious and of sound mind. Not for nothing does one have to sign a disclaimer before an operation.

(Guardian, 8 August 1992)

ACTIVITY

- Read the letter from the Guardian reproduced in the text about the refusal of a blood transfusion.
- Then consider the following four cases and discuss what recommendations you would have made in each of them.
- Finally, compare your conclusions with the court rulings given below.

The cases:

1 A 35-year-old Jehovah's Witness gave birth to twins. To save her life she required a blood transfusion. She refused this.

2 A 16-year-old anorexic refused to undergo treatment, even though she was aware that she would die without it.

3 T, who refused a blood transfusion, was 20. Her parents separated when she was three. Her mother was a fervent Jehovah's Witness, a faith which regards blood transfusions as sinful. T's father emphatically rejected the faith.

4 A 30-year-old woman who had two other children refused to have a caesarian, although the surgeon was emphatic that the unborn child could not be delivered without the operation. The woman and her husband said the operation was against their principles as born-again Christians. Because it was an emergency, the case was brought and heard within an hour.

The court rulings:

1 The blood transfusion was not given and the woman died.

2 As the patient was under 18 her refusal was overruled.

3 It was judged that T was not in a fit state to make a decision and so her wishes were overruled; she received a transfusion. It was suggested that undue pressure from her mother had influenced her refusal.

4 The mother's wishes were overruled and the child was delivered by caesarian. The baby died. This was the first case in the UK in which the rights of the unborn baby appear to have overruled those of the mother.

Compulsory admission to hospital

As has been shown, even if the patient's life is in danger, he or she can refuse to accept treatment and doctors and nurses treating patients against their will could face criminal prosecution. However, there are two circumstances in which compulsory admission to hospital occurs.

If MENTALLY ILL, patients may be detained under certain sections of the Mental Health Act. For this to occur patients must have been SECTIONED for at least 28 days. Sectioning commits patients for treatment for their own safety or the protection of others. It requires the signature of two doctors, one of them a psychiatrist, as well as that of a psychiatric social worker or the patient's nearest relative. The patient's nursing care may include restraint or seclusion. Drug treatment can be given for up to three months, but after that a second doctor's opinion is required. Electroconvulsive therapy (ECT) also requires a second doctor's opinion. The patient's consent is required for invasive therapies, such as surgery or hormone implantation.

If patients are suspected of having a dangerous NOTIFIABLE DISEASE, for example, tuberculosis, they may be isolated from others at risk. This regulation would only be enforced if the public were at risk of infection, and although the patients would be isolated, they would still not be treated against their will.

Private self-referral

Even if a patient wants to be treated privately by a consultant, he or she must still be referred through a GP. Most complementary medical provision requires private self-referral, for example, making an appointment with an osteopath or a chiropractor.

> **ACTIVITY** W
>
> Refer back to the information obtained on voluntary organizations giving health care. How do users gain access to the provision they offer? Is it by referral through professionals, or is it by private self-referral?

ACCESS TO SOCIAL CARE

The following professionals and organizations may approach a social worker in their local Personal Social Services Department to request help for a client:

- health visitor
- district nurse
- GP
- community psychiatric nurse
- teacher
- head of year
- Education Welfare Department
- magistrate
- probation service
- solicitor
- Citizen's Advice Bureau
- police

Non-professionals, such as neighbours or parents, may also ask for help, or the person requiring help may approach social services directly.

> **ACTIVITY**
>
> Examine the list of channels of referral to social services. Can you think of situations in which each might be used?

Once a person has been referred, or referred themselves, to the Social Services Department, an ASSESSMENT of the situation takes place to determine the most suitable course of action. Figure 6.7 shows a typical example of this assessment procedure.

> **ACTIVITY**
>
> Refer back to the information obtained on voluntary organizations giving social care. How do users gain access to the provision they offer? Is it by referral through professionals, or is it by private self-referral?

ACCESS TO SOCIAL SECURITY PROVISION

There are many sources of information on Social Security payments. Any of the professionals and organizations listed above may advise a person to apply for benefits. Free leaflets are available from Social Security offices and advice centres, and the press and television sometimes carry advertisements giving details of particular benefits.

The applicants will complete the necessary forms, or this will be done for them if necessary. Their entitlement to benefit will then be assessed.

> **ACTIVITY**
>
> If a person thinks that a Social Security decision is wrong, he or she can appeal. Obtain the leaflet *How to Appeal* from your local Social Security office to find out about the appeal procedure.

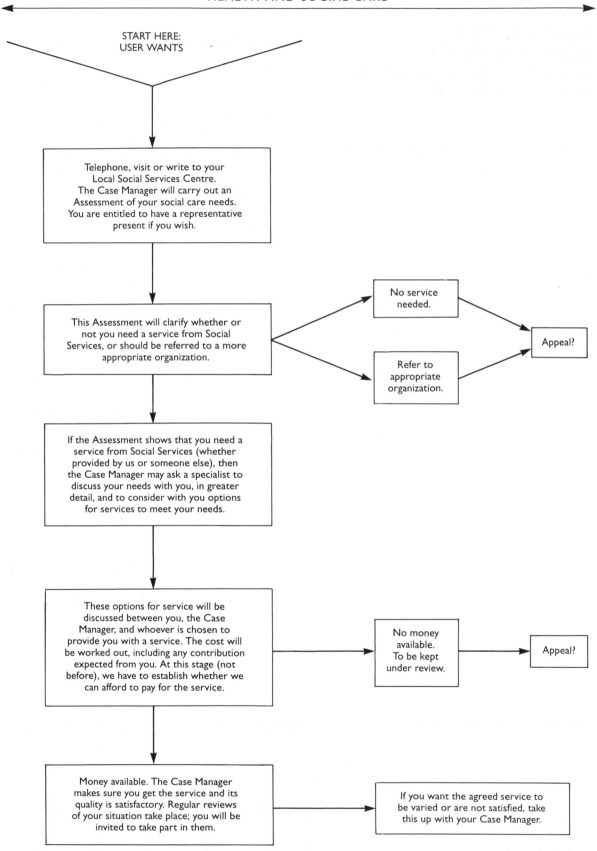

START HERE:
USER WANTS

Telephone, visit or write to your
Local Social Services Centre.
The Case Manager will carry out an
Assessment of your social care needs.
You are entitled to have a representative
present if you wish.

This Assessment will clarify whether or
not you need a service from Social
Services, or should be referred to a more
appropriate organization.

No service
needed.

Refer to
appropriate
organization.

Appeal?

If the Assessment shows that you need a
service from Social Services (whether
provided by us or someone else), then
the Case Manager may ask a specialist to
discuss your needs with you, in greater
detail, and to consider with you options
for services to meet your needs.

These options for service will be
discussed between you, the Case
Manager, and whoever is chosen to
provide you with a service. The cost will
be worked out, including any contribution
expected from you. At this stage (not
before), we have to establish whether we
can afford to pay for the service.

No money
available.
To be kept
under review.

Appeal?

Money available. The Case Manager
makes sure you get the service and its
quality is satisfactory. Regular reviews
of your situation take place; you will be
invited to take part in them.

If you want the agreed service to
be varied or are not satisfied, take
this up with your Case Manager.

Figure 6.7   The assessment procedure carried out by Social Services
Source: Surrey County Council Social Services Department.

THE IMPACT OF LEGISLATION AND FUNDING ON PROVISION AND PRIORITIES

Sources of funding in health and social care

There are four main sources of funding for health and social care. These are:

- central government
- local government
- registered charities
- commercial sources

CENTRAL GOVERNMENT

The money available for public expenditure comes from:

- taxes;
- National Insurance contributions (paid by employees, the self-employed, and employers – in fact a form of taxation);
- charges (e.g. rents, health service charges, etc.; see Table 6.1);
- government borrowing.

2 Where possible, find out the amount individuals may be asked to pay (for example, current prescription charges).

3 What exemptions are made?

4 If possible, interview a professional from each of the five areas to help you check your findings.

Figure 6.8 shows the sources of revenue and the main categories of expenditure. Figure 6.9 shows how finance flows from central government down to health and social care services.

LOCAL GOVERNMENT

Local authorities obtain their funds from the Council Tax (previously poll tax or Community Charge and, before that, Rates), and grants from central government. These grants are weighted, depending on the needs within the local authorities and financial penalties are imposed on local authorities which overspend.

ACTIVITY   W

1 Discuss what charges may be made by each of the five services listed in Table 6.1.

ACTIVITY

Discuss the arguments for and against local freedom in collecting taxes and managing services. Compile a list of each.

Table 6.1   National health and personal social services in England: charges to persons using the services (years ended 31 March)

Services	Charges (£m)							
	1981	1985	1986	1987	1988	1989	1990	1991*
All services	**524**	**808**	**930**	**925**	**1,020**	**1,072**	**1,441**	**1,606**
Hospital	54	78	86	91	97	107	399	471
Pharmaceutical	71	122	128	170	167	203	191	206
General dental	92	171	195	223	240	291	367	335
General ophthalmic	29	44	12	1	–	–	–	–
Personal social services	277	393	509	440	516	471	484	544

*1991 figures are provisional.
Source: Health and Personal Social Services Statistics for England, 1992 (HMSO).

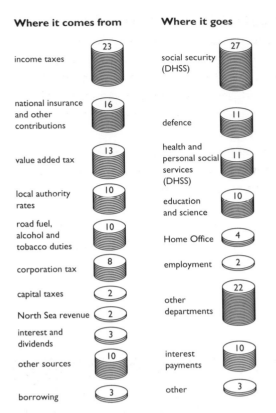

Where it comes from

income taxes ⊙ 23

national insurance and other contributions ⊙ 16

value added tax ⊙ 13

local authority rates ⊙ 10

road fuel, alcohol and tobacco duties ⊙ 10

corporation tax ⊙ 8

capital taxes ⊙ 2

North Sea revenue ⊙ 2

interest and dividends ⊙ 3

other sources ⊙ 10

borrowing ⊙ 3

Where it goes

social security (DHSS) ⊙ 27

defence ⊙ 11

health and personal social services (DHSS) ⊙ 11

education and science ⊙ 10

Home Office ⊙ 4

employment ⊙ 2

other departments ⊙ 22

interest payments ⊙ 10

other ⊙ 3

Figure 6.8 UK public income and expenditure, 1987/8, pence in every pound (to the nearest penny)
Source: G. F. Stanlake, *Introductory Economics* (Longman Group UK Ltd, 1990), using data from *Financial Statement and Budget Report 1987/8*; *Economic Progress Report Supplement, March–April 1987*.

REGISTERED CHARITIES

How are charities funded?

In the UK there are at present 175,000 registered charities, and this number is continually growing. Central government contributes a great deal to charities:

- Charitable status confers exemption from taxation, which amounts to about £3 billion of tax forgone per year.
- Various government departments may also give grants directly to charities; for example, the Department of the Environment funds many inner-city projects.

Local authorities, too, fund many charities. This may be through grants or, increasingly, with the introduction of the government's 'Care in the Community' programme, through payment for services provided.

It is often thought that charities obtain most money through donations, but in fact this accounts for less than 40% of charitable income. Donations may be gained:

- in the form of endowments;
- collected on flag-days;
- from employees at work who regularly; donate part of their wage;

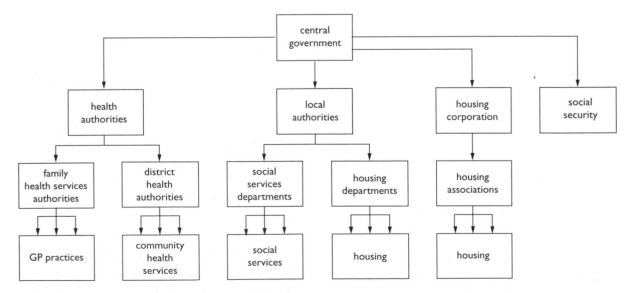

Figure 6.9 The flow of finance from central government
Source: Audit Commission, *Community Care: Managing the Cascade of Change* (HMSO, 1992) reproduced by permission of the Controller of Her Majesty's Stationery Office.

- from corporate sponsorship;
- from charity shops.

Recession hits charities hard. It means less government money and donations at a time when demand for their services is increasing.

Some fund-raisers worry that as services provided by charities replace those previously provided by the state, people will be less willing to donate money.

ACTIVITY

- Look at Figure 6.10.
- Discuss the distribution of charity donations. Why are some causes more 'popular' than others?

Charitable funding of the NHS

Charitable fund-raising is not limited to voluntary organizations. Before the NHS was founded in 1948, charity was at the forefront of health services. After this, up until 1980, charity in hospitals ceased to be of any significance.

In 1980 the Health Services Act empowered health authorities to fund-raise, and the amounts collected through this activity doubled every year throughout the late 1980s. Proceeds are now used to pay for basic patient care and hospital building, not just small comforts for patients and staff and for research.

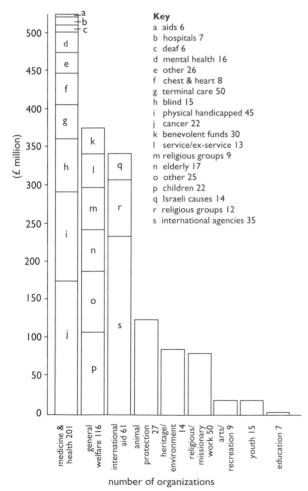

Key
a aids 6
b hospitals 7
c deaf 6
d mental health 16
e other 26
f chest & heart 8
g terminal care 50
h blind 15
i physical handicapped 45
j cancer 22
k benevolent funds 30
l service/ex-service 13
m religious groups 9
n elderly 17
o other 25
p children 22
q Israeli causes 14
r religious groups 12
s international agencies 35

Figure 6.10 Voluntary income received by the largest 500 charities by sector
Source: Charity Trends 16th edition, published by Charities Aid Foundation.

ACTIVITY   W

1 What examples can you find of charitable funding of the NHS in your area?

2 What are the merits and drawbacks of the charitable funding of health care?

COMMERCIAL FUNDING

Corporate sponsorship

An important aspect of charitable fund-raising is CORPORATE SPONSORSHIP. It is now common for local businesses to fund building programmes and pay for items of equipment in hospitals.

West Middlesex University Hospital marked its first day of NHS trust status by signing a deal for a new state-of-the-art endoscopy unit which will allow them to treat patients more efficiently.

Lister BestCare Limited are funding the building of the unit which can diagnose and treat conditions of the stomach and intestine without surgery.

(Richmond and Twickenham Guardian, April 1993)

In another example, in an effort to boost take-up of child immunization, St Helen's and Knowsley Health Authority on Merseyside struck up a deal with Iceland frozen foods to distribute £6,000 in grocery vouchers to families in the worst-performing neighbourhoods who completed all immunization courses before their child's third birthday.

ACTIVITY   **W**

1   Discuss the advantages to a business of donating funds.

2   Can you find examples of corporate sponsorship in your locality?

Selling goods and services

The selling of goods and services has been covered earlier in the chapter, in the sections on private provision.

There are increasing numbers of examples of the NHS raising funds through commercial transactions. For example, when staff at West Dorset Hospital in Dorchester found that 68% of new-born babies were being taken home by car without any form of seat restraint, they introduced the sale of baby chairs and started to provide carriers for parents to take babies from the maternity department to the car.

The private sector also invests in profit-making schemes in hospitals; for example, there are privately managed shopping malls.

Recently the use of private finance has been widened. The limit above which NHS trusts and health authorities need Treasury approval for contracts involving private finance has risen from £250,000 to £10 million. This has led to opposition from MPs accusing the Conservative government of trying to 'fudge' the difference between private and public health care.

The growing demand for health and social care

ACTIVITY

There are many factors which raise costs or create an increase in demand for health and social care. In a group, discuss what these factors may be and then compare your ideas with those given below.

POPULATION CHANGES

The population is constantly increasing (see Figure 6.11). Obviously more people mean a higher demand for health and social care.

Perhaps even more important than the change in population size is the change in AGE

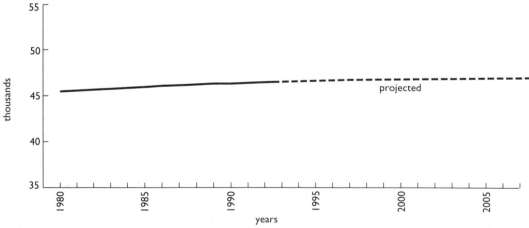

Figure 6.11   Population size in England

Source: Crown copyright. Reproduced with the permission of the Controller of Her Majesty's Stationery Office.

STRUCTURE of the population. On average, one person aged 75 or over costs the health and personal social services seven times as much as one person of working age. By the year 2001 there will be 10.6 million pensioners, and by the year 2031, 14.6 million.

ACTIVITY

Explain why we have an 'ageing population'.

ADVANCES IN MEDICAL SCIENCE

When the NHS started it was envisaged that the cost of health care would fall over the years as people became healthier. However, as medical technology advances, conditions which were previously incurable can now often be treated and improvements in treatment are continuously being made. People expect these often expensive advances to be freely available. For example, improved anti-depressants have been developed which, if taken in an overdose as a suicide attempt, are far less likely than previous ones to be fatal. However, these new drugs are over twenty times more expensive than the old ones.

INCREASED EXPECTATIONS

Just as people expect increases in their standard of health care, so increases in the standards of housing and education are also expected.

ACTIVITY

Chat to elderly relations or friends about their living conditions, and the health care and education they received, when they were young. List the improvements there have been. Have there been any deteriorations in living standards?

CHANGED FAMILY PATTERNS

Perhaps one of the most significant social changes in recent decades is the increase in the divorce rate. This has left a high number of families headed by a single parent, which has increased the demand on all the major social services (for example, housing, personal social services and social security benefits).

COPING WITH INCREASED DEMAND

In recent years the government has had to consider carefully the options open to it to cope with the increased demand for health and social care described above.

The amount of money collected (from charges, taxes and National Insurance contributions) could be increased, or the pattern of government spending could be changed (Figure 6.12).

Increasing funding

The funding available to the government is largely dependent upon the state of the economy. The higher the rate of employment, the more people are paying taxes and National Insurance contributions and the lower are social security claims.

ACTIVITY

1 Find out the current rates of the following sources of government funding and then discuss the relative advantages and disadvantages of increasing each of them:

- Charges. Consider in your discussion which charges could be increased or whether any new charges could be introduced. For example, it has been suggested that people convalescing in hospital would be asked to pay the equivalent of what they would spend at home.

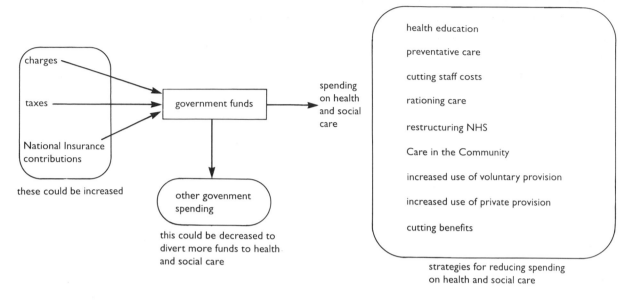

Figure 6.12 Possible strategies for coping with increased demand for statutory care

- Taxes. What taxes are currently levied in the UK? Which could be increased (e.g. income tax, VAT, council charge)?
- National Insurance contributions.

Conduct a survey to find out people's attitudes to paying each of the above.

2 Debate the advantages and disadvantages of the suggestions made in the *Observer* article reproduced here for increasing funding of the NHS through increased charges.

A MEANS-TEST FOR HEALTH CHARGES CAN SAVE THE NHS

The forecast by the architect of the modern welfare State, William Beveridge, that the cost of free health care would decline as the nation's health improved has been shown to be, in Enoch Powell's phrase, 'a miscalculation of sublime proportions'. The cost of the NHS has grown 100 times since its inception in 1949. It is now about £40 billion a year, roughly £650 for every person in the country.

Rising life expectancy, advances in high-tech treatment and an ageing population mean health expenditure is certain to continue to increase ahead of inflation. By the end of the century, there will be twice as many people aged over 80 as now, and the cost of care for this group is roughly 10 times that for those in work.

So how is this bill for an ever-expanding health service going to be met? If demand for a service free at the point of supply is almost infinite, the sums can only be made to add up by queuing, rationing or simply removing some medical procedures, such as in-vitro fertilisation, from available treatment. And that is what is happening.

Conservative governments have increased spending on the NHS by 58 per cent in real terms since 1979, but the perception of a grossly underfunded service is widespread. Hospitals unable to perform urgently-needed operations, children having to wait months for routine procedures, wards left empty because of shortages of funds are everyday occurrences.

If the NHS is to prosper, it needs additional sources of revenue, and these can only come from charges. Before howls of fury rent the land, it is worth pointing out that we already have a crude charging system. Prescription charges have been increased by more than 2,000 per cent since 1979.

A far better system would be to charge for drugs according to income, using a computerised family income coding. The poor would pay nothing; the rich would pay nearly the full cost for most drugs.

Much of this would be very unpopular. But if the NHS continues to be grossly underfunded, the result is inevitable. A two-tier, separate system of private and public health care is well established. Spending on private health care is rising three times faster than spending on the NHS; more than one in six households is covered by private health insurance.

(Observer, 28 March 1993)

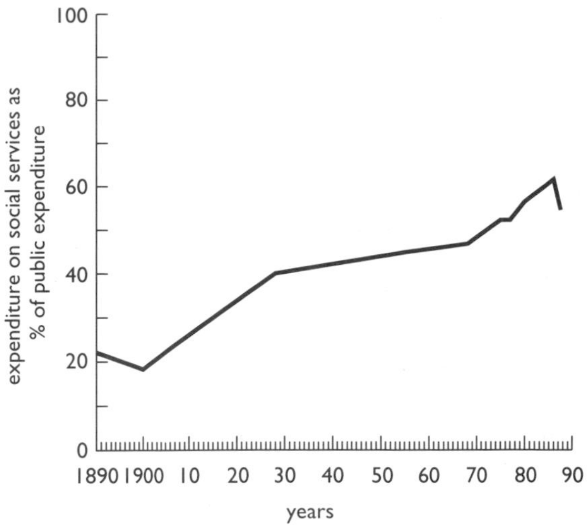

Figure 6.13 The proportion of public expenditure devoted to social services, 1890–1986
Source: Peacock and Wiseman, *The Growth of Public Expenditure*; *Annual Abstract of Statistics*; *Economic Trends* (CSO Publications).

Changing the patterns of spending

PRIORITIZATION OF GOVERNMENT SPENDING

The largest single category of public expenditure in the UK is spending on social services. Under this heading it is usual to include education, health and social security benefits, and these three items account for about 50% of total public expenditure. This expenditure has increased over the years (Figure 6.13). The decision could be taken to meet increased demand by further increasing this percentage.

ACTIVITY

1 What else accounts for government spending besides social services?

2 Discuss what expenditure could be decreased to allow extra funds to become available for social services. What opposition would the government meet?

Within the social services sector the priority given to different aspects could be changed. For example, spending on health could be increased at the expense of spending on housing.

Within one social service priorities could be changed. For example, spending on welfare services for the elderly could be increased at the expense of spending on the handicapped.

SAVINGS AND EFFICIENCY

Health education

It has been suggested that increased spending on health education would result in a healthier population, and, therefore, a decrease in demand for health services.

ACTIVITY

Visit your local Health Promotion Unit (you can find the address in the phone book). Find out:

- what services it provides
- information on its funding
- how it measure its effectiveness

Does health promotion reach the more deprived sectors of the community who suffer the worst health?

Preventative care

In 1990, the government drew up new contracts for GPs and dentists which were intended to encourage them to do more work to *prevent* disease. GPs are now expected to provide health checks for patients, and are rewarded for achieving certain targets of immunization and screening.

ACTIVITY

1 Visit your local GP's surgery to find out what health checks, screening and health promotion clinics are available.

2 Find out the levels of immunization and screening required for the GP to obtain payments.

3 If possible, interview a GP about his or her opinion of the new contracts. For example, has the amount of paperwork increased?

Dentists are now paid an annual fee for each child on their list instead of being paid for each treatment. Incentives are given for quality rather than quantity; for example, if fillings fall out within a year, they have to be replaced free of charge.

Cutting staff costs

A high percentage of the expenditure on health and social care goes on staff costs. The NHS alone is one of Europe's biggest employers, and 75% of total NHS resources are spent on paying staff. This means the government can make savings by paying staff working in statutory health and social care less than they would earn outside.

ACTIVITY

1 Find how the wages of staff in statutory care compare with the wages of the equivalent staff in private care. Do they differ significantly?

2 How do the wages of staff in the 'caring sector' compare with the wages of staff in industry?

Some government advisers have recommended that the NHS could sack at least 200,000 people (one-fifth of the workforce) without any adverse effect. This would release an extra £4.6 billion a year for patient care.

Rationing care

While reading this section, it should have become apparent to you that in many cases, because of the availability of scarce resources, care may have to be rationed. NHS waiting lists are an example of the RATIONING OF CARE. Between 1987 and 1991 the government spent an extra £156 million to reduce waiting lists dramatically. The numbers of patients waiting more than one year dropped considerably; but the numbers of those waiting less than a year shot up.

Since the 1991 NHS reforms the income of hospitals depends far more on the number of patients treated. This has encouraged measures to move patients more quickly through the system. For example, day surgery is increasing, with a subsequent drop in waiting lists. It has been predicted that further increases in day surgery could reduce waiting lists in the UK as a whole by a third.

Rationing may also be seen at work in the prescription of drugs. Some which the DoH regards as too expensive have now been placed on a 'restricted list', which means they cannot be prescribed on the NHS.

Restructuring the NHS

In the late 1980s an 'internal market' was created within the NHS by splitting the service into PURCHASERS and PROVIDERS. The aim was to make the NHS work more like private industry, where competition ideally keeps prices low and quality high. Purchasers buy treatment for patients, and providers provide the treatment. The main purchasers are the District Health Authorities, and the main providers are the hospitals and GPs.

As explained above, the District Health Authorities make annual contracts with hospitals, agreeing in advance the services the hospital will provide and the price to be paid for them.

The Family Health Services Authorities are the purchasers who make contracts with the providers of non-hospital care: GPs, dentists, pharmacists and opticians.

Fund-holding GPs are purchasers as well as providers. They have their own budget to purchase drugs and hospital care for their patients.

The main criticism of the 'internal market' is that competition does not necessarily guarantee better quality. Providers might lower their standards in order to keep prices down. GPs may base their treatment decisions on cost rather than medical need. The following newspaper articles illustrate some of the problems which have been blamed on the market system.

NHS MARKET BLAMED FOR TREATMENT DELAYS

Patients facing delays in treatment at Papworth heart hospital in Cambridgeshire have been sent to St Bartholomew's in London, even though Bart's is unable to treat many of its own patients.

This has arisen as a result of the National Health Service market system.

Earlier this week, Mary Lambert, of Buckhurst Hill, Essex, told how her husband, Bert, died after being told by Bart's he could not have a coronary arteriogram, a form of X-ray, until April.

But Bart's has been treating patients unable to be seen by Papworth. Dr Ian Cooper, a consultant cardiologist at Papworth and at

Bedford General, said he had been told to refer to Bart's 12 patients whom Papworth would not treat.

The district found it had spare cash 'on account' at Bart's. It agreed that the money could be used for coronary procedures and told Dr Cooper to refer 12 of his patients.

'The whole thing is completely stupid,' Dr Cooper said. 'We are told how the beauty of the market system is that the money follows the patient. In fact, you have got patients here being told to follow the money.'

The Department of Health has told hospitals and health districts that patients deemed urgent, like Mr Lambert, must not have treatments delayed until the new financial year.

A department spokesman said Mr Lambert's case was 'tragic' but that, at the time he was put on the Bart's waiting list, he had not been considered an emergency. 'Doctors, not administrators, are responsible for deciding which cases are emergencies.'

(Guardian, 5 March 1993)

HOSPITAL IN CRISIS AS AXE FALLS ON ROUTINE OPS

The Lister Hospital, Stevenage, in the East and North Herts health authority, will be treating 3,000 fewer patients than last year. It will be axing 40 nursing jobs and closing 50 beds because of an estimated £20 million cash squeeze in the district health authority, due to the number of GP fundholders who take money out of health authority spending budgets.

The crisis at Stevenage underlines problems facing hundreds of hospitals as the start of the financial year looms. Many may be faced with a situation where they can only operate on urgent cases because there are no funds for routine waiting list surgery.

Lister managers have blamed the health authority for their lack of cash. The authority has said the Government's financial squeeze means there is no more money to treat non-urgent waiting list patients.

(Observer, 13 March 1993)

Care in the community

Between 1979 and 1993 the cost to the state of residential care rose from £10 million to £2.5 billion. The main reason for this was that the Department of Social Security had to pay for the accommodation of anyone entitled to Income Support, which included the majority of those in residential care. For example, pensioners in private nursing homes had an automatic right to Income Support of up to £315 per week. With the increasing number of elderly people, it was apparent that these costs would continue to grow.

There were complaints that little help was available to people looking after relatives at home, and that the system therefore encouraged these carers to put their relatives into residential care.

The programme the government developed in an effort to solve these problems, CARE IN THE COMMUNITY, was introduced in April 1993 to cater for people with problems of ageing, mental illness, mental handicap, physical or sensory disabilities, or drugs and alcohol. The main change was that the money which had previously come from the DSS now goes to councils who work with local health authorities to decide who should be looked after in residential homes, who needs medical support, and who should be looked after at home, possibly with the assistance of professional carers. The councils also decide what should be paid for the various services required.

ACTIVITY

1 A 90-year-old man who has some mobility problems because of arthritis lives alone. What support is he likely to require from Social Services to allow him to continue living in his home?

2 Discuss the advantages and disadvantages (a) to the carer, (b) to the dependent relative, of care in institutions compared with care in the community.

Although there are obvious advantages to giving people the opportunity to remain living in their own homes where possible, many criticisms have been made of the Care in the Community programme.

Inadequate funding. The chief complaint is that there is inadequate funding for the scheme. For example, for 1993/4, the local authorities in England received a transfer of £399 million from Social Security, plus £140 million to get things under way. It was claimed that this falls short of what is needed by £135 million.

Good home care is at least as expensive as residential care if the necessary support is provided. However, councils are required to spend 85% of their funds in the private sector, and most private provision is in residential care and nursing homes. This means that there will be little cash left for the promised new services to help people to stay in their own homes and provide temporary care to give relatives and other carers a break.

Another possible problem leading to lack of funds is the fact that in future years the community care budgets may be raided to pay other council bills, as the money is only 'ring-fenced' for the first four years.

Although there is a cash shortage, councils could face legal action if they inform people about services and then fail to provide them because of insufficient funds. Therefore, in some circumstances, local authorities may record 'unmet choice', rather than conceding that it was an 'unmet need'. Research has also shown that on some occasions Social Services staff secretly ration the care and services available by failing to suggest services which are considered too expensive to provide.

Some clients are now contributing more to funding their care than they would have in the past. For example, the number of beds in long-stay geriatric wards in NHS hospitals (which are provided free to patients) are being cut, and the patients transferred to residential homes for which they are means-tested. It is likely that in the future there will be more emphasis on payment by the client from his or her savings or selling assets, or by payments by the relatives. This may prove to be very expensive. On average a man spends the last three years of his life, and a woman spends the last five to six years being looked after, either in nursing homes, or in their own home with nursing or community care back-up. For this reason long-term care insurance plans are becoming increasingly popular.

ACTIVITY

Find advertisements for long-term care insurance schemes. How do policies change with the age at which insurance is taken out, and what services does the insurance eventually cover?

Changes in family structure and attitude. There is a worry that the number of family carers will not increase at the same rate as the number of dependants. An increasing divorce rate means that there may be fewer people caring for spouses and parents-in-law.

Many people have grown up with the belief that the state will care for elderly relatives. For example, in a recent survey two-fifths of the people questioned said that they felt 'no obligation to care for a parent'.

Abandonment. Already there are cases which are termed by the popular press 'Granny-dumping', where stressed relatives, feeling unable to continue caring for elderly relatives at home, leave them at day centres or in hospital.

At present three-quarters of general hospitals say that this happens once a month; one-third say it happens once a week; and one-tenth say this happens every day. As more people are cared for in relatives' homes, these figures seem likely to increase.

NHS 'bed-blocking'. Hospitals may be unable to discharge patients who are otherwise ready to go because of delays in undertaking care assessments and arranging any further services they require.

Viability of 'low-priority' services. It is feared that hostels for homeless mentally ill people and residential drug and alcohol addiction clinics may be a low priority for local authorities and may, therefore, close.

ACTIVITY

Prepare a list of the advantages of the Care in the Community scheme and then debate whether, overall, these outweigh the disadvantages, or vice versa.

Increased use of voluntary provision

As you may have found through your research earlier in this chapter, an important aspect of the Care in the Community scheme is the increased role played by charities and voluntary organizations. They frequently replace and supplement some aspects of public social services.

Although local authorities will pay for services, many organizations are under financial pressure because of rising costs and cuts in local authority grants. There are complaints that by providing services for local authorities they have to operate under greater restrictions, ranging from staff qualifications to the colour of the carpets!

Increased use of private provision

Now that local authorities are playing a key role as 'commissioners' of services, they often 'contract out' to private organizations services which previously they would have supplied themselves. It is suggested that services may run more efficiently in private hands, but this opens up a debate on the question of EFFICIENCY.

If people can be persuaded to pay for their own private care this obviously saves money: examples include the use of private schools and hospitals. Commercial sponsorship will also save local authorities money.

Cutting Social Security

This is considered to be one of the most

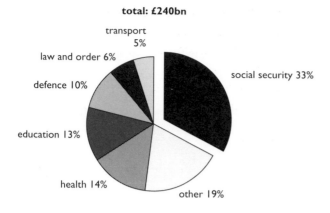

total: £240bn

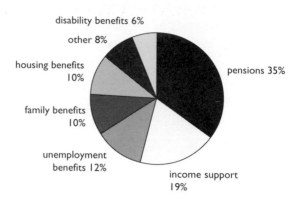

social security total : £79bn

Figure 6.14 **Where the money goes: public spending, 1992/3 (estimate, excluding debt interest and other accounting adjustments)**
Source: Economist, 13 February 1993.

likely areas of cuts in both the long and the short term, as it accounts for such a high percentage of government spending (Figure 6.14).

This may mean the extension of means-testing to target benefits where they are most needed. Younger people may become compelled to take out insurance against sickness and mortgage default, which will mean lower payments of state benefits. Employers will also be required to take greater responsibility for sick pay and maternity benefit.

The retirement age for women is to be raised by five years so that there is a common retirement age of 65. This change will be phased in over 10–15 years. Eventually the savings from this alone will be worth about £4 billion per year to the government.

Political priorities

SUMMARY OF LABOUR PLANS FOR HEALTH CARE (1992)

- More services outside the hospital by community health teams or GPs.
- Care of elderly or chronically ill patients must get a higher priority.
- Mental health services must get a fairer share of resources.
- Quality of treatment and services must be recognized as equally important as quantity.
- A permanent Cabinet committee on health promotion to be created.
- Tobacco advertising to be banned.
- Random breath-testing to be introduced.
- Nutritional guidelines for school meals to be restored.
- Free eye tests to be restored.
- GPs to be helped to make more time available for health promotion.

ACTIVITY

Recently a government brainstorming seminar took place on how to contain the growing financial burden of looking after a population that is living longer. Organize a similar activity to produce a list of suggested options.

ACTIVITY

1 Examine the list describing some of the plans for health care produced by the Labour Party prior to the 1992 election. Discuss the funding implications.

2 What are the present priorities for health and social care of the main political parties? If possible, divide into three groups, each of which should report back on the priorities of one of the parties. Present your findings to the class as a whole and discuss the relative merits and practicalities of the proposed priorities. (Use newspapers and journals such as *The Economist*, and write to your local MP and party headquarters for information.)

Legislation

Carers need to be aware of the legal aspects of their work in order to perform their duties correctly and to avoid potential legal pitfalls.

Broadly, two types of law exist: STATUTORY PROVISION and COMMON LAW.

STATUTORY PROVISION

This consists of statutes written in Acts of Parliament – for example, the Race Relations Act 1976; the Sex Discrimination Acts 1975 and 1986 (refer back to Chapter 1). Breaches of this mandatory legislation will result in a criminal trial.

Acts may also provide ENABLING LEGISLATION, which allows organizations to follow certain courses of action at their discretion. For example, the NHS and Community Care Act 1990 supplied the enabling legislation for:

- The establishment of a purchaser/provider split in the health-care services and the creation of an internal market, with the purchasing authority buying services supplied under contract by hospitals, community health services, ambulance services and other provider bodies.
- The creation of self-governing provider units, called NHS trusts, each managed by an independent body of trustees accountable directly to the Secretary of State and capable of owning (and disposing of) assets, setting staff pay levels and

conditions of service, borrowing money and preparing its own business plan, contracts and capital development programme.
- Some larger general practices to become fund-holding practices, able to buy hospital and other services directly for their patients.
- A transfer of responsibility for some long-term care services from health authorities to the Social Services Departments of local authorities, with a corresponding shift in the emphasis from institutional care to care 'in the community'.

COMMON LAW

This consists of unwritten rules which have evolved from previous judgements in similar cases. Breaches of common law usually involve infringement of an individual's rights for which compensation is sought in civil courts. For example, individuals could bring charges of noise pollution against their neighbours under the common law.

ACTIVITY

Investigate one area of legislation in a health and social care context.

For example, you could look at the effects of one of the following:

- Health and Safety at Work Acts;
- Employment Acts;
- Children Act 1989 (and previous legislation referring to children and young people);
- NHS and Community Care Act 1990;
- Child Support Act 1993;
- Education Acts (e.g. Education Act 1981; Education Reform Act 1988).

The actual Acts are long and complicated, so it is best to find a summary. You may find this through:

- relevant journals;
- voluntary organizations;

- trade unions (e.g. UNISON, NUPE, NUT, GMB);
- appropriate government departments (e.g. Departments of Health, Education, Social Security, Trade and Industry);
- newspapers on CD-Rom (e.g. *The Times*, *Guardian*);
- HMSO.

1 Outline the main points of legislation contained in one Act.

2 Interview a professional to find out how this legislation affects provision and priorities of care.

3 If possible, cite examples of court cases in which this legislation has been tested (see the weekly 'Law Reports' in quality national newspapers).

WAYS IN WHICH SERVICES WITHIN HEALTH AND SOCIAL CARE OPERATE

Service provision

ACTIVITY

At the start of this chapter the current system of health and social care provision was described, and you investigated the various services operating within this system.

In a group, discuss briefly the provision of the following services within your locality:

- community and hospital health
- social work
- social care
- early education

Broadly, what are the functions of each of these systems? Do their functions overlap?

Strategies for service delivery

Within each service a variety of methods or strategies may be used to deliver care.

INTERVENTION

Generally the main aim of a social worker is to help clients to help themselves. To do this the social worker INTERVENES in the life and situation of the client.

ACTIVITY

Look up 'intervene' in a dictionary to check that you are clear as to the word's meaning.

To help enable the social worker to find out which particular elements of practice are helpful, and which are not, the following categories of intervention are sometimes used:

1 *Authoritative*:
- *Prescriptive*: Giving advice, being critical or judgemental to direct the client's behaviour.
- *Informative*: Giving new information or advice to the client.
- *Confronting*: Challenging the client, perhaps by giving direct feedback about his or her behaviour.
2 *Facilitative*:
- *Cathartic*: Helping the client to release emotion.
- *Catalytic*: Enabling the client to develop through self-discovery and self-direction.
- *Supportive*: Affirming the worth and value of the client as an individual.

All categories are equally important and a skilled social worker should possess expertise in all.

ACTIVITY

1 In pairs, think of examples of situations in which a social worker might use each

of the six interventionist approaches listed in the text. Briefly role-play these situations. Which did you find difficult and why?

2 Examples of areas of social work intervention include:

- counselling
- behaviour modification
- task-centred case work
- group work
- life-skills training
- welfare rights/financial counselling

Find out what each of these involves and then decide which of the six categories of intervention listed above might be involved in each area.

REMEDIAL

Remedial treatment involves the rehabilitation of a client. The person is returned to as near normal a state of health as possible. Although the organic disease process cannot be stopped, the effects can be offset by giving remedial care, for example, physiotherapy, occupational therapy or speech and language therapy.

PREVENTATIVE

Preventative health care is aimed at keeping people healthy. Examples of this, such as health education, immunization and screening have been mentioned earlier (see Chapter 5). Further examples include fluoridation, chiropody and compulsory seat belts.

ACTIVITY

1 Can you think of preventative health measures other than those mentioned in the text?

2 The restriction of some advertisements is considered to be an aspect of

preventative health care. Find out what products have restrictions placed on their advertisements and what these restrictions are. Do you agree with them?

3 What are the advantages of preventative care?

THERAPEUTIC

A therapeutic strategy involves giving clients treatment in the expectation of a particular outcome. Very often the treatment given is in the form of drugs. Examples of therapeutic care include chemotherapy and radiotherapy.

HOLISTIC

Holistic care involves the treatment of the whole person. It takes into account the social, psychological and environmental influences, including nutrition, exercise and mental relaxation, that affect health. The individual is encouraged to take responsibility for his or her own well-being. Complementary medicine is often linked to the holistic approach.

MULTIDISCIPLINARY

A multidisciplinary approach involves a whole range of disciplines working together to provide care. A multidisciplinary team may consist of physiotherapists, occupational therapists, doctors, dieticians, domestics, nursing auxiliaries, porters and many more (for an example see Figure 6.5 on page 210). Although all are working towards the same broad aim, each occupational and professional group will have a different focus.

ACTIVITY W

If you can observe a patient or client being cared for by a multidisciplinary team, carry out the following tasks:

- List the occupations involved in delivering care.

- What are the major functions of each of these occupations in the care delivery?
- Who is the team leader? Why?
- Is communication good between team members?
- How could communication be improved?

ACTIVITY W

Choose one of the following services to study:

- Community and hospital health
- Social work
- Social care
- Early education

Within your chosen service investigate which strategies of care and care delivery are employed. (It is probably best to do this during a period of work experience.)

In practice there are many ORGANIZATIONAL CONSTRAINTS which prevent the delivery of care from being ideal. Examples of such restraints include:

- limited budgets;
- limited resources;
- difficulties caused by decision-making processes;
- difficulties caused by organizational and management structures.

For example, in a nursery, it may be considered ideal for each child to spend some time each day reading a book on a one-to-one basis with a carer. However, limited resources (carers' time) may mean this does not happen.

In your investigation note any specific examples of organizational constraints you come across. Can you suggest ways in which the impact of the constraints could be minimized?

Present the results of your investigation to the rest of the group.

REFERENCES AND RESOURCES

Byrne, Tony and Padfield, Colin (1993), *Social Services*. Oxford: Butterworth-Heinemann.
Today's Health Services: A User's Guide (1993). London: Channel Four Television Publications.
Tossel, David and Webb, Richard (1986), *Inside the Caring Services*. London: Edward Arnold.

In this rapidly changing area there are often relevant articles in the quality daily newspapers.

USEFUL ADDRESSES

Council for Complementary and Alternative Medicine
Suite 1
19A Cavendish Square
London W1M 9AD
Tel.: 071 409 1440

Institute for Complementary Medicine
PO Box 194
London SE16 1QZ
Tel.: 071 737 5165

NHS Trusts Unit
NHS Management Executive
Department of Health
Richmond House
79 Whitehall
London SW1A 2NS
Tel.: 071 210 3000

USEFUL SOURCES OF CAREERS INFORMATION IN THE UK

Care assistant: see Social worker

Chiropodist:
Society of Chiropodists
53 Welbeck Street
London W1M 7HE
Tel.: 071 486 3381

Institute of Chiropodists
91 Lord Street
Southport
Merseyside PR8 1SA
Tel.: 0704 546141.

Dietitian:
The British Dietetic Association
7th Floor
Elizabeth House
22 Suffolk Street
Queensway
Birmingham B1 1LS
Tel.: 021 643 5483

Health Service Manager:
National Health Service Training Directorate
St Bartholomew's Court
18 Christmas Street
Bristol BS1 5BT
Tel.: 0272 291029

The Scottish Health Service Management
Development Group
Scottish Health Service Centre
Crewe Road South
Edinburgh EG4 2LF
Tel.: 031 332 2335

Homoeopath:
British Homoeopathic Association
27a Devonshire Street
London W1N 1RJ
Tel.: 071 935 2163

The Society of Homoeopaths
2 Artizan Road
Northampton NN1 4HU
Tel.: 0604 21400

Housing officer:
Institute of Housing
Octavia House
Westwood Business Park
Westood Way
Coventry
Warwickshire CV4 8JP
Tel.: 0203 694433

Institute of Housing in Scotland
6 Palmerston Place
Edinburgh EH12 5AA
Tel.: 031 225 4544

District nurse, health visitor, hospital nurse, midwife:
English National Board for Nursing,
Midwifery and Health Visiting
ENB Careers Service
PO Box 356
Sheffield S8 0SJ

National Board For Nursing Midwifery and
Health Visiting for Scotland
22 Queen Street
Edinburgh EH2 1JX
Tel.: 031 226 7371

Occupational therapist:
The College of Occupational
Therapists/Occupational Therapy Training
Clearing House/British Association of
Occupational Therapy
6/8 Marshalsea Road
London SE1 1HL
Tel.: 071 357 6480

Physiotherapist:
The Chartered Society of Physiotherapy,
Central Applications Office for Diploma
Courses in Physiotherapy
Room 422
Fulton House
Jessop Avenue
Cheltenham
Gloucestershire GL50 3SH

North London School of Physiotherapy for the
Visually Handicapped
10 Highgate Hill
London N19 5ND
Tel.: 071 288 5959

Probation officer:
Central Council for Education and Training in
Social Work (CCETSW)
Derbyshire House
St Chads Street
London WC1H 8AD
Tel.: 071 278 2455

Probation Service Division
Room 442
Home Office
50 Queen Anne's Gate
London SW1H 9AT
Tel.: 071 273 2675

Psychologist:
British Psychological Society
St Andrews House
48 Princess Road East
Leicester LE1 7DR
Tel.: 0533 549568

Social worker (field/residential)/care assistant:
Central Council for Education and Training in
Social Work (CCETSW)
Derbyshire House
St Chads Street
London WC1H 8AD
Tel.: 071 278 2455

CCETSW Information Office
78–80 George Street
Edinburgh EH2 3BU
Tel.: 031 220 0093

Speech and language therapist:
The College of Speech and Language
Therapists (CSLT)
Harold Poster House
6 Lechmere Road
London NW2 5BU
Tel.: 081 459 8521

Teacher: special educational needs:
Teaching as a Career (TASC)
Publicity Unit
Elizabeth House
39 York Road
London SE1 7PH
Tel.: 071 925 6617/8

Scottish Office Education Department
Careers Service Branch
Room 5/32
New St Andrews House
St James Centre
Edinburgh EH1 3SY
Tel.: 031 224 4692/8

Volunteer organizer:
Volunteer Centre UK
29 Lower King's Road
Berkhamsted
Hertfordshire HP4 2AB
Tel.: 0442 873311

Volunteer Development Scotland
80 Murray Place
Stirling FK8 2BX
Tel.: 0786 79593

Youth and community worker:
National Youth Agency
17–23 Albion Street
Leicester LE1 6GD
Tel.: 0533 471200

Scottish Community Education Council
West Coates House
90 Haymarket Terrace
Edinburgh EH12 5LQ
Tel.: 031 313 2488

CARE PLANS

◄──►

An important aspect of many professional carers' work is the development of care plans. This involves:

- assessing the client's needs;
- setting goals;
- listing the necessary action to meet the goals set;
- if necessary, justifying the actions set.

Once the care plan has been developed it is then implemented and regularly monitored and evaluated. Figure 7.1 shows an example of the stages in the development and implementation of a care plan by social workers involved in protecting children. Refer back to this for examples of the phases described throughout the chapter.

In Chapter 2, assessment of clients and the development of care plans were considered using the case studies of Mrs Ivy Trent and Tracy Congdon. What follows in this chapter is a reiteration of the main stages in care plan development.

PHASE 1: INITIAL ASSESSMENT OF NEEDS

ACTIVITY

1 Refer back to Chapters 1, 2 and 4, where the following needs of clients were identified:

- physical (Chapter 2)
- emotional (Chapter 2)
- cognitive (Chapter 2)
- identity (Chapter 4)
- cultural (Chapter 1)

Check that you understand the meaning of each of these terms.

2 Refer back to the case histories of Ivy Trent and Tracy Congdon in Chapter 2. Remind yourself of their needs, dividing your list up into the five categories shown above.

There are many METHODS OF ASSESSMENT of client needs (refer again to Chapter 2). Any or all of the following methods may be used by a professional assessing a client:

- observation of
    physical condition
    behaviour
    personal circumstances
- Questioning
- Use of secondary sources, including
    relatives
    advocates
    support networks
    medical records

When using any of these methods, the professional carer must bear in mind CLIENT RIGHTS with respect to assessment. The client has the right to:

- independence
- identity maintenance
- choice and control
- confidentiality

ACTIVITY

1 Refer back to Chapter 2:

- What methods were used to assess Ivy

STAGE	Time scale	Key activities	Areas for decision-making	Framework
STAGE 1 **Recognition...** (*referral or suspicion of abuse*)	24 hours	Discuss with referrer. Consult (where possible) with supervisor. Gather information from other key professionals. Involve other investigating agencies e.g. police, doctors, the Reporter (in Scotland). See child/other children/parents/carers/ alleged perpetrator as soon as possible if urgent. Evaluate initial data.	Is there cause for concern? Is action needed to protect the child? Protection in the family (or wider family) possible? Placement outside the family needed? Place of safety order? Access arrangements.	Legal. Children's Hearing system (in Scotland). Agency and inter-agency policies and procedures.
... and investigation (*initial assessment*)	Up to 1 week plus	Continue to gather information from child/other children/family members. Evaluate data. Consult with supervisor. Continue discussion and co-operation with other key professionals.	Emergency protection now, or still, needed? Maintain child in family with intervention? Call case conference? No further action needed? Care proceedings?	Legal. Children's Hearing system (in Scotland). Agency and inter-agency policies and procedures. Initial case conference arranged.
STAGE 2 **Assessment and Planning**	Up to 12 weeks maximum. (*preferably less*)	Following case conference, decide if comprehensive assessment is needed. If so: gather information/ direct work with child/ family unit/wider family. Liaison with management and professional network. Evaluate data. Formulate action plan.	Care proceedings? Short-term separation continues? Access arrangements? Long-term separation indicated? Child stays in family with intervention? Long-term plan formulated?	Legal. Children's Hearing system (in Scotland). Agency and inter-agency policies and procedures. Review machinery: statutory (where appropriate) and inter-agency.
STAGE 3 **Implementation and Review**	6–12 months	Implementing action/ treatment plan. Reviewing progress. Direct work with child/parents/ family unit/wider family. Consult with supervisor and professional network.	If child is at home: No further action? Continued treatment? If child is in temporary, substitute care: Rehabilitation? Long-term separation and permanent substitute care?	Legal. Children's Hearing system (in Scotland). Agency policy and procedures. Review machinery: statutory (where appropriate) and inter-agency.
Leads to Rehabilitation	Can occur any timescale	Preparation for return: direct work with child and family. Protection plan/contract regarding treatment and monitoring after child's return, including child's health and development. Consult with supervisor and others in professional network.	What are the conditions of the return home? Is there a renewed need to intervene to protect?	Legal. Children's Hearing system (in Scotland). Agency policy and procedures. Review machinery: statutory (where appropriate) and inter-agency. Protection plan agreed with parents.
Leads to Separation (*permanent*)	Decision can be at any time but often after assessment or period of unsuccessful treatment.	*Child* – bereavement and separation work, life story book, selection of and introduction to new family, continuing direct work. *Family* – bereavement, separation work, continued help and support where necessary.	Long-term family placement: adoption or long-term fostering placement? Alternative residential provision for child who cannot yet be placed in substitute family home? Access arrangements.	Legal. Children's Hearing system (in Scotland). Agency policy and procedures. Review machinery: statutory (where appropriate) and inter-agency.
Disengagement	At any timescale.	Consult and review progress with supervisor, management and others in professional network. Careful planning and preparation for disengagement with child and family.	Can parents care safely for child without further social work help? Are other support networks needed? Should any court order be revoked? Should (in Scotland) any supervision requirement be terminated?	Legal, Children's Hearing system (in Scotland). Agency policy and procedures. Review machinery: statutory (where appropriate) and inter-agency.

Figure 7.1   Stages in the development and implementation of a care plan

Source: Crown copyright. Reproduced with the permission of the Controller of Her Majesty's Stationery Office.

Trent's and Tracy Congdon's needs?

- Check that you understand the meaning of each of the client rights listed on page 235.

2 Read through the two accounts of clients below. For both Rajpreet and Helen:

- suggest the methods of assessment that would be used to identify their needs;
- identify the needs that will have to be met;
- note any particular precautions for maintaining client rights that would have to be observed when using your suggested methods of assessment.

CASE HISTORY A

A young child, **Rajpreet** (five years), is admitted to a hospital paediatric ward via the Accident and Emergency department with asthma. She has been treated for asthma for six months but, on this occasion, the medication had not relieved her wheezing and difficulty in breathing. She is very distressed when her parents have to leave.

(If possible, watch the film made in the 1960s of children being admitted to hospital and separated from their parents: J. and J. Robertson, *Young Children in Brief Separation*, Ipswich: Concorde Films, 1969.)

CASE HISTORY B

A young mother, **Helen**, is referred to a voluntary agency because it is feared she may have a nervous breakdown as has happened in the past.

Helen's only income comes from Supplementary Benefit and she complains that her housing conditions are very bad. She is also worried because her 14-year-old son is getting into trouble with the police for shoplifting and she is unwilling to let her 13-year-old daughter out with her friends because the area is so 'rough'. A six month old baby completes the family.

You may wish to repeat the activity suggested above and the two following activities using the case histories of Ivy Trent and Tracy Congdon from Chapter 2.

PHASE 2: DEVELOPMENT OF THE CARE PLAN

Once the needs of the client have been assessed, and the needs which are not being met (i.e. the problems) identified, goals can then be set (i.e. the required outcome). The action required to meet these goals should then be identified and implemented.

Figure 7.2 shows an example of a table used by nurses to develop a care plan. Figure 7.3 shows an example of a table used by social workers involved in the protection of children to help with the development of a care plan.

ACTIVITY

Figure 7.4 shows a care plan for Rajpreet. Using the same format, develop a care plan for Helen.

- In the 'problem' column fill in all the needs you identified which were not being met.
- In the 'goal' column identify for each of the problems the desired outcome.
- In the 'action' column identify the action which must be taken by professionals to bring about the desired outcome.

PHASE 3: IMPLEMENTATION AND MONITORING

You will notice in Figure 7.4 a column headed 'Review date'. Throughout the implementation of a care plan there should be

NURSING ASSESSMENT
Usual routines, what s/he can and cannot do independently. (*delete as appropriate.)

DATE: TAKEN BY:
SIGN:

LABEL

Patient Perceived Problem
Nurse Perceived Problem
GOAL 1. Who 2. What is to be achieved 3. When
Nursing Action Review Date & Signature

	Assessment details
1. MAINTAINING A SAFE ENVIRONMENT	*INFECTIOUS ALLERGIES IMMUNOSUPPRESSED
2. COMMUNICATING	HEARING _____ AID USED YES/NO* SPEECH _____ SIGHT _____ GLASSES YES/NO* LANGUAGE _____ LENSES YES/NO* present on ward YES/NO*
3. MENTAL ORIENTATION	*ANXIOUS/CHEERFUL/EUPHORIC/ORIENTED/DISTRESSED/CONFUSED/CO-OPERATIVE UNCO-OPERATIVE/RESPONDS TO COMMANDS/RESPONDS TO PAIN STIMULI UNRESPONSIVE TO PAIN STIMULI
4. BREATHING	COUGH PRODUCTIVE YES/NO* SMOKES: YES/NO* Number per day _____
5. NUTRITIONAL NEEDS	DIET _____ APPETITE _____ MEALS per day _____ FOOD PREFERENCES _____ ORAL DRUGS: YES/NO* Present on Ward. YES/NO*
6. FLUID NEEDS	DRINK PREFERENCES _____ NORMAL DAILY FLUID INTAKE _____ mls. ALCOHOL DRUNK: YES/NO* Amount per week _____
7. PERSONAL CLEANSING	ORAL HYGIENE _____ DENTURES TOP/BOTTOM* on ward? YES/NO* *NO HELP REQUIRED/ASSIST/TOTAL HELP
8. DRESSING	*NO HELP REQUIRED/ASSIST/TOTAL HELP
9. BODY TEMPERATURE/ CIRCULATION	*NORMAL LIMITS/HYPOTHERMIA/PYREXIA
10. MOBILISING	WALKING: IMMOBILE/NEEDS ONE PERSON/CAN MANAGE STAIRS/ INDEPENDENT. *USES AID: TYPE: _____
11. LIFESTYLE/CULTURE	
12. SLEEPING/REST	HOURS PER NIGHT: _____ from: _____ to _____ SEDATION: YES/NO* WHAT HELPS _____
ELIMINATING	*CONTINENT/CATHETER/STRESS INCONTINENCE/INCONTINENT BOWEL HABIT _____
13. CONDITIONS OF SKIN	PRESSURE AREA _____ COMMENTS WOUND LESIONS RASH
14. SPECIAL PSYCHOLOGICAL NEEDS	

Figure 7.2   Table used by nurses to develop a care plan

Nursing Action
Sign and Date when completed

Nursing Action
Sign and Date when completed

Nursing Action
Sign and Date when completed

Nursing Action
Sign and Date when completed

PLANNING MODEL TABLE: ACTION BASED ON ASSESSMENT

IMPORTANT: The items listed on the table are examples only

Section	Main features a) positive	Main features b) negative	Changes needed	Factors helping change	Factors blocking change	Timescale	Resources needed	Action plan Goals to be achieved and action for achieving them
CAUSES FOR CONCERN		Neglect. Abuse: Repeated. Serious. Bizarre. Sadistic. Sexual. Emotional. Premedited etc. Poor standards of care.						
ATTITUDE OF PARENTS TO PROBLEMS	Shows remorse. Concerned for child. Sought help quickly.	Denies or projects blame. Concerned for self. Little concern for child.						
ATTITUDE OF PARENTS TO INTERVENTION	Accepts need for change. Genuinely co-operates. Some insight.	Rejects need for help. Superficially co-operative.						
THE CHILD	Generally well cared for. Health and development satisfactory.	Neglected. Failing to thrive. Poor general health. Young and vulnerable child						
FAMILY COMPOSITION	Information openly shared. Clear boundaries. Straightforward, stable structure.	Secretive. Difficult to obtain information. Confusing, blurred, ever-changing boundaries.						
INDIVIDUAL PROFILE OF PARENTS/CARERS	Good experiences in childhood. Come to terms with negative experiences in childhood. Able to make and sustain deep and warm relationships. Able to control behaviour and tolerate some frustration. Open and honest.	Poor experiences in childhood. Unresolved emotional issues in childhood. Coldness & superficiality. Authoritarian attitudes. Manipulative & plausible. Previous family violence. Alcohol to excess.						
COUPLE RELATIONSHIP and...	Stable sustained relationship. Complementary. Healthy mechanisms for resolving conflict. Evidence of trust. Sexual warmth, love. Sexual needs met.	Multiple partners. Unrealistic expectations of partner. Collusive. Violent. Mistrusting. Sexual frustrations.						
FAMILY INTERACTIONS	Child's needs put first. Realistic expectations of child. Loving, can have fun.	Parents needs first. Unrealistic expectations of child. Views child as naughty, powerful. Scapegoats child. Cold with child.						
NETWORKS	Supportive but separate. Good networks and lifelines.	Interfering. Enmeshed. Distant. Isolated. Unsupported.						
FINANCE	Manages financial affairs adequately. Acute problem – willing to seek help and accept advice.	Many debts. Impulsive with money. Chronic problems. Unwilling to follow advice.						
PHYSICAL CONDITIONS	Basic needs of child for shelter, warmth, food, sleep etc. adequately met.	Chronic problems. Basic needs of child unmet or vulnerable.						

Figure 7.3 Table used by social workers to develop a care plan
Source: Crown copyright. Reproduced with the permission of the Controller of Her Majesty's Stationery Office.

Name of client: Rajpreet Patel			Name of primary carer:	

Date	Problem	Goal	Action	Review date
	Difficulty breathing	Restore normal breathing	Observe condition Medication	
	Anxiety	Relieve anxiety	Reassure child Provide facilities for parents to stay with child	

N.B. Only the broad principles of care have been considered, not the actual physical care (for example, oxygen and ventolin).

Figure 7.4 **Example of a care plan form**

both repeated assessment of the client's needs and constant MONITORING of progress so that the care plan can be adapted if necessary.

Monitoring can be defined as checking care and performance with criteria against agreed standards to produce a measurement of quality.

The Royal College of Nursing defines a STANDARD as 'a professionally agreed level of performance appropriate to the population addressed, which is observable, achievable, measurable and desirable'. In simple words, standards are statements of intent.

CRITERIA are the means of measuring whether a standard has been reached or not. For example:

• *Standard*: The cultural needs of all hospital patients will be met.

• Examples of *criteria*:
    an appropriate menu is offered;
    religious needs are considered;
    cultural practices involved in childbirth, washing, family planning, etc. are considered.

Once standards and criteria have been set a tick list or similar form can be designed and the care plan monitored.

A variety of sources of information can be used to enable the professional to monitor a care plan, for example:

• client interview;
• carer interview;
• client's records;
• observation of client, his or her care and environment;
• examination of support services.

ACTIVITY

1 Look back at the care plans you developed for Rajpreet and Helen. List the sources of information you would use to monitor these care plans.

2 Why is it important to ensure that the client (or the client's representative) is consulted throughout the monitoring process?

PHASE 4: REVIEW AND EVALUATION

Evaluation is a means of finding out whether the carer, or team of carers, has achieved what they set out to do when they developed the care plan. It is important that evaluation is OBJECTIVE and not SUBJECTIVE. For this reason, where possible, standards and criteria are needed to guide the evaluator.

In the light of the evaluation, shortcomings can be identified and, resources permitting, improvements made to subsequent care plans.

ACTIVITY **W**

You may be able to observe directly the processes involved in developing, implementing, monitoring and evaluating a care plan. If this is not possible, interview a professional to obtain the information.

1 Describe the development of a care plan for a client.

- How are the client's needs assessed?
- What precautions are taken to protect the client's rights?
- What needs were identified?
- Is a standard assessment form used?
- Is a standard care plan form used?

2 Describe how the care plan is monitored and evaluated.

- Are standard forms used?
- What sources of information are used?
- For what purposes is the care plan monitored and evaluated?

NB: Remember to observe confidentiality in writing up your notes.

If possible carry out the above in both a health care and a social care setting. This will allow you to compare and contrast the methods used.

REFERENCES AND RESOURCES

Department of Health (1988), *Protecting Children: A Guide for Social Workers Undertaking a Comprehensive Assessment*. London: HMSO.

Kemp, Nan and Richardson, Eileen (1990), *Quality Assurance in Nursing Practice*. Oxford: Butterworth Heinemann.

RESEARCH IN HEALTH AND SOCIAL CARE

Health and Social Care embraces a variety of disciplines, drawing from the natural, behavioural and social sciences to cover health care issues. Although the subject matter of these different sciences may vary considerably, they all share a need to have defined investigative procedures, which are known as METHODS OF ENQUIRY. These methods may involve re-analysing data which already exist, such as statistics and historical documents, which are known as SECONDARY DATA, or alternatively methods may be used to produce PRIMARY DATA, which are then analysed.

METHODS OF ENQUIRY USING PRIMARY SOURCES

Experimentation

Experimentation is the method of enquiry most widely used by natural scientists. It is also frequently used by behavioural scientists. The process in which experimentation is used can be broken down into stages (Figure 8.1).

The first stage involves the researcher making an OBSERVATION. For example, you may notice that, even if the water from a certain tap is always at the same temperature, if your hands are cold, it may feel hot, and yet if your hands are warm, it may feel only lukewarm.

From the researcher's observation, a HYPOTHESIS or an educated guess can be made to explain the observation. Using the example given, the researcher might guess 'skin receptors detect *changes* in temperature rather than *actual* temperature'. This is the hypothesis which the experiment will test.

In a CONTROLLED EXPERIMENT only one condition at a time should be changed. The conditions which can change are known as VARIABLES. Those remaining constant are FIXED VARIABLES, and that being changed by the experimenter is the MANIPULATED VARIABLE.

ACTIVITY

1 Think of observations that you have made in your everyday surroundings.

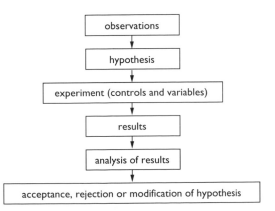

Figure 8.1 Stages involved in the process of experimentation

Can you suggest hypotheses to explain these observations?

2 Design a simple experiment to test the hypothesis: 'Skin receptors detect *changes* in temperature rather than *actual* temperature.'

ACTIVITY

1 In the experiment you were asked to design in the previous activity, apparatus could be set up as shown.

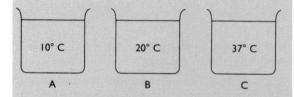

The subjects could then put one hand in A and the other in C for one minute, then place both hands in B; and then record their observations.

2 Which of the following are fixed variables and which is the manipulated variable?

- volume of water;
- temperature of water;
- time hand is placed in initial temperature.

3 Carry out the experiment shown above for testing the hypothesis 'Skin receptors detect change in temperature rather than actual temperature.' For accuracy, test at least three people, preferably more. From your results do you accept or reject the hypothesis?

The observations made in an experiment may be QUALITATIVE or QUANTITATIVE.

- A qualitative observation describes without measurement.

- A quantitative observation involves measuring an amount or quantity (such as length, volume, mass or time).

The observation made in the experiment above is qualitative, as the subject would just be recording whether the water felt hot, cold, tepid, etc. This is a DESCRIPTION and not a MEASUREMENT.

ACTIVITY

The observations below were recorded by a nurse working in the casualty department in a hospital. Which of her observations are quantitative, and which are qualitative?

At 23.00h a young man was brought in. He was semi-conscious and incoherent, but from his driving licence he was found to be 23 years old. His temperature was 36°C, but his skin was sweaty. His lips had a bluish tinge. His pulse rate was 120 per min., and his blood pressure 90/50 mm/Hg. His breath smelt quite strongly of pear drops.

Refer to a first aid book, and you should be able to make a diagnosis.

WRITING UP AN EXPERIMENT

An important part of research is communicating your findings to others. The following guidelines will help you produce a comprehensive written report of your experiment.

- Use an informative title, e.g. 'Experiment to investigate the detection of temperature by skin receptors'.
- Write a short summary of the investigation, briefly outlining the aims, methods and main conclusions. This is known as the *abstract*.
- State your *hypothesis*.
- Explain your experimental *method*.
- Record your *results*. This might be in the form of, for example, a table, graph, bar

chart, pie chart, drawing or written description (see section on 'Data handling').

- In your *discussion*:
  - (a) draw your *conclusions*, i.e. explain whether your results mean that you are accepting, rejecting or modifying your hypothesis;
  - (b) Write a critical *evaluation* of your results. Addressing the following questions may help you to do this.
    - Are your results *valid*, i.e. has the method measured what it set out to measure?
    - Are your results *reliable*, i.e. would the method used give consistent results?
    - Did you have any unexpected results?
    - If so, can you explain them?
    - Were there any sources of inaccuracy?
    - How could you improve your method?
    - How could you extend your research?
- List your *references*. Any information you have given from other sources, or direct quotes, should be followed by the name of the author and the year of publication. For example: 'It is considered that by 1991 the Health Service had spent around 2 billion pounds in computer developments and is currently spending 50 million pounds a year buying in computer and information technology consultancy to develop and rectify computer systems' (Proctor, 1992).

  At the end of your report you should list the authors alphabetically, and include the following details so that the reference may be found by the reader.

  For books, give:
  - author's surname, followed by initials
  - date of publication
  - title
  - place of publication
  - publisher

  For example: Procter, P. (1992), *Nurses,*

Computers and Information Technology, London, Chapman and Hall.

For journal articles, give:
- author's surname, followed by initials
- date of publication
- title of article
- name of journal
- volume number
- issue number
- page range

For example: Weedon, P. and Curry, M. (1992), 'Diabetes: Switching to Insulin', *Nursing Times*, vol. 88, no. 49, 34–36.

Some do's and don'ts for writing your experimental method:

- DO write in sufficient detail for someone unfamiliar with the method to repeat the experiment exactly.
- DO write in short, simple sentences.
- DON'T use long words if short words will do.
- DO write in the past tense, for example: 'The test tubes were placed in a water bath.'
- DON'T write as a list of instructions – NOT, for example: 'Place the test tubes in a water bath.'
- DON'T use personal pronouns – NOT, for example: 'I placed the test tubes in a water bath' or 'We placed the test tubes in a water bath.'

ACTIVITY

1 Look in journals to find lists of references. Can you find variations in the ways in which these are given?

2 How does a bibliography differ from a list of references?

Correlation

A CORRELATION STUDY is a method of enquiry widely used by natural and behavioural scientists.

In the experimental method of enquiry described earlier, generally the scientist manipulates one variable, and observes the response of a second variable.

However, it is often not possible to do this, and so observations must be made of two variables, neither of them manipulated.

To see if there is a relationship between the two variables, the results should be plotted on a SCATTERGRAM. For example, in an investigation to find whether there is a relationship between shoe size and height in females, the following data were obtained from eight women:

Height (cm)	Shoe Size
158	4
162	3
161	5
162	5
162	6
164	7
168	6
166	7

To plot these data on a scattergram, create a graph with one variable measured on the vertical (*y*) axis and the other on the horizontal (*x*) axis; then enter a point on the graph for each pair of data.

In a correlation study you can put each variable on either axis as neither is manipulated; in a controlled experiment it is conventional to put the manipulated variable on the *x* axis.

If there is a relationship (correlation) between two variables, the points will lie along an imaginary line. The more scattered they are, the less likely there is a correlation between the two variables.

ACTIVITY

1 Plot the height/shoe size data given in the text on a scattergram.

2 From the scattergram, say whether you think there is a correlation between height and shoe size or not.

3 Study Figure 8.2. In which graph, (a) or (b), is a correlation more likely to exist?

If there is a correlation, to show the line around which the points are scattered, the LINE OF BEST FIT can be drawn. Although statistical methods can be used to find out where this straight line lies, it is often satisfactory to judge this by eye. (A transparent ruler helps, as this enables the points on both sides of the line to be seen at once.)

If the line of best fit slopes upwards from left to right, as shown in Figure 8.3(a), we say that there is a POSITIVE CORRELATION. If it slopes downwards from left to right, as shown in Figure 8.3(b), we say that there is a NEGATIVE CORRELATION.

(a)

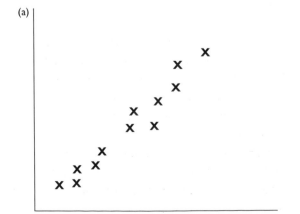

(b)

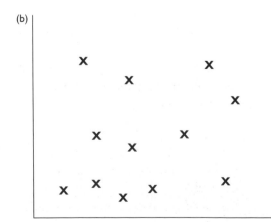

Figure 8.2

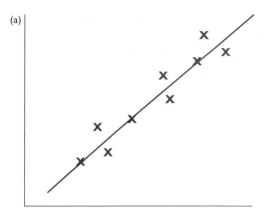

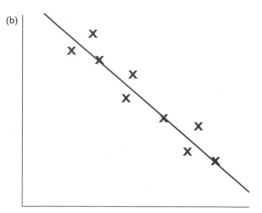

Figure 8.3   (a) positive correlation; (b) negative correlation

ACTIVITY

1 Using the information given on positive and negative correlation, select the correct alternative in each of the following statements:

*   When there is a positive correlation, as measurements of one variable increase, the measurements of the other variable tend to *decrease/increase/stay the same.*
*   When there is a negative correlation, as measurements of one variable increase, the measurements of the other variable tend to *decrease/increase/stay the same.*
*   When there is no relationship between the measurements of two variables, the variables show a *positive/negative/zero correlation.*

2 Did your first scattergram (of height and shoe size) show a positive or negative correlation?

3 Which of the following pairs of variables do you think would show a positive correlation, which do you think would show a negative correlation and which would show no correlation?

*   cost of 100 g of a food and energy content (kJ) of the food (you may find this an interesting topic to research).
*   length of gestation and birth-weight of baby.
*   number of cigarettes smoked per week by pregnant women and length of gestation.
*   age of a person and skin elasticity.
*   breathing rate and pulse rate in a number of people performing a standard exercise (research this yourself using at least 10 volunteers).

4 Try to think of one further example of your own of positive correlation, one example of negative correlation and one example of zero correlation.

A word of warning: Even if a correlation can be shown between two variables, it does not necessarily mean that one *causes* the change in the other. There may be another variable (or variables) involved which causes the correlation. This is illustrated by the following example.

Over the past 40 years there has been a steady trend to hospitalise all mothers in labour. In Britain, 99 per cent of mothers now deliver in hospital. This shift away from home has coincided with a steady drop in the perinatal mortality rate (meaning the percentage of babies who are stillborn or who die shortly after birth). But just because two things happen simultaneously doesn't mean that one causes the other. Reduced perinatal mortality reflects all sorts of things, such as improved maternal health, smaller family size and better nutrition. Exactly where people give birth may be irrelevant. Currently, a third of all Dutch mothers deliver at home, and the perinatal mortality in Holland is roughly the same as ours.

(Observer Sunday Magazine, 25 October 1992)

And a more trivial example:

Between 1981 and 1988, consumption of white bread in the UK fell by 29 per cent.

Between 1981 and 1988, convictions for bigamy in the UK fell by 29 per cent.

Eating white bread causes marital complications.

(Observer Sunday Magazine, 6 November 1992)

ACTIVITY

Suggestion for an investigation using a correlation study

It is widely accepted that smoking has a negative effect on health, though demonstrating this is not always easy.

How does smoking actually affect the physical condition of people? Is there a relationship between the number of cigarettes smoked and indicators of physical fitness?

A correlation study could be used to investigate this issue, and your task is to design and execute a study to determine whether there is a relationship between cigarette smoking and one or more health indicators of your choice. (For example, the number of step-ups done in one minute; pulse rate after a short period of vigorous exercise; time for this pulse rate to return to the resting rate.) Write:

- your hypothesis;
- methods (including precautions taken to fix as many variables as possible);
- results (plot a scattergram with line of best fit if appropriate);
- conclusions (is a correlation likely? If there is, is it negative or positive?);

- discussion (i.e. consider the limitations of your methods and suggest improvements).

Quantitative methods in social science research: surveys and field research

Is it appropriate for social scientists, in their study of human behaviour, to use the experimental and quantitative methods of research employed by natural scientists such as physicists and chemists? Can social scientists be *objective* (free of any subjective elements, desires, biases and preferences) when they choose areas of research and carry out and interpret the results of their studies? Is it possible for social scientists to explain and predict, with levels of certainty equivalent to those claimed by natural scientists investigating non-human or biological phenomena, reasons for human behaviour?

This debate can be studied in more depth by reference to most A Level or undergraduate textbooks in sociology or psychology. What we can highlight here are the *possibilities* and *problems* associated with the use of quantitative methods by social scientists. These can be briefly outlined as follows.

POSSIBILITIES

- Through the use of social surveys researchers can gain information from a large number of people. From this information, generalizations about the population as a whole can be made.
- Questions can be pre-set and, since everyone can be asked the same questions, answers can be compared. If respondents fill in their own answers, there is no problem of interviewer bias.
- The form of a survey can vary widely, ranging from, at one extreme, a long list of closed, short-answer or multiple-choice questions to, at the other, a fairly brief list of structured but 'open-ended' questions forming an 'interview schedule'.

- A pilot survey can be carried out to test the appropriateness, validity and wording of the questions asked.
- Surveys can be administered relatively cheaply and easily. With the aid of computers, the results can be collated swiftly and accurately.
- Large-scale surveys such as the ten-yearly Census can generate massive amounts of vital information for use by government departments, social scientists and others.

PROBLEMS

- Choosing a representative sample is not always straightforward. If samples are biased in a particular direction, the results of the survey may be open to criticism.
- The wording of questions in surveys can be extremely difficult to get right. Ambiguous questions can lead to confusion on the part of the respondent and to non-comparable answers.
- The answers to open-ended questions are often difficult to classify and interpret. Closed questions do not always allow the respondent to answer in the way he or she would want. All questions can be interpreted differently by people. They may not be answered honestly or with much care or thought.
- Information from surveys can 'date' very quickly. Large-scale analysis of a mass of complex data may not, in the end, prove much use if events have outstripped the findings of the survey.
- A legally enforceable survey, such as the Census, may ensure a high response rate. Other researchers may be less successful in finding people willing to complete their surveys.

In practice, many social scientists use a wide range and variety of methods of research, both quantitative and qualitative. Some social scientists find this distinction between types of research in itself limiting. Quantitative research in the natural and social sciences often has a higher status and prestige than qualitative research, despite the fact that many researchers find that different methods of research can complement each other by compensating for the inadequacies in any single methodology. Others suggest that the use of observation or interviews in field research can also involve rigorous and careful collection and analysis of data. In the study of health and illness, social scientists often work closely with natural scientists, sharing and combining methods and approaches.

Quantitative methods in social science research therefore usually involve several of the following elements.

- Sampling, i.e. careful consideration of the representativeness of the group of people/documents/situations chosen for study.
- Counting, i.e. precise enumeration of a particular phenomenon recorded by answers to survey questions, observed in field research or a laboratory: for example, how often and why a person takes vigorous physical exercise per day.
- A comparative method, i.e. the comparison and/or contrast of two or more similar or different variables occurring in the sample in question: for example, how often *men* and *women* (the variable being sex) take physical exercise per day and the different reasons they may have for doing so.
- The generation and testing of hypotheses and/or generalizations about the group of people being studied, i.e. suggesting and checking theories to account for existing or to predict future social phenomena. For example, a survey might indicate that if people take little vigorous physical exercise, they are more likely to be overweight and unhealthy and enjoy life less.

HALF OF ADULTS IN ENGLAND 'LIKELY TO FAIL FITNESS TEST'

Eighty per cent of people believe themselves to be fit, about half of them wrongly, according to a survey published yesterday.

In addition, Dr Jacky Chambers, director of

Public Health at the Health Education Authority, said that half of the male population was now overweight, compared with four out of ten in 1982, and four out of ten women were overweight compared with three out of ten, 10 years ago.

'If we continue at this rate the majority of the adult population will be overweight by the year 2000,' she said.

Nearly 4,500 adults took part in the survey which involved questions about lifestyle, diet, and physical activity and their attitude to it. Then researchers measured their fitness.

The report defines levels of fitness into five grades; from exercising vigorously on more than 12 occasions in the previous four weeks to deliberately not taking any exercise.

It defines vigorous activity as brisk hill-walking, playing squash and running; or tennis, football and cycling provided the participant got a bit sweaty and out of breath.

Moderate activity would be heavy housework or heavy gardening, swimming, tennis, football or cycling if not out of breath; or a long walk at a fast pace. Light activity would include long walks at a slow pace, DIY, fishing or darts and social dancing and 'exercises', if not out of breath.

ACTIVITY LEVEL SCALE

Level	Activity of 20 minutes in previous 4 weeks
Level 5	12+ occasions of vigorous activity
Level 4	12+ occasions of moderate/vigorous activity
Level 3	12+ occasions of moderate activity
Level 2	5–11 occasions of moderate/vigorous activity
Level 1	1–4 occasions of moderate/vigorous activity
Level 0	None

TARGETS

Age	Target levels
16–34	Activity level 5
35–54	Activity level 4
55–74	Activity level 3

The Independent, 16 June 1992

MOST ADULTS TOO UNFIT FOR A HEALTHY LIFE

Seven out of 10 men and eight out of 10 women in England do not take enough exercise to keep themselves healthy, according to the largest ever survey into activity levels.

The survey, published yesterday by the Health Education Authority and the Sports Council, interviewed 4,316 adults over the age of 16 about daily activity including sports and recreation pastimes, with two-thirds of the group being given laboratory assessments of fitness levels.

Among 16–24 year olds, 70 per cent of men and 91 per cent of women were below activity levels necessary for a fit and healthy life.

Professor Peter Fenton, head of physiology at Nottingham University, who acted as scientific adviser to the survey, said although the levels of unfitness came as no surprise, they had to be scientifically quantified, if policies were to be formulated to improve activity levels.

The survey divided activity levels into five categories, with level five being people who exercised vigorously at least 12 times for 20 minutes or more in the previous four weeks, and level zero those who took no exercise.

	Men (%)	Women (%)
Level 5	14	4
Level 4	12	10
Level 3	23	27
Level 2	18	25
Level 1	16	18
Level 0	17	16

Guardian, 16 June 1992

ACTIVITY

Look at the two newspaper reports of a survey carried out by the Health Education Authority and the Sports Council on fitness levels among the adult British population. Then answer the following questions.

1 What was the size of the sample chosen for the study?

2 Would you describe this as a large-scale or small-scale sample. Why?

3 Which methods of research did the study choose to use in attempting to measure fitness levels?

4 What variables among the overall sample were the researchers comparing?

5 What elements of this study could be described as:
(a) mainly of interest to biologists
(b) mainly of interest to sociologists and psychologists?

6 An hypothesis (in this case a future prediction) is suggested by the Director of Public Health for the HEA as a result of this survey. What is it?

7 Briefly summarize the results of this survey. Given the information you have about the survey in the extracts above, how reliable and valid do you think this survey is?

Sampling

Once a particular research problem has been identified, the question of WHOM TO STUDY arises. Defining the population to be studied usually involves deciding upon a SAMPLE. There are various methods for choosing the type of sample most appropriate to the research in question.

The SAMPLING FRAME is a list of every member of the population from which the sample is chosen. Some examples are:

- The Small User Post Office Address File (PAF), which gives addresses and postcodes of all domestic residences in the UK.
- The Electoral Register, which lists names and addresses of all registered voters in the UK.
- A list of all schools, colleges, institutes of higher education in a particular area.
- A list of all students enrolled in an institution.

ACTIVITY

As you have seen, sampling frames can be large-scale or small-scale. What other sampling frames might researchers into health and social care issues use?

TYPES OF SAMPLING

Random sampling

A random sample ensures that every member of the sampling frame has an equal chance of selection. This can be done by:

- Selecting every, for example, fifth name on a list.
- Putting each name on the list on a slip of paper and drawing the required number from a closed box, as in a raffle.
- Using tables of random numbers. By numbering the members of the sampling frame, the tables then indicate to the researcher which numbers to select for interview. There are computer facilities for this procedure if very large samples are used.

In general, the larger the sample, the more likely it is that 'randomness' is achieved. However, this method can be expensive and must be strictly adhered to if it is chosen. If the random numbering has indicated that the resident of number 10 Tree Walk is to be interviewed, but he/she is then found to be unavailable or will not co-operate, residents in numbers 8 or 12 will not 'do' instead. The respondent is 'lost' from the survey.

If applied carefully to large samples, this method is the most likely to ensure that the sample is representative of all sections of the wider population.

Stratified random sampling

This method is used when researchers want to 'match' the sub-groups in their overall sample with the size of particular sub-groups in the population studied.

For example, a researcher wishes to study the attitudes towards trade unions among the whole staff of a particular hospital. Having consulted her sampling frame, which in this case might be a list of all hospital employees, the researcher calculates that 60% of the hospital staff are women and that 40% are men.

When choosing her sample of hospital staff to interview, she therefore randomly selects from this staffing list a sample made up of 60% women and 40% men. She has thus matched the proportions in her sample with the proportions existing in the staff as a whole.

ACTIVITY

The main problem with stratified random sampling is how to ensure that the sampling frame used can be divided into the categories or sub-groups the researcher requires. It might be easy, for example, to work out the sex of employees from a list such as the one mentioned in the case above; but what difficulties might a researcher face in dividing up a list of hospital employees by:

- ethnic origin?
- social class?
- age?
- type of job?

Quota sampling

In this type of sampling, a 'sampling frame' is often unnecessary. Quota samples are often used when the researcher wants a certain number of people in a number of defined categories. Filling a quota sample therefore involves deciding upon what numbers of respondents to include in any category and then interviewing those respondents until the quota is 'full'.

For example, an interviewer may have been given instructions to interview twenty people aged over 65 and twenty people aged 45–64 on their attitudes towards diet, health and lifestyle. Standing outside a local supermarket, she gradually fills up her 'quotas' in each age category.

However, her final sample may be unrepresentative of these age-groups in the population as a whole. Two ways in which this could come about are:

- A special offer at the supermarket for cut-price cigarettes that day may have attracted relatively more smokers than usual into her quota sample.
- The people who actually agree to stop and answer her questions may have a particular interest in the topic she is researching.

How might this lack of genuine randomness affect the study?

Non-representative or convenience sampling

There are occasions when the researcher cannot or does not wish to ensure representativeness in the sample. It is not always easy to gain access to the people you wish to study and contacts might have to be built up tentatively and as the opportunity arises. An initial contact with one interviewee might lead him or her to suggest other suitable people to interview and the sample may be built up in that way ('snowballing'). Often a sample may be made up of subjects who are simply available in a convenient way to the researcher. This is often the case when 'sensitive' subjects are being researched. The following extract from Mary Eaton's book *Women after Prison* illustrates this process:

At this stage I was fortunate in receiving encouragement and help from Women In Prison, particularly from the director. She contacted a number of women on my behalf and asked if they would be willing to be interviewed. All agreed – I do not know whether this was a result of the director's skill in choosing possible subjects or her persuasive powers when explaining the project. I then telephoned each woman and arranged to meet her. In most cases the interviews took place in the woman's home, usually within the following two days. Five women were interviewed at their place of work in a voluntary sector organization. Three women were interviewed at the offices of WIP. One woman was interviewed at my office in Central London. One interview was conducted in a pub but later followed up at the offices of WIP.

When I first described the project to the director of WIP I said that I was interested in the prison experiences and post-prison experiences of all women and I asked that none should be excluded on the grounds of the untypicality of her crime or her circumstances. There was a deliberate decision at this stage to include four women imprisoned for action at Greenham Common. Three of these women (Barbara, Judith and Martha) felt that their experiences were too unlike those of other prisoners to be useful. However, there was in these differences the source of useful comment on the more usual experiences of other women prisoners. Throughout their sentences, members of the Greenham Common peace camp received letters and flowers from those outside. This lessened their sense of separation from the wider world. Indeed, these women were not excluded by their community and were continually reminded, through the letters and flowers, of their inclusion, by their actions, in the aims and objectives of camp members. However, even though prison was a rational choice, made to further the cause, and even with the extraordinary level of support that these women received, it was not enough to counteract the impact of prison on their sense of self. With less support and longer sentences other women are likely to be even more susceptible to the influences of the prison regime.

(Eaton 1993)

In practical terms this is likely to be the method of sampling most used in student research. This is perfectly acceptable as long as the risk of bias is duly noted.

Question wording

This is a surprisingly difficult part of constructing a questionnaire or interview schedule. If a large-scale piece of research is being carried out and the reliability of the data generated is therefore an important feature of the research, it is vital that the wording of questions is clear, unambiguous and likely to mean the same to researcher and respondent. This is also true of smaller-scale, face-to-face, less structured interviewing; but in this case there is at least the possibility of explaining, elaborating upon and probing further into the initial questions asked.

SOME TECHNIQUES IN QUESTION WORDING

Closed questions

The simplest method of asking questions is to give the respondent the choice of a fixed and limited number of pre-set possible answers. Closed questions can vary from a simple:

Have you ever been in hospital for an operation?

YES ☐   NO ☐

to a more complex series of options, such as:

What were your immediate feelings when waking up after your hospital operation? Please tick any which apply.

Drowsiness	
Nausea	
Disorientation	
Dizziness	
Panic	
Thirst	
Pain	
Discomfort	
Need to urinate	
Other (please state)	

The obvious advantage of closed questions is that the responses can be easily and quickly collated and analysed, perhaps using a computer. The disadvantage is that the respondent's range of possible replies are structured in advance and may therefore be unrepresentative of his or her 'true' feelings, or may fail to convey any complexity or ambiguity within them.

ACTIVITY

1 Suggest areas of research where closed questions might be useful and effective.

2 Design a short questionnaire using only closed questions.

Rating scales/semantic differential technique

Social scientists (in particular social psychologists) may use these question-wording techniques as part of a larger questionnaire or interview schedule or as a complete piece of research in itself.

RATING SCALES are used to ascertain the respondent's attitudes across an established range of positions set by the researcher. They are useful for making comparisons across large samples of respondents relatively quickly and cheaply. They can take a variety of forms and combinations of forms.

Numerical rating scales explore ways in which people can use numerical measures to assess situation of feelings. For example:

If 1 = low satisfaction and 10 = high satisfaction, on a scale of 1–10, how would you rate:

(a) the hospital care you received prior to your operation?
1   2   3   4   5   6   7   8   9   10
(please ring)
(b) the hospital care you received after your operation?
1   2   3   4   5   6   7   8   9   10
(please ring)

Written/verbal rating scales explore ways in which people can use words to assess and describe situations. For example:

How would you rate the hospital care you received prior to your operation?

(a)   excellent

(b)   good

(c)   adequate

(d)   poor

(e)   very poor

SEMANTIC DIFFERENTIAL TECHNIQUE is a specialized method which:

allows a researcher to explore the similarities and the differences between perceptions of situations, people and things. It is an underlying assumption of the technique, that certain words have similar meanings for different individuals.

The technique offers subjects a series of bipolar dimensions along which they rate themselves, other people or activities. For example, a subject may be asked to consider his/her ability to care. This is done by placing a tick on a scale like the one below. Ratings along the scale can be compared.

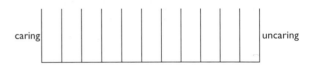

(Burnard and Morrison 1990)

CHARTS or other GRAPHICAL methods may be used to provide respondents with a means of rating attitudes, ideas, feelings, etc. For example, the respondent may be asked to use the chart shown in Figure 8.4 to rate the general state of his/her health at different life periods.

Open questions

These are simply open-ended questions to which respondents are invited to reply in any way they wish. For example:

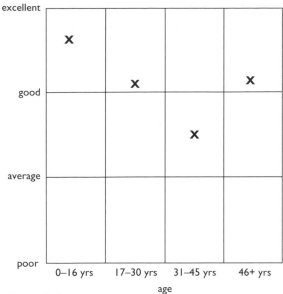

Figure 8.4

Do you regard yourself as a healthy person? Why or why not?

The answers to open questions can provide more detailed and interesting answers but can prove difficult to analyse.

ACTIVITY

Write an open-ended question on any subject which interests you and ask everyone in your class or your family to write an answer. How can the answers you received be analysed and summarized?

Leading questions

Questions which, through the use of emotive language or suggestiveness, 'lead' to a certain type of response should be avoided. An example might be: 'Do you think that dentists are completely wrong to refuse absolutely to take new adult NHS patients?'

Administering questionnaires in survey research

All research costs money and researchers have to consider the most effective way of using the money available to them. Spending much time and effort constructing a survey which then achieves a LOW RESPONSE RATE is disappointing for all concerned.

A range of factors can affect the likelihood of achieving a high or low response rate to a piece of research. A study carried out by Kay Wellings *et al.* (1994), *Sexual Behaviour in Britain: The National Survey of Sexual Attitudes and Lifestyles*, is used here to illustrate the range of factors involved in choosing a method of delivery for a piece of research.

This study, sponsored by the Wellcome Trust, was interested in two broad questions:

- What patterns of sexual behaviour exist in the population of the UK, and how might these contribute to the spread of HIV/AIDS?
- What patterns of sexual behaviour exist in the population of the UK, and how might these contribute to an understanding of the ways to prevent the spread of HIV/AIDS?

The researchers wished to choose a method of delivery for their research which would:

- achieve a very large overall random sample and therefore ensure representativeness and the sampling of sufficiently high proportions of minority, uncommon sexual behaviours;
- overcome the problems in administering a survey on very sensitive, personal issues associated with sexual practices, experience and behaviours.

POSTAL QUESTIONNAIRES were therefore rejected. Although sending questionnaires through the post and requesting that respondents post them back when completed is a relatively cheap and straightforward method, other studies using postal questionnaires have found that the response rate is often as low as 30%. In the sensitive subject area of this survey, the response rate was likely to be even lower – or might only reflect a 'self-selected sample' of those who had a particular interest in the subject matter of the survey.

TELEPHONE INTERVIEWS were also rejected. Again, these are convenient and relatively easy to carry out, but in this sensitive area the interviewer could not be sure who might be in the same room as any interviewee and what inhibiting effect this might have on interviewees' responses.

Finally it was decided to employ and train a team of 500 interviewers who would VISIT and attempt to interview people aged between 16 and 59 in their homes. Fifty thousand names and addresses were selected from the PAF (see the section on 'Sampling'), covering 100 electoral wards representative of metropolitan, urban and rural areas in the UK.

Figure 8.5 shows the response rate to this survey.

ACTIVITY

1 Make a list of reasons why researchers may not achieve a 100% response rate to their research.

2 What methods could researchers employ to minimize the risks of a low response rate?

Interviews

For many people the word 'interview' conjures up two types of image. On the one hand there is the stressful, very formal and often highly structured situation of a job interview or, for children, an interview with a headteacher. On the other hand there is the

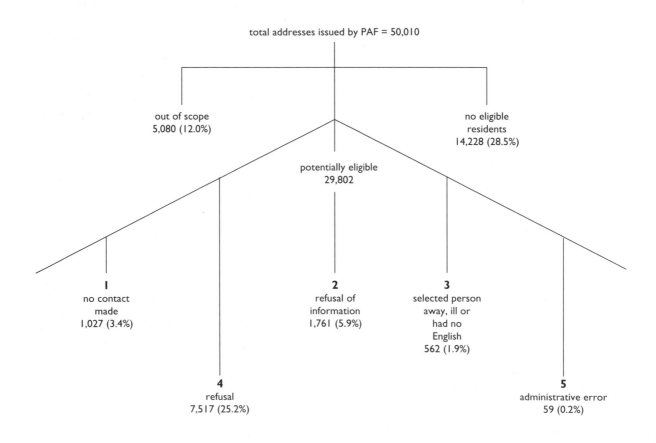

Figure 8.5

seemingly relaxed, spontaneous, jokey and conversational interviewing of the famous or not so famous by television or radio presenters such as Terry Wogan or Chris Tarrant. Some people may also have experienced MARKET RESEARCH, where they have been interviewed by someone employed by a company or agency and asked for their opinion on and consumption patterns of a specific product or service.

TYPES OF INTERVIEW

Social scientists use a similar range of types of interview with individuals or groups of people. There are some situations where highly structured interviews using pre-set lists of questions and a fairly formal relationship between interviewer and interviewee may be more appropriate and may suit the research aims of the study. For example, if the researcher wishes to interview a fairly large number of people reasonably quickly to compare their experiences, attitudes, beliefs or intentions, it may be more practical, financially and methodologically, to conduct a structured interview. The researcher may use a pre-designed QUESTIONNAIRE (a list of questions for self-completion by the respondent) or an INTERVIEW SCHEDULE (a list of questions to be asked by the interviewer, face to face or on the telephone).

AMBIGUITY

The structured interview is most successfully used where there is likely to be the least ambiguity over the wording and possible interpretations of the questions.

Problems arise when interviewees experience difficulty in understanding the intended meaning of a question. Interviewers may then have to prompt or explain questions and in so doing may unintentionally 'steer' the respondent towards a particular response to a question.

ACTIVITY

Study the following interview schedule.

Which of the following questions might raise problems of interpretation?

1 Are you a
   (a) vegetarian or
   (b) a non-vegetarian?
   (Please tick)

Questions for vegetarians

2 How long have you followed this healthy lifestyle?

3 Are you a vegetarian
   (a) for health reasons
   (b) for political reasons
   (c) for social reasons
   (d) for religious reasons
   (e) other (please state)
   Please tick the one above that applies to you.

4 How do you think most other people react to you being a vegetarian?
   (a) very positively
   (b) regard you as 'deviant' or 'strange'

Questions for non-vegetarians

5 How many times have you eaten meat today?

6 How do you feel about people who kill animals?

Try rewriting this short interview schedule on vegetarianism and non-vegetarianism, making the questions as unambiguous and as clear as possible.

Some social scientists believe that if an interviewer does intentionally or unintentionally prompt or steer respondents towards certain answers, the research data are then invalidated, because one can never be really certain that the interviewee's 'true' feelings, beliefs, attitudes and intentions have been established. There is the suspicion that the research data have become 'tainted' by the values, perspectives and approach of the interviewer and is thus no longer objective.

INTERVIEWING TECHNIQUE

Other social scientists suggest that this issue is less important than using an interview technique which is designed to elicit the most detailed and insightful information about the lives of the people being studied. Unstructured, informal, open-ended interviewing encourages the interviewer:

- to be flexible;
- to respond to what the interviewee is saying;
- to probe a little deeper than surface attitudes and beliefs;
- to establish a relationship of mutual trust and confidence;
- to encourage the interviewee to relax and talk freely and thus allow the conversation to develop naturally.

In their study of mixed-face relationships, *The Colour of Love*, Yasmin Alibhai-Brown and Anne Montague say that the aim of the interviews they conducted with people (and their children) in mixed-race relationships was to gain insights by:

asking people with immediate personal experience to talk about the subject – people who, through their relationships with partners, parents and children, have insights that no neat journalistic analysis or ponderous research tome can hope to capture ... The conversations were unstructured in a formal sense and self-determined by our interviewees. Their views were taken on board, they had access to us and we did not impose any pre-packaged notions on the people we spoke to.

(Alibhai-Brown and Montague 1992)

As with the more formal, structured interview, the open interview requires considerable care in preparing the ground to be covered in the interview and the range of possible questions/approaches to be taken, and the establishing of trust and a relaxed context in which to carry out the interviews.

Sometimes the interviewer may feel the need to interview the same person or group of people several times over a certain period, to allow time for ideas to develop or to note changes in attitudes and experiences during a particular period in the person's life.

The interviewer also has to make decisions about what might be the most appropriate techniques to 'get people talking'. Should the researcher:

- be non-directive?
- refrain from offering personal opinions?
- avoid approval or disapproval of what is said?
- be disingenuous and pretend to know less than he or she does?
- be aggressive and provocative?
- be sceptical?
- be totally honest about the aims of his or her questioning?

Alibhai-Brown and Montague (1992) made it clear that their approach to interviewing was NON-DIRECTIVE. Other sociologists have found problems in establishing a relationship with interviewees if the issue under discussion frequently turns into argument rather than discussion. Signifying understanding of what the interviewee is saying, rather than agreement or disagreement, may ease the progress of the interview, even if in practice this may give the impression that the interviewer agrees with what is being said when he or she does not. This technique may be useful where there are relatively minor areas of disagreement. Where potentially explosive areas of conflict might arise between the interviewer's own social, political, religious and moral perspectives and those of the interviewee, it makes more sense to avoid this method of research altogether or deliberately to choose issues more likely to coincide with the researcher's own interests. Many social scientists have noted that women find it easier to interview women, men to interview men. As Ann Oakley, a feminist sociologist, has said: 'The point is that academic research projects bear an intimate relationship to the researcher's life; however, 'scientific' a sociologist pretends to be, personal dramas provoke ideas that generate books and research projects.' (Oakley 1991)

'PUBLIC' AND 'PRIVATE' ACCOUNTS

Some of the very complex and less immediately obvious problems with interviews are discussed by Jocelyn Cornwall in her book *Hard-Earned Lives*, an enquiry into people's experiences of health and illness and health services which focuses upon the lives of twenty-four people who live in East London (Cornwall 1984).

Cornwall used interviews which were constructed around a schedule of topics. She included some standard questions which were put to everyone and also questions developed specifically for each individual each time he or she was interviewed. All were recorded on tape and took place in people's homes. She interviewed the same people repeatedly and took her cue from them, 'to let them direct the course of the interview and to follow their interest in the topics proposed to them'.

The problem with interviews which Cornwall highlights is that differences in social class, gender, race and educational background between interviewer and interviewee, as well as the artificial situation of the interview itself, can result in the interviewees giving what Cornwall describes as 'public accounts' rather than 'private accounts' of situations they experience or ideas and beliefs they hold. By this Cornwall means that people tend to give the answers they feel would be acceptable to other people, not what they really think themselves. When Cornwall asked people to 'tell stories' about their experiences rather than answer questions, she found that interviewees could more readily control what they said and were less self-conscious and more likely to give both 'public' and 'private' accounts of

experience. This helped Cornwall to explore the difference between the two and link her findings to the major theme of her book: the relationship between medicine and the medical profession on the one hand and society – 'ordinary people' – on the other.

Despite these and other problems with interviewing, there is no doubt that many interviewees, given the opportunity to reflect upon, explore and analyse their beliefs and ideas in a relatively systematic way, find the experience extremely positive. Alibhai-Brown and Montague (1992) claim that:

The people we talked to gave us endless amounts of time and coffee and allowed us intimate access to their lives, even when it was incredibly painful or when, as well-known figures, they could so easily have held back. Some people found the conversations cathartic after years of burying feelings about the issue. Others talked to each other as we talked to them, often for the first time, about their worries and realisations. Some claim to have found renewed joy and vigour by being forced to excavate the past and remember what they gave up in order to be with one another. Theirs were exceptional insights.

ACTIVITY

In practice, social scientists adapt the interview method (open or more formal) to the particular situation to be researched. Discuss which types of interview might work best in the following research projects:

1 A study of nurses' experiences of sexual and/or racial discrimination in the NHS.

2 A study of refugees in Britain to establish their health needs and the use they make of the health services.

3 A study of returning overseas travellers to investigate the range of health-related

problems they experienced while abroad.

4 A study to compare the experiences of fund-holding GPs with those who are not fund-holders. (In 1991, 1,720 GPs in 306 practices became fund-holders.)

5 A study looking at the causes of Sudden Infant Death Syndrome (SIDS). In England and Wales about two infant deaths per 1,000 live births are attributed to SIDS.

Case studies

Case studies are most commonly used when the researcher wishes to focus, in depth, upon individual people, small groups, an organization, a community, a nation or an event. The aim of the case study is usually to throw light on wider issues by studying carefully the case in question. Factors which exist in one case may need to be taken into account when explaining others. The researcher recognizes that the case chosen may not be typical (and would therefore have to exercise caution in making generalizations) but may use the case study to:

- Study the lives of particular individuals – particularly if they have made a significant political, historical or social impact upon the world. For example, studying the life of Marie Stopes would reveal social attitudes towards contraception, sex and abortion in the late nineteenth and early twentieth centuries.
- Develop a better professional under-standing of a client, group of clients or institution (the method here being more akin to a case history).
- Provide a base or 'trial run' for larger-scale research by generating hypotheses and indicating at least some of the facts and situations which will need to be taken into account.
- Give a basis for comparison between two

or more similar cases (NHS trust and non-trust hospitals) or between two or more apparently different cases (NHS and private-sector hospitals).

- Look at the lessons which could be learned from an apparently 'deviant' or 'atypical' case. The film *The Silence of the Lambs* illustrated the way in which psychologists, criminologists and psychiatrists are cur-rently interested in studying the individual cases of serial killers and psychopaths in the hope that this will lead to an understanding of the pathologies of other killers and make detection and arrest easier.
- 'Balance' or 'give colour to' a large-scale quantitative study by selecting cases which graphically illustrate some of the issues in question. For example, a researcher studying the extent to which an 'alternative' therapy, such as homoeopathy or acupuncture, is used in Britain may illustrate any statistical data generated by the study with a number of detailed, descriptive cases of the users of such therapies. This technique is often used in the 'investigative reporting' of TV documentaries such as *Panorama*, *Public Eye*, etc., and in print journalism.

The key problem with case studies is the question of the VALIDITY of wider generalizations based on the often rich and detailed insights generated by this method. Therefore case studies are often best used in conjunction with other methods of research.

ACTIVITY

1 Consider the GP surgery you use. If you were asked to carry out a case study of the way this surgery was run, how might you approach this task? What factors do you think might make it typical or atypical of other GP surgeries in your area?

2 What useful insights might a case study of this kind give you?

3 How might the ideas generated from this case study be used in a larger-scale piece of research?

Observation

Of all the research methods mentioned in this chapter, observation is possibly the most difficult to carry out skilfully. This may seem strange, since we spend our lives observing, using a variety of senses, albeit with very different and constantly changing levels of attention and perception. For example, what different kinds of observation might be involved in the following situations?

- a mother or father looking at their newly-born child;
- a teacher watching and listening to children in his or her class discuss a project in a lesson;
- staring out of the window of a bus;
- noticing your friend has had a haircut;
- meeting your girl or boyfriend's parents for the first time.

To each of these situations we bring feelings, emotions, memories of past experiences and knowledge. We make judgements on the basis of our observations and these ideas go on to structure the way we continue to 'see' situations or people. For much of the time we do not question or doubt our observations – although we can be discomfited if someone 'sees' a situation differently from us, as this reminds us that our perceptions are not necessarily the only ones possible.

For those working in the caring professions, whether they are carrying out 'research' or not, careful observation becomes a vital skill, one which is practised and improved. Social workers may need to make careful and sensitive observations about people's circumstances and behaviour, for example in assessing whether a child should remain in the care of his or her parents. Residential workers and foster-parents may have to look out for signs of distress or unhappiness. Nurses will become skilled in

detecting physical and psychological changes in the patients in their care. The professional practice of observation is similar to the social science use of observation as a research tool, in that both are conscious and deliberate 'ways of looking': there are specific reasons for the observation.

REASONS FOR OBSERVATION

Perhaps the researcher wishes deliberately to take part in a social situation or join a social group which has previously been unfamiliar to him or her. The aim of the study is to understand and attempt to explain to others how the people the researcher is studying 'see' the world from their PERSPECTIVE. Sociologists have studied the behaviour and attitudes of groups of people 'from the inside' either by joining them COVERTLY (i.e. by deception and pretending to be 'one of them' and/or by joining them but not revealing the nature of the research which is being carried out) or OVERTLY (by openly joining groups and getting to know the people involved extremely well). Here social scientists aim to remind us about what we in our everyday lives can easily forget, ignore or misunderstand; what it might be like to 'be' other people in social situations very different from our own. Observational studies of the mentally ill, of criminals and deviants, of gangs and of religious sects have frequently been carried out for this reason.

Or a researcher may wish to observe others systematically, over specific periods of time, to 'test' whether a usual, taken-for-granted or common-sense perception of a situation is actually accurate. Most people do not have time for such systematic observation, but social scientists are interested in the ways patterns of interaction and behaviour develop and come to define and structure particular situations. Some social scientists, for example, are interested in the differences between what people say happens, or what they think will happen, in certain situations and the actual events which occur – including apparently unintended consequences.

In this context, there have been studies of classroom behaviour – looking for patterns in the interactions observed and asking questions which seem to arise from these observations, e.g.

- Do boys receive more attention than girls from teachers?
- In what ways does the behaviour of boys and girls in classes differ?
- What consequences do these patterns appear to have for the lives of the individuals involved?

There are also occasions when researchers wish to record and analyse their observations of particular situations or behaviours in an extremely structured way. Here social experiments (in 'the field' or in a laboratory) may be set up in a way very similar to experiments used by natural scientists (see the section on 'Experiments' earlier in this chapter). Some examples of experiments of this kind are discussed throughout this book.

DIFFICULTIES IN OBSERVATION

There are two key difficulties in using observation as a method of research, each of which you can test out for yourself by trying out the Activity in this section:

- Does the presence of the observer (covert or overt) alter the behaviour of those observed in any way? Does this make a difference to the situation he or she is observing? Does it matter?
- Is it possible to observe situations objectively, without any preconceptions or prejudices which might alter the way you 'see' things?

ACTIVITY

1 When next using a bus or a train, spend a few minutes actively observing the people around you. Do not read or look out of the window but instead closely observe the passengers. You could (mentally) count them; try to put them into categories; decide what they might have been doing and where they might be going; observe who is talking to who, and so on.

Did your active observation of the passengers make any difference to them? Can you think of situations where observation may make a difference?

2 Observe any situation with which you are very familiar – a family meal, for example. First write a paragraph describing this situation. Then write a paragraph trying to describe this situation as if you and the person reading your description had never seen or experienced that situation before.

Do your accounts differ? If so, why might this have happened?

METHODS OF ENQUIRY USING SECONDARY SOURCES

Secondary sources of data are very useful in identifying patterns and trends over time. They can be used in two contrasting ways:
- They can be examined and then a hypothesis can be formulated.
- They can be used to test an existing hypothesis.

Official statistics

Advantages:

- Statistics are readily available on a wide range of issues (see suggestions of sources on page 263).
- Research based on secondary data is cheaper than that involving collection of primary data.

Disadvantages:

- Not all statistics are reliable. They may include biases and inaccuracies.

Table 8.1 Population age and sex structure 1991, and changes by age, England, 1981–91

Age (in years)	Resident population at mid-1991 (thousands)			Percentage changes (persons)			
	Persons	Males	Females	1981–91	1988–89	1989–90	1990–91
Under 1	663	339	324	10.8	−0.8	0.9	2.3
1–4	2,575	1,318	1,257	15.2	2.5	1.1	1.3
5–15	6,465	3,318	3,147	−13.2	−0.6	0.6	0.9
16–29	10,206	5,191	5,016	3.5	−0.5	−1.1	−1.6
30–44	10,153	5,084	5,069	10.7	0.7	1.0	1.2
45–64/59*	9,122	5,138	3,984	0.2	0.8	0.8	0.9
65/60–74**	5,436	1,897	3,539	−3.7	−0.5	−0.4	0.1
75–84	2,618	968	1,650	16.4	1.4	0.6	−0.2
85+	770	199	571	50.6	5.0	3.9	4.1
All ages	48,008	23,451	24,557	2.5	0.3	0.3	0.4

*45–64 years for males and 45–59 years for females.
**65–74 years for males and 60–74 years for females.
Notes: i. Figures may not add precisely to totals due to rounding.
  ii. These estimates are based on the 1981 Census with allowance for subsequent changes. Revised estimates will be prepared, first for mid-1991 and eventually for earlier years, when 1991 Census results become available.
Source: OPCS.

Table 8.2 Mean age of women at first live birth within marriage, according to social class of husband, England, 1981, 1990 and 1991

Social class of husband	Mean age of women at first birth within marriage		
	1981	1990	1991
All social classes	25.4	27.2	27.5
I and II	27.6	28.7	29.0
III Non-manual	26.1	27.4	27.7
III Manual	24.5	26.4	26.7
IV and V	23.4	25.3	25.8

Note: Figures for social class are based on a 10% sample.
Source: OPCS.

• The researcher must find out how concepts have been defined and measured. This might have changed over time.

Tables 8.1 and 8.2 give examples of information published by the Office of Population, Censuses and Surveys (OPCS).

ACTIVITY

1 Study Table 8.1. Then answer the following questions:

• Which age group has shown the most rapid increase in number?
• Suggest possible reasons for this increase (i.e. formulate hypotheses to account for the increase).
• If you were to test these hypotheses, what statistics would you require access to?
• Do these statistics support the hypothesis 'Women are more likely to live longer than men'.

2 Formulate two hypotheses supported by observations made from Table 8.2.

• Can you think of possible explanations for these trends?
• On what basis are people allotted to a social class?

USEFUL SOURCES OF OFFICIAL STATISTICS

Official reports and other government documents are available from HMSO (for address see list at end of chapter).

The DEPARTMENT OF HEALTH produces:

• *The Health Service in England* (annual report).

- *On the State of the Public Health* (the annual report of the Chief Medical Officer of the Department of Health).
- Health and Personal Social Services Statistics for England.

The OFFICE OF POPULATION CENSUSES AND SURVEYS (OPCS) publishes annual medical and population tables published in separate, topic-oriented volumes on: family statistics, deaths, morbidity, population estimates and projections, births, cancer, communicable diseases, congenital malformations, demographic review, general household survey, hospital in-patient enquiry, labour force, longitudinal study, marriage and divorce, abortion statistics, migration, local authority vital statistics and electoral statistics.

Content analysis

Content analysis is most commonly used when studying the output of forms of the mass media (television, radio, newspaper, magazines, books, film, music on disc/tape/LP etc.), although the content of other documents may also be worthy of systematic study. Photographs, letters, official documents, reports and pictures/drawings can all be used to look at the ways in which *issues*, *groups of people* (such as those with mental disorders, drug users or AIDS sufferers) or *images* are most commonly represented. Different forms of content can be compared and the question of BIAS can then be raised. Because reporting in television and newspapers has been shown to be biased, it is more useful to use them to show *how an item is reported*, rather than as a *source of information*.

CARRYING OUT A CONTENT ANALYSIS

The first step is to identify an area of concern to investigate and then to establish the purpose of the investigation: for example, the ways in which tabloid and broadsheet newspapers report cases of AIDS sufferers could be compared. A clearer 'picture' of the

range of images most commonly shown makes it possible to go on to discuss the potential impact of these images on audiences and the public.

ACTIVITY

Think of other issues related to health and social care which could be explored through content analysis. How many can you list? Why do you think this form of investigation is suitable for them?

The next task is to devise a SCHEME OF ANALYSIS. Depending upon the issue and form of content chosen to study, this would usually involve:

- a QUANTITATIVE ASSESSMENT of the content examined (i.e. counting the number of times a theme or issue appears and recording the form in which it does so);
- the subsequent construction of THEORIES to interpret and explain the findings.

AN EXAMPLE OF CONTENT ANALYSIS

Hypothetical task: '*Examine the influence of the mass media upon the socialization of young children, choosing a theme related to a health and social care context.*'

One possibility here would be to carry out a content analysis of children's TV programmes and/or advertising, choosing to focus upon one or more of the following issues which have prompted general public concern over the past decade or so:

- How do children interpret and react to violence on television? What implications does exposure to screen violence have for children's health and development?
- Are children absorbing sexist and/or racist images from children's television?
- In what ways might children's television programmes and advertising be influencing

their families' consumption of toys and games (e.g. video games)?

- Are standards of literacy and numeracy 'declining' because children are watching too much of the 'wrong' sort of television programmes (e.g. animation and cartoons, which may encourage more passive viewing, rather than programmes like Blue Peter, which encourage more active involvement)?

While content analysis in itself cannot provide a complete answer to any of these questions, it can be used to establish possible trends, effects and influences. Depending, therefore, upon the emphasis chosen for the investigation, the content analysis itself might involve one or more of the following elements over a specified period of time (a week, a month, longer . . .):

- An analysis of the hours devoted to children's programming on each television channel, including an assessment of the time devoted to each different type of programme (drama, animation, 'factual' programmes, etc.).
- An analysis of the timing of these children's programmes and/or advertising.
- An analysis of the age-ranges catered for by the programmes.
- An analysis of comparisons between the content of specific programmes/adverts for their approach to issues of gender, race, disability, etc.

After carrying out such an analysis, some INTERPRETATION of the results needs to be carried out. This could lead to a theory or hypothesis explaining the phenomena/trends observed which may, in turn, be tested choosing different methods of research.

The crucial limitation of content analysis is that, in itself, it tells us nothing about how audiences might be interpreting or reacting to the media content or form of content chosen as the subject of study. It is a very useful method of research, however, for generating theories and hypotheses and is most

productively employed in association with other methods of research.

Below is a report of the content analysis carried out by the Broadcasting Standards Council, published in the *Guardian*:

CHILDREN'S TV 'LEANS MORE ON CARTOONS'

The factual content of children's television has declined in favour of cartoons and entertainment formats, the Broadcasting Standards Council said yesterday.

It warned of a further creeping erosion, caused by the squeeze on funds, more severe competition for ratings and the reduced power of regulators to defend quality.

A council report reveals that ITV has cut spending on children's programmes by 40 per cent over the past five years – from £50 million to £30 million – and the BBC has cut its children's budget by 5 per cent a year over the past two years.

By 1991, more than half of BBC1's and ITV's children's hours were devoted to animation and other predominantly entertaining formats, up from between a quarter and a third in 1981.

One of the report's researchers, said that drama like the BBC's Chronicles of Narnia were high quality and sold well, but there was a danger that contemporary drama, without an overseas market, was at risk.

(Guardian, 10 December 1992)

ACTIVITY

Study the extract from the *Guardian* on children's television.

1 What broad conclusions did this analysis reach regarding the content of children's television programming in 1991?

2 If you were asked to check whether these findings of the BSC still applied, using a fortnight's television programming for children over the next month, how would you go about this task?

3 Given the conclusions reached in the BSC study, can you suggest any possible hypotheses about how current children's programming might be affecting the children who watch? What other research methods could you employ to test your hypothesis?

Documents

A document is, broadly speaking, any written or graphic material which can generate data for research. The use of books, statistics and the media as secondary sources and for the purposes of content analysis has been discussed earlier in this chapter; here we will be concentrating upon the almost endless variety of other documents which can prove useful to researchers. These include:

- official and unofficial reports;
- minutes of meetings;
- memos and other records of the business and administration of organizations;
- publicity and promotional material;
- leaflets;
- diaries;

. . . and many others.

ACTIVITY

1 You have been asked to compare the way truancy is approached and dealt with in two secondary schools in your area.

What documents might you wish to study and analyse? Give reasons for your choices.

2 A student health visitor is carrying out research into how effectively new parents use the 'Personal Child Health Record' books issued in several health authorities to enable parents to record developments in their children's health – dates of vaccinations, visits to the GP, major illnesses, treatments, medicines prescribed, etc. (see Figure 8.6).

Assuming that the student has sought and gained permission from a sample of parents to look at their use of these Child Health books, how might she go about analysing the information within them? What trends or patterns in their use might she look for? To what use might the information she collects be put?

There are often problems associated with the use of documents. Medical records, which could prove an invaluable source of research material in the study of health and illness, are of course confidential while the person to whom they relate is still alive. The secrecy and non-availability in whole or in part of some documents is therefore a potential obstacle to research.

Researchers also need to check whether the documents they use are:

- complete and reliable;
- written with sincerity or written with the intention to mislead;
- representative.

WRITING UP A RESEARCH REPORT

Whatever your method of research, an essential element is communicating your findings to others.

For the basic guidelines on writing a research report, refer back to the section on 'Writing up an experiment' earlier in the chapter. These principles apply whether you are describing a simple experiment or a complex survey project – although for more involved pieces of research you will probably want to add an introduction after the abstract before you go on to describe your research method. This introduction should state your hypothesis and outline succinctly any relevant background information, for example, previous research that has been conducted on the same topic.

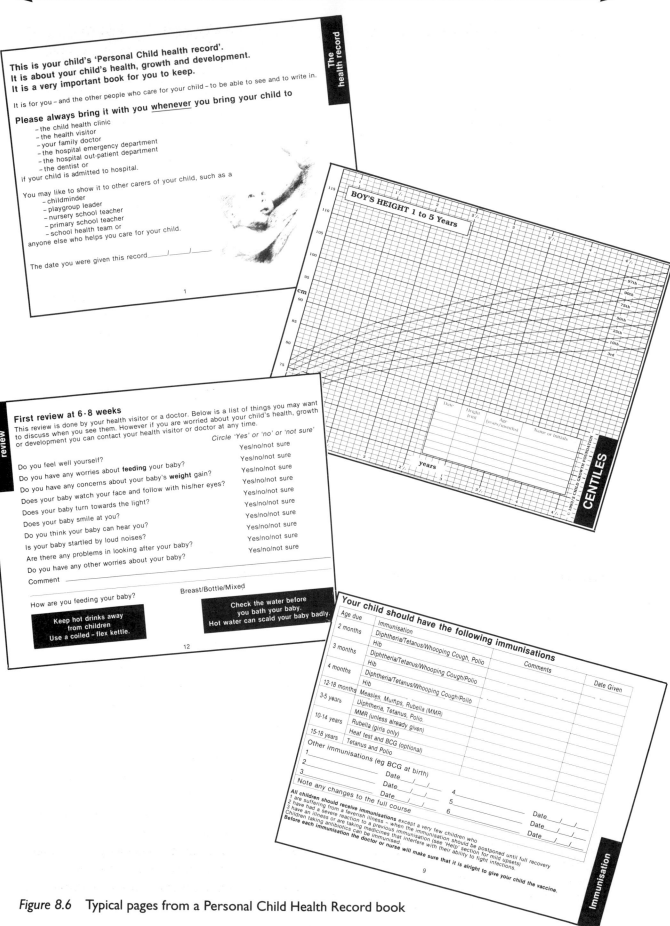

Figure 8.6   Typical pages from a Personal Child Health Record book

DATA HANDLING

Arithmetical techniques

You will need to understand the following:

- addition
- subtraction
- multiplication
- division
- fractions
- decimals
- percentages
- ratios
- means
- range
- plotting coordinates

It is not within the scope of this book to cover these techniques; if you need further help with them, refer to *Calculations for Health and Social Care* by Gordon Gee, or other appropriate maths books.

Data presentation

Unless results are very clear-cut, it can be difficult to draw conclusions from raw data. However, if data are presented in the correct way, patterns, trends and relationships can become obvious.

TABLES

Generally, the first way in which you will organize your data is in the form of a table. Essential points about tables are:

- Each table should have a title.
- Don't include too much information on one table.
- Label columns and rows clearly (include any units of measurement used).
- Construct your table *before* you start recording any results.
- Do not leave blanks. Show a zero value as 0, and a missing observation as −.

ACTIVITY

Refer back to the experiment described at the beginning of this chapter for investigating temperature detection by the skin. Design a table which would be suitable for recording the results from ten subjects.

LINE GRAPHS

Two variables can be plotted on a line graph, which will show any relationship existing between them.

Points to remember when plotting a graph:

- The values for the *manipulated variable* (i.e. the variable controlled by the experimenter) go on the horizontal or *x* axis. The values for the *dependent variable* (i.e. the 'unknown quantity') go on the vertical or *y* axis.
- Each axis should be labelled, including the unit of measurement.
- A scale should be used which is simple and produces a graph large enough to be clear. (The axes do not have to begin at 0.)
- The co-ordinates should be marked by an X or ⊙, not just a dot, as a dot is not visible when a line passes over the point.
- Points may be joined by a series of straight lines (i.e. from point to point), a smooth curve, or a 'line of best fit' (see the section on 'Correlation').
- The graph should have a full title, such as 'Graph Showing the relationship between . . .'
- Two or more lines can be plotted on the same axes, but you must label each line clearly. For example, use an X to mark each point on the line, and join them with a solid line, and use a ⊙ for each point on another line, joining the points with a broken or dashed line (- - - - - -). Show these symbols clearly in a key.

ACTIVITY

Practise constructing a line graph by plotting the data in the following table.

Prevalence of cigarette smoking in adults (aged 16 years and over) in England and Wales, 1974–90

	Men %	Women %
1974	51	41
1976	46	38
1978	45	37
1980	42	37
1982	38	33
1984	36	32
1986	35	31
1988	33	30
1990	31	29

Source: OPCS

- Consider whether to join the points with a series of straight lines, to draw a curved 'line of best fit' or to draw a straight 'line of best fit'. Use the most appropriate method. Which do you consider the least appropriate method?
- During this time period (i.e. 1974–90), is the rate of decrease in smoking faster in men or women? (NB: the steeper the graph, the faster the rate of decrease.)
- INTERPOLATION is the estimating of other values by reading off co-ordinates at any point along the line. What percentage of women would you estimate were smokers in 1983?
- EXTRAPOLATION involves extending the line outside the range of the graph to estimate further values. Use this method to estimate the percentage of male smokers in 1992.
- Compare your answers to the last two questions with others; it must be emphasized that these interpolated and extrapolated values are only estimates, so that it is likely you will not agree on identical figures.

HISTOGRAMS

In a FREQUENCY TABLE the data are grouped in some way, and the number in each group (frequency) is recorded. For an example, see Table 8.3, recording an experiment in which

Table 8.3   The initial capacity of 50 male subjects

Vital capacity (dm^3)	Tally chart	Frequency
2.80–2.99	II	2
3.00–3.19	HHT	5
3.20–3.39	HHT HHT	10
3.40–3.59	HHT HHT HHT I	16
3.60–3.79	HHT HHT I	11
3.80–3.99	IIII	4
4.00–4.19	II	2

the VITAL CAPACITY (i.e. the maximum amount of air exchanged during forced breathing) was recorded for 50 males. These data can be plotted in the form of a HISTOGRAM, where the areas of the bars represent frequency.

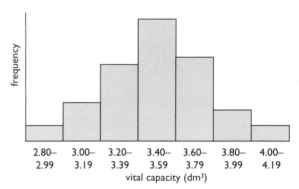

Figure 8.7   Histogram displaying data shown in Table 8.3

If a curve is joined to link the mid-points of the top of each rectangle in Figure 8.7, a 'bell-shaped' curve is seen. This is known as a NORMAL DISTRIBUTION CURVE, which will generally be found whenever the frequency distribution of a physical parameter such as height or weight is displayed.

ACTIVITY

1 Measure the length of the index finger of 20 people. Record your results in a tally chart, and draw a histogram to show frequency distribution.

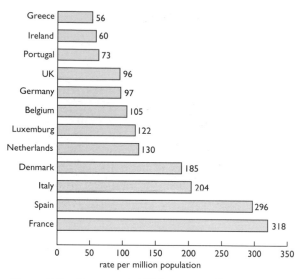

Figure 8.8 Reported AIDS cases in Europe: cumulative rates to December 1991
Source: Crown copyright. Reproduced with the permission of her Majesty's Stationery Office.

2 The most common value, or range of values, is known as the MODE. The MEDIAN is obtained by arranging the values in order and taking the 'middle' value. What are the mode and median values of your data?

BAR CHARTS

Bar charts are essentially the same as histograms, but are used when one variable is not numerical, and the height rather than the area of each 'bar' represents the frequency. As the groups are quite distinct (i.e. not on a scale of measurements as with histograms), the bars have gaps between them. For examples, see Figure 8.8.

A variation of the bar chart is the PICTOGRAM, where the length of each bar is represented by an appropriate pictorial image. For an example see Figure 8.9.

ACTIVITY

Look for examples of pictograms illustrating health-related statistics in newspapers and magazines.

THE WORLD'S HEAVIEST SMOKERS

Annual cigarette consumption per country (millions). All figures are for 1991

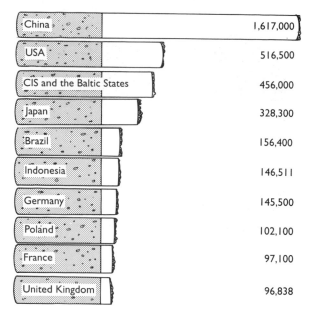

Daily cigarette consumption per man, woman and child. All figures are for 1991

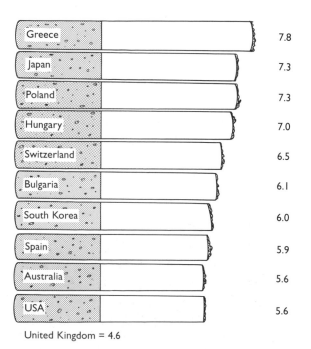

United Kingdom = 4.6

Figure 8.9 Pictogram showing cigarette consumption per country, 1991
Source: *Sunday Observer Magazine*, 8 November 1992.

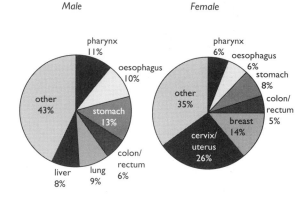

Figure 8.10 Pie charts showing distribution of cancer incidence by type and level of development for males and females, 1980
Source: UNEP, *Environment Data Report 1989* (Blackwell, 1989).

PIE CHARTS

Pie charts can be used as an alternative to bar charts to display data. For examples see Figure 8.10.

	Total	Females	Males
Medical (e.g. consultants, registrars, house officers)	48,018	12,951	35,067
Dental	2,051	524	1,527
Nursing	385,878	341,629	44,250
Midwifery	22,606	22,539	67

Source: Health and Personal Social Service Statistics for England, 1992 (HMSO).

ACTIVITY

1 Study Figure 8.10 and then answer the following questions.

- In developed countries, which cancers are most common in:
  (a) males?
  (b) females?
- In developing countries, which cancers are most common in:
  (a) males?
  (b) females?
- Overall, the *number of cases of cancer* were divided almost equally between developed and developing countries. Can the pie charts show this information?

2 The following table shows the numbers of staff in four hospital occupations in the UK in 1990.

From the table:

- Find the total number of people employed in the four occupational areas.
- Draw a pie chart to show the proportions of staff employed in each of the four occupational areas.
  Calculate the angle of each sector by using the equation:

  Number of people in an occupation
  × 360 = total number employed

- Now draw two separate pie charts, to show the relative proportions of males and females.

- There are far more females (377,643) compared with males (80,911) employed in these four occupational areas. Do your pie charts show this difference in total number?

TEXT

Very often data will not be displayed in a figure (e.g. table, graph or pie chart), but will be included in the text. For example: 'Currently 65% of children and 58% of adults are registered with a dentist. Most adults, except those on Supplementary Benefit, pay 80% of the cost of dental treatment.'

ACTIVITY

Find care-related newspaper articles which include data in the text. Convert this data into a diagrammatic form (e.g. table, graph or pie chart). Which is the most effective form of communication? What are the advantages and disadvantages of presenting data in text?

Conveying messages with statistics

How data are presented can affect the messages conveyed. There are various ways in which statistics can be presented in a form which, although not incorrect, is misleading.

USE OF A 'FALSE ORIGIN'

Take the following data:

Total NHS expenditure (£ millions):
1991/2   1992/3
23,260   24,430

The most obvious way of expressing this data is shown in Figure 8.11(a). However, if a politician wanted to make the point that there had been a large increase in spending, most of the vertical scale could be deleted, as shown in Figure 8.11(b).

To the casual reader the clear conclusion would seem to be that there was a huge increase in expenditure from one year to the next.

BARS OF DIFFERENT WIDTHS

Although it is the *height* of a bar on a bar chart

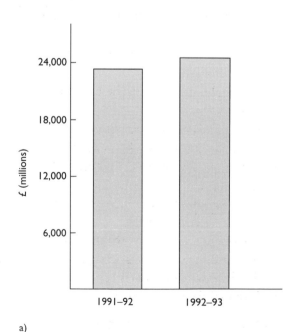

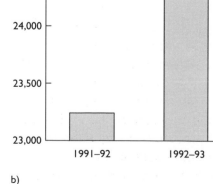

a)   b)

Figure 8.11

which gives information, different widths may be used to mislead the reader.

For example, the manufacturer of a low-fat yogurt, Brand A, may produce the advertisement shown in Figure 8.12 in a slimming magazine. Without careful inspection of the bar chart, Brand A would appear to the casual reader to have less fat than the other brands shown.

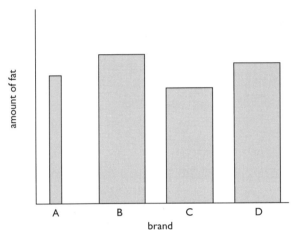

Figure 8.12

SELECTION OF FIGURES

Data to illustrate a point are often chosen very selectively. Although the data used are themselves accurate, this can give a misleading impression.

For example, a £2 million government campaign, introduced in December 1991, to reduce cot deaths by putting babies to sleep on their backs, was judged to be a huge success. The death rate dropped by 50%, and the Health Department held a press conference to call attention to its success. What it failed to point out was that the rate of cot deaths was already falling, before the campaign was introduced (see Figure 8.13).

Although the campaign advice is obviously very sound, it was felt by many researchers that further lessons could be learned by endeavouring to explain the drop in cot death rate prior to the campaign.

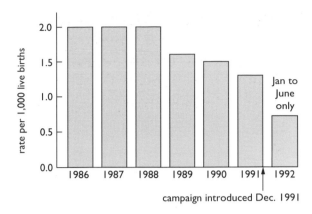

Figure 8.13   Sudden infant death syndrome ('cot death'), England and Wales, 1986–92
Source: Observer, 30 May 1993.

Data processing and computers

Computers are often used to help collect, store and analyse data. However, it must be remembered that there is legislation which restricts the storage and access of data on computer.

The DATA PROTECTION ACT, which was passed by Parliament in 1985, has eight main principles. These are:

- Personal data (i.e. information about a living individual) must be obtained fairly and the data user must register the source of such data.
- Personal data must be held for specified purposes only.
- Personal data must not be held for any other purpose.
- Personal data must be both relevant and adequate to the specific purpose.
- Personal data must be accurate and updated as necessary.
- Personal data must not be held for any longer than is necessary.
- Personal data must be made available to the data subject on request and provision made for the correction of data.
- Personal data must be kept securely.

In May 1987 the ACCESS TO PERSONAL FILES ACT was introduced. This complements the Data

Protection Act, and gives people the right to see their own records kept on computer. This may include, for example, records kept by Social Services, banks and doctors.

ACTIVITY

Read the section on 'Data processing and computers'.

What are the possible advantages and disadvantages of giving people access to their files?

ACTIVITY W

Talk to professionals working in health and social care about the Data Protection and Access to Personal Files Acts, to find out how this legislation affects their work.

ETHICAL ISSUES IN RESEARCH

Neither natural nor social scientists can avoid considering ethical issues when carrying out their research.

In MEDICAL SCIENCE ethical issues often arise as a result of the widespread use of CLINICAL TRIALS for new drugs or treatments. To test the effectiveness and safety of such new drugs and treatments, patients or volunteers participating in trials may not know whether they are part of a CONTROL GROUP receiving the PLACEBO or standard conventional treatment, or whether they are part of the TREATMENT GROUP receiving the new drug or treatment. Occasionally, and very controversially, clinical trials are conducted without the consent or knowledge of the participants.

Using people as 'human guinea pigs' does raise questions about the risks to those people exposed to new drugs and treatments, and these risks have to be set against the potential benefits for a particular group of people in the population as a whole.

Interestingly, it might be argued that using people in clinical trials receives less publicity, and appears to arouse less concern, than the use of ANIMALS IN EXPERIMENTS — another ethical issue which there is not space to discuss here.

The article from the *Guardian* reproduced here describes the clinical trials for the hormone drug tamoxifen.

WOMEN AT RISK FROM BREAST CANCER PIN HOPES ON HORMONE DRUG STUDY

The Royal Marsden Hospital, in London, announced that it had just recruited its 2,000th volunteer into a study it has been running since 1986 into possible protective effects of tamoxifen against breast cancer.

The drug has been used as back-up therapy for women with breast cancer since 1971, but the Marsden study is the first in the world to try to investigate whether tamoxifen can prevent the disease in the first place.

It is planned to recruit another 500 women to the study. All receive six-monthly check-ups, with breast X-rays each year. The screening costs about £500 a year each, with the drug costing about £7 a month and the placebo £2.

If there is a marked protective effect it should be possible to detect it sometime between 1996 and 1998, Dr Powles, the study co-ordinator, said.

Dr Powles said so far 11 cancers had been spotted, all at an early stage. It was not possible to say yet if these had occurred in the tamoxifen or the placebo women, but the number was smaller than might have been expected in a high-risk group.

Some 20 to 25 cancers might have been expected in such a group, but it was too early to say if the drug was successful.

The women all have a family history of breast cancer, with a close relative affected. Most are aged between 35 and 70.

Plans for a national tamoxifen trial involving 15,000 women are being delayed while the Department of Health makes a decision about possible side effects. The Committee on Safety of Medicines has approved the national study, but the Medical Research Council has raised questions because some rats given the drug developed liver cancer.

Yesterday Dr Powles said no liver cancer had been seen in his group, or in the 6 million women around the world given the drug as part of breast cancer therapy. Side effects were either non-existent or mild.

Dr Powles said 15 per cent of women experienced hot flushes, and 10 per cent had some irregularity of periods. There was no evidence it caused an early menopause, and no medical reason why it could not be taken by women receiving hormone replacement therapy.

(Guardian, 22 April 1993)

ACTIVITY

Study the *Guardian* article on the clinical trials for tamoxifen.

1 What is the purpose of this clinical trial?

2 How is the clinical trial being carried out?

3 What special characteristics apply to the group of women who are involved in this trial?

4 What possible risks in taking tamoxifen have been suggested?

5 Ask other people whether they would be prepared to be involved in a clinical trial such as this? What kinds of responses did you find?

6 Do you think that it can ever be justifiable to involve someone in a clinical trial without their consent or knowledge?

In SOCIAL SCIENCE ethical (and sometimes legal) dilemmas arise precisely because social research intrudes into the lives of those studied. For some, completing a questionnaire or participating in an interview may be an interesting, perhaps even a rewarding or enlightening, experience. For others, especially those involved in research into 'sensitive' issues or subject to a prolonged period of observation or case study, the experience may be less positive. People may feel that their privacy is being invaded. Feelings or thoughts suppressed for a long time may be uncomfortably re-awoken and prove disturbing. Some people may feel very anxious about the uses to which the research data will be put. Covert participant observation raises serious questions about whether researchers should always be honest and open with the people and organizations they are studying.

There are occasions when social scientists (and other professionals, such as journalists) have used covert participant observation to uncover injustices or to investigate what would otherwise be closed and secret areas of social life. However, there are considerable practical risks to the researcher using this method and many social scientists suggest that more open forms of observation study can engender a trust and acceptance of the researcher which allows him or her to gain an intimate and privileged insight into the lives of the people being researched.

In general, as a STUDENT RESEARCHER, if you have the opportunity to carry out research of your own, consider the following points.

- Try to obtain and consult any statement of ethical practice issued by academic associations in the particular field of research you are considering; for example, the British Sociological Association issues its own 'Statement of Ethical Practice'.
- Always obtain consent from the people you involve in your research. If observing or interviewing children, ensure you obtain consent to do so from the adults responsible for them.
- Ensure that the participants in your research are aware of the true nature of your research.

- Be sensitive to the privacy and feelings of the participants in your research. Even if you involve people you think you know well in your research, you may be taken by surprise at an unexpected reaction to a particular question asked.
- Reassure your participants that they will be afforded anonymity and confidentiality and that they will not be identified by name. Ensure that this is the case when writing, recording and presenting your research. Consider using pseudonyms when referring to organizations and institutions studied in a project.
- For your own personal safety, never agree to interview anyone whom you do not know if you are at all unsure about the circumstances and location of the interview.

PRACTISING RESEARCH SKILLS: IDEAS FOR RESEARCH ASSIGNMENTS

1 Design a piece of research (including any questionnaires, interview schedules, document analysis, etc.), covering community, GP, hospital inpatient and outpatient services, to:

- determine ethnic group, sex and age of respondents;
- identify whether respondents can speak, read, write in English;
- identify health needs of respondents;
- identify health services used by respondents;
- determine levels of satisfaction with services used;
- identify possible improvements to services as suggested by respondents;
- identify how respondents would like health information communicated.

This project is adapted from the research brief of Nirveen Kalsi when, as a development worker in health and racial equality, she carried out research into the health needs and experiences of ethnic minorities in the London Borough of Haringey in the late 1980s. While it would be unrealistic to expect students, in designing an appropriate piece of research, to carry out much more than a hypothetical exercise here, there might be practical opportunities to try out at least some sections of the overall research plan in their local community.

2 You will probably be able to think of areas that you wish to research, using the methods described in this chapter. If you need help, the suggestions below may help you to get started.

- provision for working parents, including childcare facilities;
- public perception of AIDS/HIV;
- the role of alternative/complementary medicine;
- the role of a professional (for example, midwife);
- provision of care (for example, for elders).

There are many other suggestions made throughout the book.

REFERENCES AND RESOURCES

Alibhai-Brown, Yasmin and Montague, Anne (1992), *The Colour of Love*. London: Virago.

British Sociological Association, 'Statement of Ethical Practice'. Durham: BSA.

Burnard, Philip and Morrison, Paul (1990), *Nursing Research in Action: Developing Basic Skills*. London: Macmillan.

Cornwall, Jocelyn (1984), *Hard-Earned Lives*, Social Science Paperbacks.

Eaton, Mary (1993), *Women after Prison*. Milton Keynes: Open University Press.

Gee, Gordon (1994), *Calculations for Health and Social Care*. London: Hodder and Stoughton.

Kalsi, Nirveen, and Constantinides, Pamela (1989), *Working towards Racial Equality in Health Care: The Haringey Experience*. London: King's Fund Centre for Health.

Oakley, Ann (1981), *From Here to Maternity*. London: Penguin.

Reid, Norma G. and Boore, Jennifer R. P.
(1987), *Research Methods and Statistics in Health
Care*. London: Edward Arnold.
Sapsford, R. and Abbott, P. (1992), *Research
Methods for Nursing and the Caring Professions*.
Oxford: OUP.
Wellings, Kay *et al.* (1994), *Sexual Behaviour in
Britain: The National Survey of Sexual Attitudes and
Lifestyles*. London: Penguin.

USEFUL ADDRESS

HMSO
49 High Holborn
London
WC1V 6HB
Tel.: 071 873 0011

Appendix

EXPERIENCE IN THE WORKPLACE

An important part of a vocational health and social care course is one or more work placements.

FUNCTIONS OF A WORK PLACEMENT

1 It allows a student to find out first-hand about various careers. Many students find their true vocation on a work experience placement. (Equally some students find that their chosen career is not, after all, for them!)
2 The work placement is a 'learning experience'. Not all learning has to take place in the classroom.
3 The work placement allows students to put into practice the theory learnt in the classroom – for example, assessment of client needs (Chapter 7).
4 Students can develop skills in the workplace, for example, communication.
5 Students may have the opportunity to carry out research in the workplace.
6 Positive comments on a student's performance on a work placement are viewed favourably in references or Records of Achievement. In an interview the student will have an advantage if he or she can talk knowledgeably about practical work experience.

ACTIVITY

Study the list of functions of a work placement. Can you think of any others?

SUGGESTIONS FOR HEALTH AND SOCIAL CARE PLACEMENTS

Your choice of placement(s) will obviously be limited to those within an acceptable travelling distance, your previous experience and your future aspirations. The following list should help you consider some of the options:

- hospitals (private, NHS trust/non-trust)
- community health clinics
- probation service
- education welfare department
- social services
- public health authorities
- Citizens Advice Bureaux
- other voluntary agencies
- nurseries/playgroups
- schools (including special schools, day or residential)
- probation hostels
- day care centres for physically or mentally handicapped people
- residential homes for physically or mentally handicapped people
- day care centres for elders
- residential homes for elders

To find these establishments locally check libraries, Yellow Pages, and the CAB.

PLANNING YOUR PLACEMENT

An important aspect to be planned is the LENGTH OF TIME you spend at your placement.

This may be beyond your control, but if you have the choice it requires careful consideration.

Some colleges send their students out on a BLOCK of work experience (for example, four continuous weeks per year); others send them out for SINGLE DAYS (for example, a day a week throughout the course).

ACTIVITY

1 What do you consider to be the advantages and disadvantages of the two work experience schemes, block and single day?

2 On a full-time, two-year health and social care course, what would you consider to be an adequate length of time to spend in the workplace?

If a student is to have more than one block of work experience, he or she may find it useful to progress on to a different establishment where clients have greater needs.

PERMISSION TO VISIT an establishment can be requested by letter or telephone. Be willing to give a concise description of your course, your intended career, and what you hope to achieve from the placement.

Confirm in writing when you will be visiting and, if possible, arrange a PRELIMINARY VISIT. Obviously you will find out all you can about the placement before this first visit, but actually going there will allow you to meet staff and to find out:

• how to get there;
• the hours you will be working;
• likely tasks you will be involved in;
• what style of dress will be suitable;
• practical arrangements, for example, where to have lunch.

You should take a copy of the TASKS you are required to do during your placement, and explain the assessment procedure.

Check with your school or college that the necessary INSURANCE has been arranged.

WORK EXPERIENCE TASKS

Tasks to be carried out prior to the placement

To gain the maximum benefit from the work placement it is important to be well prepared. The following tasks are suggestions to help you with this preparation.

1 Following your preliminary visit discuss your feelings and reactions with other students. The following areas should be covered:

• your initial impressions;
• the atmosphere;
• the clients;
• the staff involved in the care of the patients/clients;
• Your expectations of your future placements in terms of self-development, job satisfaction and problem areas.

2 Copy the 'skills checklist' in Figure A.1 and use it to make a self-appraisal before you go to visit your workplace. Grade yourself on each skill: 4 for very good; 3 for good; 2 acceptable and 1 poor.

From the completed skills checklist you will see that you have positive attributes to offer the workplace. If there are any areas you've identified that you feel might cause some problems at the workplace, DISCUSS these on a one-to-one basis with your tutor to enable you to plan strategies on how to deal with them before you go to the workplace.

Make a list of the practical skills you have already acquired on your course so far, or on previous courses you have followed. Be proud of your accomplishments so far, and use this recognition as a basis for starting a PRACTICAL SKILLS PROFILE which can be added on to throughout the whole course, including

Skill	Score			
	1	2	3	4
Motivation				
Effort				
Self-confidence				
Enthusiasm				
Ability to follow instructions				
Ability to assess when to ask for help				
Listening skills				
Co-operation				
Relationships with colleagues				
Accuracy in practical work				
Punctuality				
Attendance				
Time management				
Ability to take criticism				
Ability to present written reports				
Ability to handle calculations				

Figure A.1   Checklist for scoring relevant skills

subsequent work placements. This will give you valuable information to put into your curriculum vitae or future applications for further training or jobs.

Write a statement of your PERSONAL CAREER AIMS identifying the career you might want to follow and the progression route which you think you will follow to this career. You can get advice from the local careers service and your teachers or lecturers.

How do you think the workplace that you are going to could help you acquire the practical and personal skills that you will need in the career you want to follow?

3 Before you go into the workplace it is important that you are aware of CONFIDENTIALITY issues (see Chapter 2).

Tasks to be carried out in the workplace

Throughout this book many suggestions have been made for activities which either can or should be carried out in the workplace. In addition, the following written tasks may be carried out to help you benefit from your work experience.

1 Keep a DIARY or LOG BOOK on your work experience.

- Note activities undertaken each day and the time spent on them.
- Record your feelings and reactions to your experiences.

2 Describe:

- The SERVICE(S) provided by your work experience establishment.
- The needs of the CLIENTS using these services.
- The work of the PROFESSIONALS with whom you come into contact.

What do you think are the main qualities/skills they each require?

3 Conduct one or more of the following CASE STUDIES. NB: This task should be carried out only after a preliminary discussion with placement staff as to what aspects of the task are considered to be both permissible and possible. Confidentiality and respect for the individual and family should be maintained.

(a) Conduct a case study on one employee/pupil/client, to include:
- reasons for selection;
- personal details of the individual, such as age, sex, family situation, special interests and abilities, etc.;
- an analysis of the role of the individual in the establishment and the demands made on him/her by the establishment.
(b) Make brief notes on different attitudes patients/clients have to themselves and their care, focusing on two case studies.
(c) Make notes on cases you observe where professionals influence the way in which patients/clients view their own identity.
(d) Examine and record one example of group interactions and dynamics.

4 Investigate and comment on the following aspects of HEALTH AND SAFETY in your workplace:

- fire prevention and drill;
- safety policy, officers, first aiders;
- actual/potential hazards to staff and clients;
- provision of rest/recreation areas for clients.

5 Evaluate the role of COMPUTERS in the workplace: how they are used, the tasks they perform and the software used. Consider other tasks being performed that could be computerized and assess how valuable the computer is as a work aid.

6 Throughout your work experience period make a note of any issues arising that you wish to discuss, or any questions that arise and are unanswered. You can then raise these issues later with your visiting tutor or other students.

Tasks to be carried out following the placement

1 Produce an ASSESSMENT OF YOUR OWN STRENGTHS AND WEAKNESSES during your placement. Refer back to your 'skills checklist' completed prior to the time spent in the workplace.

- Has your self-appraisal changed?
- Have your career aims changed?
- Have you gained skills which will be necessary for your chosen career?

Update your CV and, if possible, plan strategies for overcoming any remaining areas of weakness.

2 Give an ORAL PRESENTATION of your work experience to other students. Your presentation should include:

- an outline of the organization/s and type of work;
- your own role and tasks;
- the challenges and problems you faced;
- an assessment of what has been learned and the personal development that has taken place.

There should also be an opportunity for a more informal debriefing session to allow discussion of any points raised in Task 6 which was completed during the placement.

3 Write a LETTER OF THANKS to the employer(s) at your placement.

4 EVALUATE the usefulness of your placement.

- What aspects were most satisfactory?
- What aspects were least satisfactory?
- Do you have any suggestions for improvements?
- Would you recommend the placement to another student?

This feedback should be used to help students with organization of future work placements.

ASSESSMENT

It will be useful for you to receive as much feedback as possible on your performance in the workplace. The possible sources of assessment will be:

- yourself
- your placement supervisor and colleagues
- your visiting tutor
- your written work

It is advisable to give your supervisor in the workplace a standard form to enable him or her to comment on your performance. Figure A.2 shows an example of this.

Your supervisor should also be encouraged to give feedback on the organizational aspects of the work experience. These comments should then be considered when planning future placements.

Student's name --

Name of establishment --

Employer's Comments

Please comment on the following:

1. Student's attitude with reference to attendance, punctuality, etc.

2. Student's interest and enthusiasm.

3. Ability to work and co-operate with others.

4. Suitability of the student for this type of work.

5. Any other comments.

Signed --- Date ---

Position ---

Figure A.2   Example of employer's comment form

ROLE OF THE VISITING TUTOR

Although assessment by your visiting tutor was mentioned above, the main role he or she will have is to support you and if necessary help solve any problems you may encounter. He or she may also give feedback on the suitability of the workplace for student placements. Make sure you know how to contact the visiting tutor if the need arises.

AND FINALLY . . .

Many workers in caring professions are under a great deal of pressure, perhaps because of understaffing, or perhaps because of the nature of the job. It may be an added pressure for them to work with a student. If you observe the following points it will help your working relationship to flourish:

- Find out as much as you can about the placement before you arrive.
- Be punctual.
- Inform your supervisor and college tutor of any unavoidable absences.
- Be prepared for shift-work hours.
- Be co-operative.
- Treat clients and staff with respect.
- Observe confidentiality.
- Show an interest by asking questions at convenient times.

Remember, the impression you give may affect the employer's willingness to offer students placements in the future, and, you never know, you may eventually return for an interview for a full-time post!

INDEX